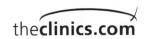

SURGICAL CLINICS
OF NORTH AMERICA

Vascular Surgery: New Concepts and
Practice for the General Surgeon

GUEST EDITOR
Benjamin W. Starnes, MD

CONSULTING EDITOR
Ronald F. Martin, MD

October 2007 • Volume 87 • Number 5

SAUNDERS

An Imprint of Elsevier, Inc.
PHILADELPHIA   LONDON   TORONTO   MONTREAL   SYDNEY   TOKYO

W.B. SAUNDERS COMPANY
A Division of Elsevier Inc.

1600 John F. Kennedy Blvd., Suite 1800, Philadelphia, PA 19103-2899

http://www.theclinics.com

SURGICAL CLINICS OF NORTH AMERICA
October 2007
Editor: Catherine Bewick

Volume 87, Number 5
ISSN 0039–6109
ISBN-10: 1-4160-5126-0
ISBN-13: 978-1-4160-5126-8

The ideas and opinions expressed in *The Surgical Clinics of North America* do not necessarily reflect those of the Publisher. The Publisher does not assume any responsibility for any injury and/or damage to persons or property arising out of or related to any use of the material contained in this periodical. The reader is advised to check the appropriate medical literature and the product information currently provided by the manufacturer of each drug to be administered to verify the dosage, the method and duration of administration, or contraindications. It is the responsibility of the treating physician or other health care professional, relying on independent experience and knowledge of the patient, to determine drug dosages and the best treatment for the patient. Mention of any product in this issue should not be construed as endorsement by the contributors, editors, or the Publisher of the product or manufacturers' claims.

Surgical Clinics of North America (ISSN 0039–6109) is published bimonthly by Elsevier Inc., 360 Park Avenue South, New York, NY 10010-1710. Months of publication are February, April, June, August, October, and December. Business and Editorial Offices: 1600 John F. Kennedy Blvd., Suite 1800, Philadelphia, PA 19103-2899. Customer Service Office: 6277 Sea Harbor Drive, Orlando, FL 32887-4800. Periodicals postage paid at New York, NY and additional mailing offices. Subscription prices are $220.00 per year for US individuals, $347.00 per year for US institutions, $110.00 per year for US students and residents, $270.00 per year for Canadian individuals, $424.00 per year for Canadian institutions, $286.00 for international individuals, $424.00 per year for international institutions and $143.00 per year for Canadian and foreign students/residents. To receive student/resident rate, orders must be accompanied by name of affiliated institution, date of term, and the *signature* of program/residency coordinator on institution letterhead. Orders will be billed at individual rate until proof of status is received. Foreign air speed delivery is included in all *Clinics* subscription prices. All prices are subject to change without notice. POSTMASTER: Send address changes to *Surgical Clinics*, Elsevier Periodicals Customer Service, 6277 Sea Harbor Drive, Orlando, FL 32887-4800. **Customer Service: 1-800-654-2452 (US). From outside of the US, call 1-407-345-1000.**

The Surgical Clinics of North America is also published in Spanish by McGraw-Hill Interamericana Editores S.A., P.O. Box 5-237 06500 Mexico D.F. Mexico; and in Portuguese by Interlivros Edicoes Ltda., Rua Comandante Coelho 1085, CEP 21250, Rio de Janeiro, Brazil; and in Greek by Paschalidis Medical Publications, Athens Greece.

The Surgical Clinics of North America is covered in *Index Medicus, EMBASE/Excerpta Medica, Current Contents/Clinical Medicine, Current Contents/Life Sciences, Science Citation Index*, and *ISI/BIOMED.*

Printed in the United States of America.

CONSULTING EDITOR

RONALD F. MARTIN, MD, Staff Surgeon, Marshfield Clinic, Marshfield; and Clinical
Associate Professor of Surgery, University of Wisconsin School of Medicine and Public
Health, Madison, Wisconsin; Lieutenant Colonel, Medical Corps, United States Army
Reserve

GUEST EDITOR

BENJAMIN W. STARNES, MD, FACS, Chief, Division of Vascular Surgery, University
of Washington, Seattle, Washington

CONTRIBUTORS

CHARLES A. ANDERSEN, MD, FACS, Chief, Vascular/Endovascular Surgery Service,
Department of Surgery; and Director, Wound Care Clinic, Madigan Army Medical
Center, Tacoma, Washington

CPT ZACHARY M. ARTHURS, MD, Department of Surgery, Madigan Army Medical
Center, Tacoma, Washington

KRISTEN L. BIGGS, MD, Fellow in Vascular Surgery, UCLA Division of Vascular Surgery,
Los Angeles, California

W. DARRIN CLOUSE, MD, Director, Endovascular Surgery, Division of Vascular Surgery,
Wilford Hall Medical Center, San Antonio, Texas; Assistant Professor of Surgery,
Uniformed Services University of the Health Sciences, Bethesda, Maryland

JONATHAN L. ELIASON, MD, Assistant Professor, Vascular Surgery, Department
of Surgery, The University of Michigan Health System, Ann Arbor, Michigan

BRIAN L. FERRIS, MD, Lake Washington Vascular Surgeons, Kirkland, Washington, DC;
and Lake Washington Vascular Surgeons, Bellevue, Washington, DC

LTC CHARLES J. FOX, MD, US Army Medical Corps, Walter Reed Army Medical Center,
Vascular Surgery, Washington, DC; Assistant Professor of Surgery, Department of
Surgery, Uniformed Services University of Health Sciences, Bethesda, Maryland

KATHLEEN D. GIBSON, MD, Lake Washington Vascular Surgeons, Kirkland,
Washington, DC; and Lake Washington Vascular Surgeons, Bellevue, Washington, DC

BRIAN GRANVALL, MPH, PA-C, Divisions of Thoracic and Vascular Surgery, Heart and
Vascular Institute, Southwest Washington Medical Center, Vancouver, Washington

GARTH S. HERBERT, MD, Madigan Army Medical Center, Department of Surgery, Fort Lewis, Tacoma, Washington

RIYAD KARMY-JONES, MD, Divisions of Thoracic and Vascular Surgery, Heart and Vascular Institute, Southwest Washington Medical Center, Vancouver, Washington

SEAN P. LYDEN, MD, Assistant Professor, Department of Vascular Surgery, Cleveland Clinic Foundation, Cleveland, Ohio

LTC MATTHEW J. MARTIN, MD, FACS, Assistant Professor of Surgery, Uniformed Services University of Health Sciences, Bethesda, Maryland; Trauma Director and Chief of Surgical Critical Care, Department of Surgery, Madigan Army Medical Center, Tacoma, Washington

JEROME M. McDONALD, MD, FACS, Stockton Cardiothoracic Surgical Medical Group, Stockton, California

MARK MEISSNER, MD, Department of Surgery, Division of Vascular Surgery, University of Washington School of Medicine, Seattle, Washington

WESLEY S. MOORE, MD, Professor and Chief Emeritus, UCLA, Division of Vascular Surgery, Los Angeles, California

STEPHEN NICHOLLS, MD, Divisions of Thoracic and Vascular Surgery, Heart and Vascular Institute, Southwest Washington Medical Center, Vancouver, Washington

DANIEL PEPPER, MD, Lake Washington Vascular Surgeons, Kirkland, Washington, DC; and Lake Washington Vascular Surgeons, Bellevue, Washington, DC

GANESHA B. PERERA, MD, Department of Vascular Surgery, Cleveland Clinic Foundation, Cleveland, Ohio

CPT JASON T. PERRY, MD, Division of General Surgery, Department of Surgery, Madigan Army Medical Center, Tacoma, Washington

STEVEN M. ROTH, MD, MS, Vein Care Pavilion of the South, Evans; and University Surgical Associates, Augusta, Georgia

THOMAS S. ROUKIS, DPM, FACFAS, Chief, Limb Preservation Service, Vascular/Endovascular Surgery Service, Department of Surgery; and Director, Limb Preservation Complex Lower Extremity Surgery and Research Fellowship, Madigan Army Medical Center, Tacoma, Washington

ALI SALIM, MD, FACS, Assistant Professor of Surgery, Division of Trauma and Surgical Critical Care, University of California Keck School of Medicine; and Surgical Critical Care Residency Director, Los Angeles County Hospitals and USC Medical Center, Los Angeles, California

ALAN SIMEONE, MD, Divisions of Thoracic and Vascular Surgery, Heart and Vascular Institute, Southwest Washington Medical Center, Vancouver, Washington

NITEN SINGH, MD, Assistant Professor of Surgery, Uniformed Services University of the Health Sciences, Bethesda, Maryland; Chief, Endovascular Surgery, Vascular Surgery Service, Madigan Army Medical Center, Tacoma, Washington

CPT VANCE Y. SOHN, MD, Department of Surgery, Madigan Army Medical Center, Tacoma, Washington

BENJAMIN W. STARNES, MD, FACS, Chief, Division of Vascular Surgery, University of Washington, Seattle, Washington

LTC JOHN D. STATLER, MD, Division of Interventional Radiology, Department of Radiology, Madigan Army Medical Center, Tacoma, Washington

SCOTT R. STEELE, MD, FACS, Chief, Colon and Rectal Surgery, Department of Surgery, Madigan Army Medical Center, Fort Lewis, Tacoma, Washington

NAM T. TRAN, MD, Assistant Professor, Division of Vascular Surgery, University of Washington, Seattle, Washington

CONTENTS

plays an important role, and that the data that define indications and outcomes are still emerging.

Hybrid Approaches to Repair of Complex Aortic Aneurysmal Disease

Benjamin W. Starnes, Nam T. Tran, and Jerome M. McDonald

With the endovascular revolution upon us, the management of aortic aneurysmal disease has changed dramatically. Since 1991, more than 100,000 aneurysms worldwide have been repaired using early-generation and current-generation standardized grafts and this has dramatically reduced the 30-day mortality rates associated with open aortic surgery. A new phenomenon has also arisen from this wonderful technology. The term hybrid means "of different origins" and hybrid approaches to vascular disease involve open and endovascular techniques to achieve a common goal, namely, to prevent death caused by aneurysmal rupture. This article reviews novel approaches to the repair of complex aortic aneurysms and provides several illustrative examples.

Ischemic Colitis Complicating Major Vascular Surgery

Scott R. Steele

Ischemic colitis is a well-described complication of major vascular surgery, especially following open abdominal aortic aneurysm repair and endovascular aneurysm repair, but also with aortoiliac surgery, aortic dissection, and thoracic aneurysm repair. Following its onset, mortality remains high, highlighting the need for rapidly identifying the onset of symptoms and, perhaps more importantly, those patients at risk, in an attempt to prevent its onset. In this article, the authors review the causes, presentation, and diagnostic strategies of colonic ischemia. They also cover the operative management and outcomes for bowel resection and vascular repair. Finally, they evaluate some of the newer options for diagnosing this condition.

Acute and Chronic Mesenteric Ischemia

Garth S. Herbert and Scott R. Steele

This article briefly reviews the various etiologies, presentation, and diagnosis of different types of mesenteric ischemia. Operative management techniques and the applicability of percutaneous endovascular intervention are discussed. Finally, the authors explore emerging technologies that have the potential to further improve diagnosis and treatment of this frequently lethal disease process.

For this reason, this technology has had limited utility for trauma patients who have moderate to severe injuries. Now that vascular surgeons have incorporated endovascular techniques into their practice, the operating room is a radiology suite, and the surgeon is the interventionalist. Endovascular techniques provide an opportunity to improve trauma care by either temporizing a life-threatening injury or serving as the primary treatment. Using endovascular adjuncts does not preclude standard open surgery, nor does it prohibit an immediate or delayed surgical repair.

Management of traumatic vascular injury can offer special challenges even to experienced surgeons who are functioning in resource-limited situations. Lessons learned from past conflicts have advanced the practice of vascular trauma surgery on the battlefield and in urban trauma centers. Current conflicts provide a fresh opportunity to examine those recent advancements that have improved surgical capability and as a result have changed the practice of vascular surgery on the modern battlefield. This article provides an overview of the contemporary management of vascular injuries in combat casualties during recent United States military operations.

Surgery for hemodialysis access is the most commonly performed vascular surgical operation in the United States, predominantly because of a steady increase in the prevalence of end-stage renal disease. Multiple studies have confirmed the improved patency rate and lower infection rates for native arteriovenous fistulae compared with prosthetic arteriovenous grafts. In formulating a strategy for successful dialysis access a comprehensive approach should be undertaken. The preoperative planning, as with any surgical procedure, is the most important aspect, followed by the postoperative maintenance of the access.

Vena cava filters are widely used to prevent pulmonary embolic events in patients who have known venous thromboses, or in select patients deemed to be at high risk for these events. There are few prospective or well-controlled data regarding the efficacy and appropriate indications for vena cava filter use in surgical patients. High-risk surgical patients such as those who have multiple injuries, malignancy, and those undergoing bariatric procedures may benefit from vena cava filter placement. The authors discuss the available data regarding indications, efficacy, and outcomes to assist the surgeon in deciding when to use this technology.

Endovenous laser treatment (EVLT) has become a standard therapy for the treatment of superficial venous insufficiency. It offers a rapid, office-based therapy with minimal patient downtime and an easier recovery than traditional surgical treatment. EVLT is effective and durable and can successfully treat saphenous truncal insufficiency and accessory branches with low complication rates. EVLT can increase patient satisfaction and enable the treatment of a wider variety of patients with a more efficient procedure compared with traditional techniques.

Radiofrequency ablation of superficial and perforator veins for venous insufficiency has emerged as a leading alternative to traditional vein stripping operations. This percutaneous technique can be performed in less than an hour using local anesthetic or sedation. The VNUS Closure catheters (VNUS Medical Technologies, San Jose, California) work by resistive heating in the vein wall that is constantly monitored through a feedback loop to the VNUS Closure generator. Side effects are less than with other endovenous ablation techniques and patients resume normal activity immediately. The new ClosureFAST catheter is an important advancement that combines the speed of endovenous laser ablation with the expected fewer side effects of radiofrequency ablation.

Foam sclerotherapy has been refined over the past decade to become a safe and effective treatment for varicose veins and venous insufficiency. Using duplex ultrasound guidance, it can be used to treat large and small varicosities, saphenous trunks, incompetent perforating veins, and venous stasis ulcerations.

Serious complications are rare, and in experienced hands, efficacy rivals that of traditional surgical ligation and stripping. Disadvantages of the technique are the need in many cases for more than one treatment session, and lack of US Food and Drug Administration approval of all currently available sclerosants. Foam sclerotherapy offers advantages of low cost, quick patient recovery, and ease of use; as such, it is an important tool for modern vein treatment.

FORTHCOMING ISSUES

RECENT ISSUES

The Clinics are now available online!

www.theclinics.com

SURGICAL
CLINICS OF
NORTH AMERICA

Surg Clin N Am 87 (2007) xv–xvii

Foreword

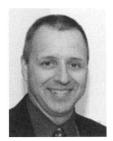

Ronald F. Martin, MD
Consulting Editor

The continuing mission of this series is to inquire into and discuss the topics that are relevant to general surgeons. One of the more ever present themes is what is it that makes a general surgeon a general surgeon. In previous issues, we have presented topics that one could argue represent specialized skills and others could state represent a limitation of scope of practice. In this issue, we come back to this dynamic of what "belongs" to general surgery and what doesn't.

My original mentors in surgery were vascular surgeons. Surgeons such as Dr. H. Brownell Wheeler and Dr. Clement Hiebert made the beginnings of their very successful careers by operating on arteries. They were in the mix when the first carotid endarterectomies were done and coronary artery bypass grafting was coming into wide use. The discipline of vascular surgery, as we were taught it, was exciting and terrifying, and it was (and still is) extremely demanding and fairly unforgiving. Also, it was a timed game; neither bleeding nor ischemia is particularly understanding of our prior time commitments. This added another layer of challenge and reward to these operations.

The field of vascular surgery is virtually unrecognizable in practice compared to those days but its fundamental principles remain beautifully similar. The concepts of "inflow, outflow, conduit" and "achieve proximal and distal control" will still carry you a long way, no matter where you are and what you have to work with.

Which brings us to the original point: what does vascular surgery have to do with general surgery? Is it a completely separate specialty or a basic

0039-6109/07/$ - see front matter © 2007 Elsevier Inc. All rights reserved.
doi:10.1016/j.suc.2007.09.005

component of general surgery? The answer, as it turns out, is probably yes. And the reason the answer to an "either /or" question is yes is because the answer changes upon local workforce structure and health care integration policies and arrangements. It may also change with weather and geopolitics.

We continue to face a debate in the United States about how to deliver health care and how to pay for it. In my opinion, the debate is being poorly conducted and mostly consists of obfuscation in order to preserve temporary perceived advantages; but that is one surgeon's opinion and I have been known to be wrong before. The parts of the story that are somewhat beyond debate is that we have a nonhomogenous distribution of resources and a disconnect between risk sharing and cost sharing. Some of this disconnect is economic, some is geographical/spatial, and some is political.

Vascular surgery is an excellent example of a tiered response system. It has a range of services from very basic repair of acute minor vascular injuries and straightforward restoration of blood flow that could be done in a tent, to complicated interventional techniques requiring expensive dedicated procedure suites that require highly specialized personnel and broad system support such as intensive care units, dialysis capability, and "open" operative support. Also, the range of costs of recruiting and retaining personnel to these differing centers is very broad.

We in the military have a significant history of managing widely varied levels of resources in various spatial configurations, from state of the art facilities in peaceful, secure areas to barely sheltered soft "facilities" in extremely austere environments. Despite an extremely gifted and dedicated transport system of air evacuation in hostile environments, time still dictates that life and limb salvage must be undertaken with limited resources and with great frequency. For those of us who were a little older, it was clear under those conditions that the comfort level of recently graduated trainees with vascular surgery being a part of general surgery was a bit less than with those who trained prior to the creation of the American Board of Surgery Vascular Surgery Board as a separate board.

The flip side of this coin is the disparity in training required to be maximally effective in an environment that has every resource. By way of example, I was recently asked to see a patient in an emergency room because he had a rigid abdomen and was in shock. I took him to the OR and started the operation to control and repair his ruptured abdominal aortic aneurysm while our vascular surgeon came in and we finished it together—good fun actually; it went well, and my colleague was responsible for the postoperative care. Our editor for this issue, Dr. Starnes, and I were talking on the phone a day or two later and I relayed the story to him. He asked me if I had considered fixing the aneurysm endovascularly. I told that even if I had wanted to, I would not have known how. And since the patient was fairly close to dying, I did not think that was a good time to learn.

Our conversation made it clear to me that state-of-the-art vascular surgery has become so evolved that it cannot be just a "part" of general surgery. Yet basic "keep them alive with their limbs on" vascular surgery probably has to remain an important part of general surgery. We simply cannot afford nor would we probably accept a system that would have to change adequately to respond to the global needs of our patients if we limited vascular surgery to surgeons who only perform vascular procedures. Furthermore, we could not project this level of sophistication to every acute facility and expect enough clinical volume to maintain system and individual proficiency.

I can think of no more qualified person to have edited this issue. Dr. Starnes has extensive experience in working in environments as austere as Forward Surgical Teams in Afghanistan to the cutting edge environment he currently works in at the University of Washington. He and his colleagues have assembled a truly magnificent collection of articles that should be relevant to any general surgeon.

Ronald F. Martin, MD
Department of Surgery
Marshfield Clinic
1000 North Oak Avenue
Marshfield, WI 54449, USA

E-mail address: martin.ronald@marshfieldclinic.org

SURGICAL
CLINICS OF
NORTH AMERICA

Surg Clin N Am 87 (2007) xix–xx

Preface

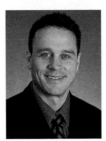

Benjamin W. Starnes, MD, FACS
Guest Editor

Vascular surgery achieved its stature as an independent and distinct specialty under the American Board of Surgery in 1982. Since its inception in the 1950s, the practice of vascular surgery has undergone dramatic changes, especially in the past ten years. With the endovascular revolution, more and more traditional vascular surgical procedures are being performed utilizing minimally invasive and endovascular techniques. This has translated into an explosion of new technologies and multiple specialties competing for the care of the patient who has vascular disease. Traditionally an integral part of general surgical training, vascular surgery as a specialty has reached yet another level of complexity that may seem out of reach to the seasoned general surgeon.

This issue of *Surgical Clinics of North America* covers many topics of interest, including current advances in vascular imaging, management of carotid disease, treatment of aortic aneurysms and dissections, and new techniques for the endovascular treatment of lower extremity ischemia. Also covered are new techniques in the management of common venous disorders. Two articles are devoted to the current management of vascular trauma, a topic of critical importance to the well-trained general surgeon, both on the modern battlefield as well as in the luxury of the modern hospital facility. Rounding out this issue are the timely topics of "The Diabetic Foot", "Successful Angioaccess", and two articles designated to mesenteric ischemia.

The authors of each of these articles are experts in their respective fields. It is my wish that this text serve as a reference for those surgeons who seek to improve their capabilities in their day to day interactions with patients harboring vascular disease. The future for vascular surgery is now the brightest it has ever been and with the current pace of transformation, it is not unlikely that this issue will be outdated in just the next five years.

Benjamin W. Starnes, MD, FACS
Division of Vascular Surgery
University of Washington
Box 359796, 325 Ninth Avenue
Seattle, WA 98104, USA

E-mail address: starnes@u.washington.edu

ELSEVIER
SAUNDERS

SURGICAL
CLINICS OF
NORTH AMERICA

Surg Clin N Am 87 (2007) 975–993

Advances in Vascular Imaging

CPT Jason T. Perry, MD[a],*,
LTC John D. Statler, MD[b]

[a]Division of General Surgery, Department of Surgery, Madigan Army Medical Center,
9400 Fitzsimmons Dr. Tacoma, WA 98431, USA
[b]Division of Interventional Radiology, Department of Radiology,
Madigan Army Medical Center, Tacoma, WA, USA

Advances in vascular surgery have mirrored advances in diagnostic imaging. Indeed, the endovascular revolution has been made possible largely by advances in computed tomography, magnetic resonance imaging, and vascular ultrasound. As technology allows better noninvasive vascular diagnosis, conventional angiography, once the gold standard for the diagnosis of vascular disease, is now reserved largely for intervention. This article discusses the current state of vascular imaging. Specific emphasis is placed on the comparative clinical utility of different imaging modalities in the detection and management of vascular disease.

Contrast media

The majority of vascular imaging involves the administration (directly or indirectly) of contrast into the vessels imaged. A brief discussion of contrast agents is included for completeness.

Iodinated contrast preparations are ubiquitous and are used in fluoroscopic examinations, angiography, and CT. Early iodinated contrast agents were both ionic and hyperosmolar. They were poorly tolerated, and associated with high rates of contrast reactions and contrast-induced nephropathy (CIN). Newer iodinated contrast preparations are nonionic and either low or iso-osmolar. Newer agents are associated with lower rates of contrast reaction and CIN. The most important risk factor in the development of CIN is pre-existing renal disease. Patients at risk include those who have

* Corresponding author.
E-mail address: jason.thomas.perry@us.army.mil (J.T. Perry).

diabetes, multiple myeloma, and those who have serum creatinine of greater than 1.5 mg/dL. Other factors contributing to CIN include use of high-osmolar contrast media, dehydration, and simultaneous patient use of nephrotoxic medications. Current recommendations for the prevention of CIN include the use of iso-osmolar contrast agents, adequate patient hydration using normal saline or sodium bicarbonate solution, and pre-medication with acetylcysteine. Patients who have pre-existing renal disease should be imaged using modalities that do not employ iodinated contrast [1].

Carbon dioxide (CO_2) is another contrast agent useful in the evaluation of arterial disease below the diaphragm. Catheter-directed injection of compressed CO_2 results in displacement of blood, creating negative contrast within the target vessel [2]. CO_2 is rapidly absorbed in the blood and is not nephrotoxic. Because of this rapid absorption, however, meaningful evaluation of the tibial vessels is impossible. CO_2 has been applied in both diagnostic and therapeutic settings [3,4]. Most recently, Chao and colleagues have demonstrated the feasibility and safety of using CO_2 in patients who have impaired renal function undergoing endovascular aortic aneurysm repair (EVAR) [5]. All of these patients, however, required general anesthesia because of significant movement associated with CO_2 injections.

Gadolinium is a noniodinated contrast agent typically used for MRI. In the past, it was used to mitigate the risks of CIN [6]. Indeed, gadolinium-enhanced magnetic resonance angiography (GE MRA), and even direct intra-arterial administration of gadolinium was thought to be the approach of choice when imaging the patient who has renal insufficiency or renal failure. Recently, this practice has been called into question [7,8]. Although gadolinium itself is thought to be nephrotoxic, it is administered in doses so low (0.05 mmol/kg–0.1 mmol/kg) that gadolinium-induced nephropathy is not a practical concern. Recently, however, several investigators have reported a disorder termed nephrogenic systemic fibrosis (NSF) as a side effect of intravenous administration of gadolinium contrast. NSF is a rare, poorly understood disorder characterized by progressive, irreversible fibrosis of skin and solid organs. It occurs weeks after gadolinium administration in patients who have pre-existing renal failure or renal insufficiency. Concern over this disease has led the US Food and Drug Administration (FDA) to recommend limiting the use of gadolinium to patients who have normal or near normal renal function [9].

The application of ultrasound contrast media to vascular disease is a new and rapidly developing field. Most ultrasound contrast agents consist of microbubbles encapsulated in a biodegradable shell, which are injected intravenously. The bubbles themselves create acoustic interfaces, which increase signal-to-noise ratio and improve conspicuity of vascular structures. Well-established roles for ultrasound contrast agents include evaluation of heart valves and intracardiac shunts. Currently, ultrasound contrast agents are not widely used in the evaluation of peripheral vascular disease.

Conventional angiography

Conventional angiography (CA) is an invasive technique that involves imaging with a radiographic source while contrast is injected directly into the vessel studied. CA is unique in that it can be both diagnostic and therapeutic. It is typically performed with the intention of treating a lesion within a vessel immediately following diagnostic evaluation [10].

Most endovascular procedures rely on digital subtraction angiography (DSA). DSA allows the operator to subtract background information, allowing high-quality depiction of vascular anatomy. The subtracted image can then be superimposed on the live fluoroscopic image, providing a vascular "road map" [11]. This decreases the amount of contrast injected during wire and catheter manipulations.

Because of its invasive nature, CA has more attendant risks than other vascular imaging modalities. These include complications caused by vessel access (hematoma and pseudoaneurysm), damage to target vessels (dissection, thrombosis, rupture), risks associated with sedation, risks inherent to the administration of iodinated contrast agents, and risks associated with ionizing radiation.

Despite these risks, DSA has significant advantages over noninvasive vascular imaging techniques. The refinement of endovascular devices has resulted in a shift toward endovascular intervention (to include angioplasty, stenting, atherectomy, and embolization) and away from open surgical procedures. Additionally, DSA yields important physiologic information—often difficult to glean from noninvasive modalities—such as the measurement of pressure gradients across lesions and the ability to observe the flow of contrast through a vessel in real time. This is particularly useful when evaluating patients who have peripheral vascular disease and poor cardiac output, or when evaluating patients for transient phenomena such as extrinsic compression (Fig. 1).

To summarize, CA retains an important role in the diagnosis and treatment of disease in all vascular territories. Advantages include its ability to provide physiologic data and to facilitate endovascular intervention. Disadvantages of CA include its invasive nature, the use of ionizing radiation, and the use of iodinated contrast agents. In the authors' practice, noninvasive imaging is routinely used for screening the patient who has peripheral vascular disease and CA is reserved for intervention once a diagnosis is established.

Multidetector computed tomographic angiography

Multidetector computed tomographic angiography (MDCTA), as its name implies, relies on multiple detectors traveling in a helical orientation about the patient to rapidly collect volumetric datasets. Once the volumetric data are acquired, they can be displayed in multiple formats, including

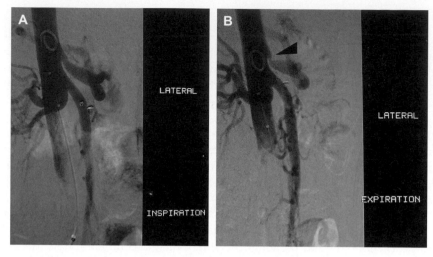

Fig. 1. (*A*) Lateral digital subtraction arteriogram of the abdominal aorta in inspiration shows mild dilatation of the celiac axis. (*B*) Lateral median arcuate ligament syndrome.

multiplanar reconstruction (MPR), maximum intensity projection (MIP), and volume rendering (VR) displays (Fig. 2) [12].

MPR refers to the ability to reformat axial data into coronal, sagittal, oblique, or even curved planes. Curved planar reformations are particularly useful for following the courses of blood vessels and assessing their patency. MIP images are generated by displaying, in planar format, only the highest

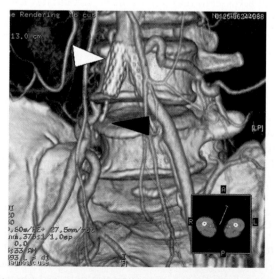

Fig. 2. Computed tomography arteriogram shows occluded right common iliac artery stent (*white arrowhead*) with lack of flow distal to stent (*black arrowhead*).

attenuation value encountered in a given volume of data, making it ideal for imaging iodinated contrast-enhanced vascular structures. A practical limitation of this technique, however, is the inclusion of bone (also high attenuation) in the final image. VR generates three-dimensional images based on differences in attenuation values of various structures. Once the image is rendered, it can be rotated to give a global overview of the anatomy of interest (Fig. 3) [13].

Because of its relative safety, excellent spatial resolution, and rapid scan times, MDCTA is becoming the preferred modality for imaging all types of aortic pathology, including dissections, aneurysms, and occlusive disease [14]. It can provide information similar to conventional angiography through MIP images, and demonstrate intraluminal thrombus and patency via MPR, and adjacent anatomy by VR [13]. As a result of this flexibility, MDCTA has assumed particular importance in the preoperative evaluation of patients for EVAR.

Early EVAR trials relied on both CT and CA for preoperative planning. Wyers and colleagues [15] demonstrated that EVAR could safely be performed with measurements obtained from reconstructed CT images without the need for preoperative CA. They used MMS, a proprietary software package (Medical Media Systems, West Lebanon, New Hampshire) to generate aortic diameter and length measurements for sizing endografts preoperatively. They found that CT reconstructions were superior to angiography in gauging graft length and adequacy of access vessels [15]. A subsequent group of investigators noted improved reproducibility when evaluating aortoiliac diameters using MMS in comparison with axial CT [16]. Parker

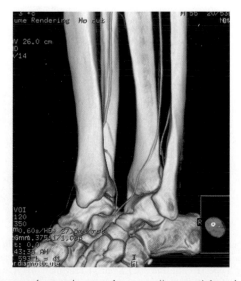

Fig. 3. Computed tomography arteriogram shows excellent spatial resolution of tibial vessels.

and colleagues [17] demonstrated similar results when comparing MMS reconstructions to axial CT combined with CA. They found, however, that clinical decision-making regarding endograft selection was similar between the two groups, calling into question the clinical utility of routine use of MMS in endograft planning.

MDCTA is the imaging modality of choice for postimplantation surveillance of endografts, specifically in the evaluation of aneurysm enlargement and endoleak [18]. A typical endograft protocol includes acquisition of unenhanced, arterial contrast, and delayed postcontrast series. Unenhanced images provide a baseline examination against which apparent abnormalities in the arterial phase can be judged. Delayed images allow for the evaluation of slow endoleaks (Fig. 4) [19].

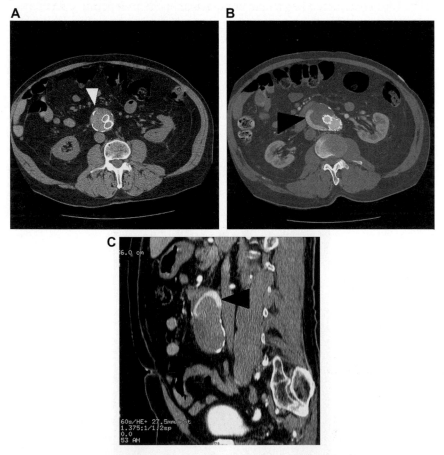

Fig. 4. (*A*) Noncontrast CT scan of patient status post EVAR. Note origin of inferior mesenteric artery (*white arrowhead*). (*B*) Delayed postcontrast CT scan shows curvilinear jet of contrast (*black arrowhead*) indicating Type II endoleak. (*C*) Sagittal reformat of CT scan showing Type II endoleak.

MDCTA is sensitive for the detection of all types of endoleaks, listed in Box 1. Stavropoulos and colleagues [20] demonstrated that once an endoleak was detected by MDCTA, CA was important, because it led to changes in classification of 11% of endoleaks. This is clinically relevant because the type of endoleak dictates the appropriate management strategy. Type I and Type III endoleaks require prompt repair. Type II endoleaks may be followed with MDCTA if the aneurysm sac diameter is stable or decreasing in size [21]. Furthermore, MDCTA can help differentiate Type II endoleaks likely to lead to aneurysm enlargement from those that are likely to remain stable [22].

MDCTA has also proven useful in the evaluation of atherosclerotic peripheral arterial disease (PAD) [23–25]. In the evaluation of severe (>75% luminal narrowing) PAD, 4-detector CTA has sensitivity of 92.2% and specificity of 96.8% in comparison with DSA. Interobserver correlation was excellent, with most disagreements between the two techniques arising in the calf vessels [24]. In comparison, 16-detector row CTA has sensitivity of 96% and specificity of 97% in detecting hemodynamically significant (>50% luminal narrowing) lesions, with similar sensitivities and specificities regardless of the arterial bed imaged [25]. MDCTA is associated with lower radiation dose than DSA, and consistency in treatment recommendations based on MDCTA is excellent [23,25].

MDCTA may play an important role in distal bypass graft surveillance [26]. Willman and colleagues [26] have demonstrated that MDCTA provides excellent graft image quality. Further, MDCTA findings correlate well with other imaging modalities used for graft surveillance, including duplex ultrasound and DSA. Compared with DSA, MDCTA has greater than 95% sensitivity and specificity for the detection of graft stenosis, aneurysm, and arteriovenous fistula formation [26].

MDCTA is proving useful in the evaluation of the cerebral circulation [27,28]. Patients presenting with cerebrovascular accidents or transient ischemic attacks will likely undergo noncontrast head CT. Contrast-enhanced MDCTA can be performed at the same time, presenting an attractive alternative to duplex ultrasound (which requires an on site vascular technician), or CA (which is invasive). CT perfusion examination can be obtained

---

Box 1. Classification of endoleaks

I. Proximal or distal seal zone leak
II. Retrograde perfusion of aneurysm sac from aortic branches
III. Component separation or graft material failure
IV. Graft porosity
V. Endotension (aneurysm enlargement without identifiable endoleak)

simultaneously, allowing assessment of end-organ perfusion. Josephson and colleagues [27] demonstrated that MDCTA has a negative predictive value of 99% and 100% for stenoses of less than 50% and greater than 70%, respectively. They also found, however, that MDCTA is less specific than carotid angiography, and may be susceptible to calcification artifact. Randoux and colleagues [28] compared MDCTA with MRA and DSA and found MDCTA to be 100% sensitive and specific for the evaluation of greater than 70% carotid stenosis, and to be better at assessing plaque irregularities and ulceration than DSA.

To summarize, MDCTA technology is exploding. As the use of 16- and 64-slice scanners becomes commonplace, MDCTA will become the standard in the diagnosis of disease in all vascular territories. Strengths of MDCTA include superb spatial resolution, widespread availability, and the ability to manipulate images in three dimensions. Data obtained from MDCTA can be used to guide selection of appropriate stents and balloons before CA, thereby limiting radiation exposure and contrast dose during intervention. Weaknesses of MDCTA include the use of ionizing radiation and iodinated contrast agents. Heavily calcified vessels and the presence of metallic foreign bodies (clips, joint replacements) can decrease diagnostic accuracy. In the authors' practice, MDCTA is the noninvasive imaging modality of choice for screening the patient who has peripheral vascular disease.

Magnetic resonance angiography

The physics of magnetic resonance are complicated and involve three major steps. First, the patient is placed in a strong static magnetic field, forcing mobile protons within soft tissue to align with the external magnetic field. Second, a given volume of tissue is pulsed with radiofrequency energy that causes transient perturbations in proton alignment, elevating protons to a higher energy state. Once the radiofrequency pulse is removed, the protons precess to their original lower energy state. Third, the energy given off by protons returning to their original energy state (echo) is recorded and localized in three dimensions.

MRA can be performed without intravenous contrast using time-of-flight (TOF) imaging sequences. This technique exploits the intrinsic motion of protons in flowing blood. The primary disadvantages of the TOF technique are poor spatial resolution and long acquisition times. Gradient imaging techniques (the so-called "white blood sequences") allow for excellent temporal resolution of moving structures, and are currently used to evaluate cardiac wall motion, as well as blood flow in large vessels such as the thoracic aorta.

MRA performed using intravenous gadolinium contrast (GE MRA) yields better spatial resolution than TOF examinations. Contrast is injected intravenously and imaging is performed as the bolus enters the target vessel.

Once acquired, three-dimensional GE MRA images can be manipulated at a workstation to yield MPR, MIP, and VR (Fig. 5) images similar to those obtained with MDCTA [29].

The primary applications of vascular MRA include the evaluation of PAD, carotid artery stenosis (CAS), and renal artery stenosis (RAS). In a meta-analysis conducted in 2000, Nelemans and colleagues [30] examined the performance of MRA (both two-dimensional TOF and three-dimensional GE) in the evaluation of PAD. They found a wide distribution of both sensitivity (64%–100%) and specificity (68%–99%) of MRA in comparison with DSA in the evaluation of PAD. Use of three-dimensional GE MRA and extensive image analysis (MIP images as well as additional formats) predicted better diagnostic yield and improved sensitivity (97%–100%) and specificity (95%–99%), making it an excellent noninvasive alternative to CA [30].

Two studies have compared clinical outcomes and costs associated with MRA, MDCTA, and duplex ultrasound (DU) in the preoperative evaluation of patients who have PAD [31,32]. In the first study, patients referred to a vascular surgeon with ankle-brachial index (ABI) less than 0.9 were randomized to preoperative imaging with either MRA or MDCTA. In the second study, they were randomized to preoperative imaging with either MRA or DU. All patients had similar postoperative outcomes, including similar improvement in ABI, walking distance, and quality of life. Both studies concluded that MRA was associated with greater cost than both MDCTA and DU. MRA was associated with higher examiner diagnostic confidence

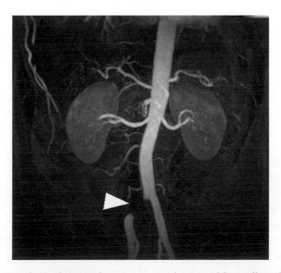

Fig. 5. Gadolinium-enhanced magnetic resonance angiogram with excellent depiction of renal arteries. Note signal dropout associated with patent right common iliac artery stent (*white arrowhead*).

than DU, which resulted in fewer subsequent vascular imaging studies. Despite the greater number of diagnostic tests in the DU group, patients undergoing MRA incurred higher diagnostic costs [32]. Another group of investigators found the use of MRA for preoperative planning to be associated with a higher surgical reintervention rate when compared with MDCTA [31]. Taken together, these studies suggest that MRA yields similar diagnostic information to MDCTA and DU, but does so at higher cost.

MRA has also been used extensively in the evaluation of CAS [28,33–35]. In a comparison of MRA with MDCTA and DSA, Randoux and colleagues [28] demonstrated that GE MRA had good sensitivity in differentiating greater than 70% stenosis, though overestimation occurred in approximately 9% of cases. MRA detected plaque irregularities less often than MDCTA, but detected ulcerations equally well [28]. Muhs and colleagues [33] found similar results when comparing MRA (both TOF and GE MRA) with DU, in that MRA agreed with DU in the evaluation of greater than 80% stenosis in 96.3% of cases. In less severe degrees of stenosis, however, concordance was much less with both TOF and GE MRA, overestimating disease in up to 86% of cases [33]. Townsend and colleagues [35] reported similar results. In their series comparing GE MRA to TOF, GE MRA overestimated clinically significant disease in 50% of arteries examined [35]. In contrast, Nederkoorn and colleagues [34], in a meta-analysis comparing MRA with DSA, demonstrated no difference in diagnostic yield between GE MRA and TOF, though the number of studies examining GE MRA was small in comparison with the number examining TOF. At this time, GE MRA cannot be recommended as the sole imaging study in the evaluation of CAS, but is complimentary to TOF and DU in the noninvasive workup of these patients.

MRA has also been used extensively in the evaluation of patients who have RAS. Leung and colleagues [36] evaluated the performance of GE MRA and DU compared with CA in the diagnosis of RAS. In comparison with conventional angiography, MRA had 90% sensitivity in the detection of hemodynamically significant RAS. Excluding patients who have fibromuscular dysplasia, sensitivity increased to 97%. Other investigators have not reported as favorable results. Patel and colleagues [37] evaluated the performance of GE MRA in the evaluation of hemodynamically significant RAS and found a sensitivity of only 87%, overestimating disease in 31% of arteries. To better delineate the role of MRA in the evaluation of RAS, Tan and colleagues [38] performed a meta-analysis and demonstrated overall sensitivities of GE MRA and nonenhanced MRA of 97% and 94% compared with CA. Taken together, these studies suggest that MRA is a reasonably sensitive screening modality for the detection of RAS. Ultimately, however, patients under consideration for percutaneous renal revascularization will undergo CA at the time of intervention.

To summarize, MRA is an excellent tool for diagnosing disease of the aorta and its major branches. Many centers consider GE MRA the procedure of choice for the evaluation of RAS. Advantages of MRA include excellent contrast resolution, excellent temporal resolution, and lack of ionizing radiation. As such, it has become a modality of choice for the evaluation of children who have cardiovascular disease. Until recently, the use of gadolinium instead of iodinated contrast was considered an advantage, and GE MRA was the procedure of choice when evaluating the patient who has renal insufficiency. Better understanding of NSF and the potential nephrotoxic effects of gadolinium compounds have led to restrictions in the use of GE MRA in this population. Other disadvantages of MRA include the restriction of some implantable medical devices (including pacemakers and some aneurysm clips). MRA tends to overestimate the degree of stenosis within a given vessel and is expensive compared with other imaging modalities.

Duplex ultrasound

DU combines two imaging modalities. Pulsed-wave Doppler ultrasound provides blood flow velocities; gray-scale ultrasound provides cross-sectional imaging based on tissue echogenicity. Duplex examination is often augmented with color Doppler to give a colorimetric analysis of flowing blood (Fig. 6). DU has been used in multiple applications to include preoperative arterial mapping of patients for peripheral artery bypass grafting (BPG); intraoperative DU to demonstrate technical success; evaluation of CAS, assessment of RAS, and endograft surveillance [39].

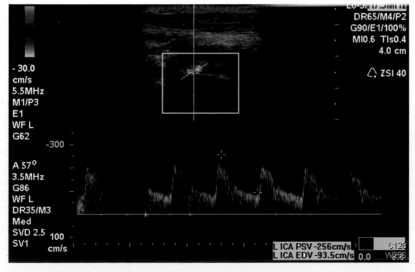

Fig. 6. Duplex ultrasound shows colorimetric analysis of turbulent flow in stenotic carotid artery as well as graphic depiction of elevated velocity (256 cm/s in this case).

Several investigators have reported the utility of DU alone when planning distal bypass in patients who have PAD [40,41]. Ascher and colleagues [40] reported outcomes from their experience with 449 revascularizations performed with this technique, and demonstrated excellent 1-year patency rates. They acknowledge limitations of this technique, citing patient factors (heavily calcified vessels, very low flow, tissue edema, ulcerations), the requirement of highly skilled vascular technologists, and the time to perform lengthy examinations (30 to 150 minutes) [40]. In a smaller study, Grassbaugh and colleagues [41] demonstrated that DU performs similarly to CA in the selection of appropriate bypass target arteries in below-knee revascularization. They noted, however, that DU detected patent peroneal arteries rather poorly. Based on these findings, they recommend a graded diagnostic approach, with CA performed only when DU could not identify appropriate distal target vessels [41].

DU can be used to demonstrate technical success and to predict 1-year patency of distal BPG. In patients undergoing below-knee revascularization, Rzucidlo and colleagues [42] demonstrated that native vessel end-diastolic velocity less than 8 cm/s was 76% sensitive in predicting graft thrombosis.

In many institutions, DU is also the imaging modality most often employed in the follow-up of BPG [26,43]. In a comparison of MDCTA, DU, and DSA in BPG surveillance, Willmann and colleagues [26] demonstrated similar sensitivity and specificity of DU in the detection of hemodynamically significant stenoses when compared with the other modalities. The routine practice of BPG surveillance with DU has recently been called into question, however. In a large prospective, randomized, controlled trial, Davies and colleagues [43] demonstrated similar patient outcomes (amputation, vascular death, quality of life) following vein BPG whether patients were followed with clinical evaluation or with routine DU surveillance. Although the clinical follow-up group did have a higher incidence of stenosis, the cost of following the duplex group was significantly higher [43].

DU is widely regarded as the procedure of choice for screening for CAS. It has been proven useful in quantifying the degree of CAS, and can be used to detect pathologically elevated flow velocities within the extracranial carotid circulation, as well as to characterize plaque morphology and composition [44]. Multiple DU criteria have been proposed to differentiate those patients requiring intervention from those who can be followed with serial examinations. Sabeti and colleagues [45] evaluated the performance characteristics of 13 different proposed DU classification schemes compared with carotid angiography. Sensitivity and specificity ranged from 77% to 98% and 60% to 82%, respectively, depending on the criteria used [45]. The three most sensitive criteria are presented in Table 1, and demonstrate that DU performs well in the evaluation of severe CAS.

In contrast, Nederkoorn and colleagues [34] performed a meta-analysis reviewing the diagnostic utility of DU and MRA in comparison with CA.

Table 1
Duplex ultrasound criteria with high sensitivity for the detection of greater than 70% carotid stenosis

Authors	Criteria	Sensitivity	NPV
Nicolaides et al [62]	PSV >250; EDV >130; $PSV_{ICA}/PSV_{CCA} >4.0$; $PSV_{ICA}/PSV_{CCA} <25$; $EDV_{ICA}/EDV_{CCA} <5.5$	98	98
Hwang et al [63]	PSV ≥200; $PSV_{ICA}/PSV_{CCA} >3.0$	98	98
Fillis et al [64]	PSV <330; EDV <130; $PSV_{ICA}/PSV_{CCA} <3.8$	98	98

Abbreviations: CCA, common carotid artery; EDV, end diastolic velocity; ICA, internal carotid artery; NPV, negative predictive value; sensitivity and NPV in percent; PSV, peak systolic velocity.

Data from Sabeti S, Schillinger M, Mlekusch W, et al. Quantification of internal carotid artery stenosis with duplex US: comparative analysis of different flow velocity criteria. Radiology 2004;232:431–9.

They found that DU had sensitivity and specificity of 86% and 96% respectively when evaluating patients who had greater than 70% stenosis [34]. Like Sabeti and colleagues [45], they acknowledged that different cutoff scores for determining greater than 70% stenosis affected the results of this analysis.

DU can also be used with high sensitivity and specificity for the detection of recurrent CAS following intervention. Using a cutoff of end diastolic velocity (EDV) greater than 70 cm/s, Telman and colleagues [46] demonstrated sensitivity and specificity of greater than 95% for the detection of recurrent CAS compared with carotid angiography. In this study, DU was more sensitive and specific for the detection of recurrent CAS than for the detection of primary CAS.

As mentioned previously, in addition to flow velocities, DU can also provide data regarding plaque morphology and composition. Lal and colleagues [47] developed a gray-scale image evaluation algorithm, called pixel distribution analysis, based on differential tissue echogenicity data derived from healthy volunteers. They then applied these criteria to patients with both symptomatic and asymptomatic CAS, identifying significant differences in plaque morphology and composition between the two groups. Plaques from symptomatic patients demonstrated more intraplaque hemorrhage, higher lipid content, larger lipid core, less distance between lipid core and flow lumen, and less calcium than plaques from asymptomatic patients. These findings correlated well with plaque histology obtained following carotid endarterectomy (CEA) [47].

Similar to the situation with BPG, DU can also be used in the intraoperative setting to demonstrate technical success following CEA. Mullenix and colleagues [48] reported their experience with intraoperative DU. They found that patients who had significant DU abnormalities that were left unrepaired were at greater risk of suffering perioperative neurologic events.

DU has long been recognized as a screening tool for the evaluation of RAS, and more recently for following patients postangioplasty and stenting

[36,49,50]. Olin and colleagues [49] demonstrated that DU could detect he-modynamically significant (>60% stenosis) lesions with sensitivity of 98% and NPV of 97% compared with CA. Leung and colleagues [36] subse-quently compared DU and MRA with CA and found only 81% sensitivity of DU in the evaluation of RAS.

Sharafuddin and colleagues [50] investigated the role of DU in establish-ing baseline examinations in patients undergoing renal artery angioplasty and stenting. They performed pre- and postprocedure DU in 22 technically successful interventions and found significant improvements in several parameters, including resistive index and waveform morphology. The utility of these indices for long-term surveillance of renal artery interventions, however, remains to be determined.

The role of DU in the assessment of endoleak and aneurysm enlargement post-EVAR is controversial [51–55]. McWilliams and colleagues [52] report ed poor sensitivity of DU in the detection of endoleak in comparison with MDCTA, but noted that the sensitivity of DU at detecting endoleak was en-hanced with the administration of intravenous sonographic contrast. Simi-larly poor sensitivity (25%–42%) in the detection of endoleaks has been reported by other groups [51,54]. In one study, nearly half of false-negative DU examinations had Type I endoleaks documented by MDCTA [54]. An-eurysm diameter change detected by DU correlated poorly with MDCTA findings, with DU showing enlarging diameters in up to 23% of cases, none of which were detected by MDCTA. In a meta-analysis, Sun [55] docu-mented sensitivity and negative predictive values of 66% and 90% respec-tively for unenhanced DU, and 81% and 95% for enhanced DU. These findings all suggest that DU is an inadequate modality to exclude endoleak or sac enlargement following EVAR.

In contrast, Napoli and colleagues [53] used DU to classify endoleaks in patients in whom other studies had failed to do so, using a more rigorous examination protocol. By incorporating contrast-enhancement and pro-longed scanning times, they found that of 10 patients who had indeterminate endoleaks (Type V), all could be classified as Type I or Type II based on DU findings. Their protocol also correctly classified 10 patients who had no en-doleak by MDCTA and 10 patients who had Type II endoleaks by MDCTA [53]. Although small, the study suggests that this emerging technology may have a role in better delineating indeterminate endoleaks.

To summarize, DU is an excellent screening modality for superficial vascular beds, including the carotids and extremities. Although DU is also excellent for the evaluation of the abdominal aorta and renal arteries, it is less reliable in obese patients. Advantages of DU include its widespread availability and lack of nephrotoxic contrast agents. In addition, DU can be performed intraoperatively to assess surgical success. Disadvantages include operator dependence and interoperator variability, as well as imag-ing obstacles presented by obese patients and those who have significant bowel gas [36,51].

Intravascular ultrasound

Intravascular ultrasound (IVUS) uses a catheter-based ultrasound transducer to provide the interventionalist with detailed endoluminal anatomic information. Specifically, IVUS can differentiate diseased from normal vessel wall, evaluate the distribution and composition of plaque, precisely define vessel cross-sectional area, and quantify degree of stenosis [56]. IVUS was first used in the evaluation of the coronary circulation and continues to be widely applied to the investigational study, diagnosis, and treatment of atherosclerotic coronary artery disease [57].

In peripheral arterial beds, IVUS is most often employed during endovascular procedures to define relevant vascular anatomy and to demonstrate technical success following intervention [58]. Renal and internal iliac artery origins (important landmarks for proper deployment of stent grafts) and aneurysm diameters and lengths obtained by IVUS correlate well with those obtained by MDCTA [59]. Despite this agreement, one group of investigators showed that IVUS prompted changes in graft selection in nearly one third of cases, most commonly because of overestimation of neck diameter by MDCTA [60]. Similar findings have been reported by other investigators [58].

Clear advantages of IVUS over MDCTA are its ability to provide real-time intraoperative imaging without the use of iodinated contrast agents or ionizing radiation. IVUS has been used in a multimodality approach to endograft implantation in patients who had contraindications to iodinated contrast media with good technical results [61].

It should be emphasized that differences in outcomes based on data derived from MDCTA and IVUS have not been rigorously examined. Consequently, the use of IVUS is left to the discretion of the operating surgeon, and is probably most useful in those patients who have challenging or unclear anatomy.

Summary

Vascular imaging has evolved to the point where the diagnosis of most vascular disease can be made noninvasively. The relative strengths and weaknesses of the various imagintbl1g modalities are summarized in Table 2. Further advancements in equipment and imaging protocols will only improve

Table 2
Relative advantages and disadvantages of vascular imaging modalities

	Ionizing radiation	Iodinated contrast	Gadolinium contrast	Cost	Availability	Intervention
DU	None	None	None	+	+	−
MDCTA	−	−	None	+	+	−
MRA	None	None	−	−	−	−
IVUS	None	None	None	−	−	−
CA	−	−	None	+	+	+

Abbreviations: +, relative strength; −, relative weakness.

the safety and reliability of noninvasive imaging. Conventional angiography has evolved as well, and is achieving an expanded role in the treatment of patients who have vascular disease.

References

[1] Tepel M, Aspelin P, Lameire N. Contrast-induced nephropathy: a clinical and evidence-based approach. Circulation 2006;113:1799–806.

[2] Hawkins IF. Carbon dioxide digital subtraction arteriography. AJR Am J Roentgenol 1982; 139:19–24.

[3] Back MR, Caridi JG, Hawkins IF Jr, et al. Angiography with carbon dioxide (CO2). Surg Clin North Am 1998;78:575–91.

[4] Frankhouse JH, Ryan MG, Papanicolaou G, et al. Carbon dioxide/digital subtraction arteriography-assisted transluminal angioplasty. Ann Vasc Surg 1995;9:448–52.

[5] Chao A, Major K, Kumar S, et al. Carbon dioxide digital subtraction angiography-assisted endovascular aortic aneurysm repair in the azotemic patient. J Vasc Surg 2007;45:451–8.

[6] Remy-Jardin M, Dequiedt P, Ertzbischoff O, et al. Safety and effectiveness of gadolinium-enhanced multi-detector row spiral CT angiography of the chest: preliminary results in 37 patients with contraindications to iodinated contrast agents. Radiology 2005;235:819–26.

[7] Morcos SK, Remy-Jardin M. Gadolinium-based contrast media for multi-detector row spiral CT pulmonary angiography in patients with renal insufficiency. Radiology 2006;238: 1077–8.

[8] Nyman U, Elmstahl B, Leander P, et al. Are gadolinium-based contrast media really safer than iodinated media for digital subtraction angiography in patients with azotemia? Radiology 2002;223:311–8.

[9] Chewning RH, Murphy KJ. Gadolinium-based contrast media and the development of nephrogenic systemic fibrosis in patients with renal insufficiency. J Vasc Interv Radiol 2007;18:331–3.

[10] Bakal CW. Advances in imaging technology and the growth of vascular and interventional radiology: a brief history. J Vasc Interv Radiol 2003;14:855–60.

[11] Katzen BT. Current status of digital angiography in vascular imaging. Radiol Clin North Am 1995;33:1–14.

[12] Hiatt MD, Fleischmann D, Hellinger JC, et al. Angiographic imaging of the lower extremities with multidetector CT. Radiol Clin North Am 2005;43:1119–27, ix.

[13] Kang PS, Spain JW. Multidetector CT angiography of the abdomen. Radiol Clin North Am 2005;43:963–76, vii.

[14] Urban BA, Fishman EK. Tailored helical CT evaluation of acute abdomen. Radiographics 2000;20:725–49.

[15] Wyers MC, Fillinger MF, Schermerhorn ML, et al. Endovascular repair of abdominal aortic aneurysm without preoperative arteriography. J Vasc Surg 2003;38:730–8.

[16] Sprouse LR, Meier GH III, Parent FN, et al. Is three-dimensional computed tomography reconstruction justified before endovascular aortic aneurysm repair? J Vasc Surg 2004;40:443–7.

[17] Parker MV, O'Donnell SD, Chang AS, et al. What imaging studies are necessary for abdominal aortic endograft sizing? A prospective blinded study using conventional computed tomography, aortography, and three-dimensional computed tomography. J Vasc Surg 2005;41:199–205.

[18] Armerding MD, Rubin GD, Beaulieu CF, et al. Aortic aneurysmal disease: assessment of stent-graft treatment-CT versus conventional angiography. Radiology 2000;215:138–46.

[19] Rozenblit AM, Patlas M, Rosenbaum AT, et al. Detection of endoleaks after endovascular repair of abdominal aortic aneurysm: value of unenhanced and delayed helical CT acquisitions. Radiology 2003;227:426–33.

[20] Stavropoulos SW, Clark TW, Carpenter JP, et al. Use of CT angiography to classify endoleaks after endovascular repair of abdominal aortic aneurysms. J Vasc Interv Radiol 2005; 16:663–7.

[21] Tolia AJ, Landis R, Lamparello P, et al. Type II endoleaks after endovascular repair of abdominal aortic aneurysms: natural history. Radiology 2005;235:683–6.

[22] Timaran CH, Ohki T, Rhee SJ, et al. Predicting aneurysm enlargement in patients with persistent type II endoleaks. J Vasc Surg 2004;39:1157–62.

[23] Catalano C, Fraioli F, Laghi A, et al. Infrarenal aortic and lower-extremity arterial disease: diagnostic performance of multi-detector row CT angiography. Radiology 2004;231:555–63.

[24] Martin ML, Tay KH, Flak B, et al. Multidetector CT angiography of the aortoiliac system and lower extremities: a prospective comparison with digital subtraction angiography. AJR Am J Roentgenol 2003;180:1085–91.

[25] Willmann JK, Baumert B, Schertler T, et al. Aortoiliac and lower extremity arteries assessed with 16-detector row CT angiography: prospective comparison with digital subtraction angiography. Radiology 2005;236:1083–93.

[26] Willmann JK, Mayer D, Banyai M, et al. Evaluation of peripheral arterial bypass grafts with multi-detector row CT angiography: comparison with duplex US and digital subtraction angiography. Radiology 2003;229:465–74.

[27] Josephson SA, Bryant SO, Mak HK, et al. Evaluation of carotid stenosis using CT angiography in the initial evaluation of stroke and TIA. Neurology 2004;63:457–60.

[28] Randoux B, Marro B, Koskas F, et al. Carotid artery stenosis: prospective comparison of CT, three-dimensional gadolinium-enhanced MR, and conventional angiography. Radiology 2001;220:179–85.

[29] Ho VB, Corse WR. MR angiography of the abdominal aorta and peripheral vessels. Radiol Clin North Am 2003;41:115–44.

[30] Nelemans PJ, Leiner T, de Vet HC, et al. Peripheral arterial disease: meta-analysis of the diagnostic performance of MR angiography. Radiology 2000;217:105–14.

[31] de Vries M, Ouwendijk R, Flobbe K, et al. Peripheral arterial disease: clinical and cost comparisons between duplex US and contrast-enhanced MR angiography—a multicenter randomized trial. Radiology 2006;240:401–10.

[32] Ouwendijk R, de Vries M, Pattynama PM, et al. Imaging peripheral arterial disease: a randomized controlled trial comparing contrast-enhanced MR angiography and multi-detector row CT angiography. Radiology 2005;236:1094–103.

[33] Muhs BE, Gagne P, Wagener J, et al. Gadolinium-enhanced versus time-of-flight magnetic resonance angiography: what is the benefit of contrast enhancement in evaluating carotid stenosis? Ann Vasc Surg 2005;19:823–8.

[34] Nederkoorn PJ, van der GY, Hunink MG. Duplex ultrasound and magnetic resonance angiography compared with digital subtraction angiography in carotid artery stenosis: a systematic review. Stroke 2003;34:1324–32.

[35] Townsend TC, Saloner D, Pan XM, et al. Contrast material-enhanced MRA overestimates severity of carotid stenosis, compared with 3D time-of-flight MRA. J Vasc Surg 2003;38:36–40.

[36] Leung DA, Hoffmann U, Pfammatter T, et al. Magnetic resonance angiography versus duplex sonography for diagnosing renovascular disease. Hypertension 1999;33:726–31.

[37] Patel ST, Mills JL Sr, Tynan-Cuisinier G, et al. The limitations of magnetic resonance angiography in the diagnosis of renal artery stenosis: comparative analysis with conventional arteriography. J Vasc Surg 2005;41:462–8.

[38] Tan KT, van Beek EJ, Brwon PW, et al. Magnetic resonance angiography for the diagnosis of renal artery stenosis: a meta-analysis. Clin Radiol 2002;57:617–24.

[39] Pearce WH, Astleford P. What's new in vascular ultrasound. Surg Clin North Am 2004;84: 1113–26, vii.

[40] Ascher E, Hingorani A, Markevich N, et al. Lower extremity revascularization without preoperative contrast arteriography: experience with duplex ultrasound arterial mapping in 485 cases. Ann Vasc Surg 2002;16:108–14.

[41] Grassbaugh JA, Nelson PR, Rzucidlo EM, et al. Blinded comparison of preoperative duplex ultrasound scanning and contrast arteriography for planning revascularization at the level of the tibia. J Vasc Surg 2003;37:1186–90.

[42] Rzucidlo EM, Walsh DB, Powell RJ, et al. Prediction of early graft failure with intraoperative completion duplex ultrasound scan. J Vasc Surg 2002;36:975–81.

[43] Davies AH, Hawdon AJ, Sydes MR, et al. Is duplex surveillance of value after leg vein bypass grafting? Principal results of the Vein Graft Surveillance Randomised Trial (VGST). Circulation 2005;112:1985–91.

[44] Tahmasebpour HR, Buckley AR, Cooperberg PL, et al. Sonographic examination of the carotid arteries. Radiographics 2005;25:1561–75.

[45] Sabeti S, Schillinger M, Mlekusch W, et al. Quantification of internal carotid artery stenosis with duplex US: comparative analysis of different flow velocity criteria. Radiology 2004;232: 431–9.

[46] Telman G, Kouperberg E, Sprecher E, et al. Duplex ultrasound verified by angiography in patients with severe primary and restenosis of internal carotid artery. Ann Vasc Surg 2006; 20:478–81.

[47] Lal BK, Hobson RW, Hameed M, et al. Noninvasive identification of the unstable carotid plaque. Ann Vasc Surg 2006;20:167–74.

[48] Mullenix PS, Tollefson DF, Olsen SB, et al. Intraoperative duplex ultrasonography as an adjunct to technical excellence in 100 consecutive carotid endarterectomies. Am J Surg 2003;185:445–9.

[49] Olin JW, Piedmonte MR, Young JR, et al. The utility of duplex ultrasound scanning of the renal arteries for diagnosing significant renal artery stenosis. Ann Intern Med 1995;122: 833–8.

[50] Sharafuddin MJ, Raboi CA, bu-Yousef M, et al. Renal artery stenosis: duplex US after angioplasty and stent placement. Radiology 2001;220:168–73.

[51] Elkouri S, Panneton JM, Andrews JC, et al. Computed tomography and ultrasound in follow-up of patients after endovascular repair of abdominal aortic aneurysm. Ann Vasc Surg 2004;18:271–9.

[52] McWilliams RG, Martin J, White D, et al. Use of contrast-enhanced ultrasound in follow-up after endovascular aortic aneurysm repair. J Vasc Interv Radiol 1999;10:1107–14.

[53] Napoli V, Bargellini I, Sardella SG, et al. Abdominal aortic aneurysm: contrast-enhanced US for missed endoleaks after endoluminal repair. Radiology 2004;233:217–25.

[54] Raman KG, Missig-Carroll N, Richardson T, et al. Color-flow duplex ultrasound scan versus computed tomographic scan in the surveillance of endovascular aneurysm repair. J Vasc Surg 2003;38:645–51.

[55] Sun Z. Diagnostic value of color duplex ultrasonography in the follow-up of endovascular repair of abdominal aortic aneurysm. J Vasc Interv Radiol 2006;17:759–64.

[56] Wilson EP, White RA. Intravascular ultrasound. Surg Clin North Am 1998;78:561–74.

[57] von Birgelen C, Hartmann M. Intravascular ultrasound assessment of coronary atherosclerosis and percutaneous interventions. Minerva Cardioangiol 2004;52:391–406.

[58] Tutein Nolthenius RP, van den Berg JC, Moll FL. The value of intraoperative intravascular ultrasound for determining stent graft size (excluding abdominal aortic aneurysm) with a modular system. Ann Vasc Surg 2000;14:311–7.

[59] van Essen JA, Gussenhoven EJ, van der LA, et al. Accurate assessment of abdominal aortic aneurysm with intravascular ultrasound scanning: validation with computed tomographic angiography. J Vasc Surg 1999;29:631–8.

[60] Garret HE Jr, Abdullah AH, Hodgkiss TD, et al. Intravascular ultrasound aids in the performance of endovascular repair of abdominal aortic aneurysm. J Vasc Surg 2003;37: 615–8.

[61] Bush RL, Lin PH, Bianco CC, et al. Endovascular aortic aneurysm repair in patients with renal dysfunction or severe contrast allergy: utility of imaging modalities without iodinated contrast. Ann Vasc Surg 2002;16:537–44.

[62] Nicolaides AN, Shifrin EG, Bradbury A, et al. Angiographic and duplex grading of internal carotid stenosis: can we overcome the confusion? J Endovasc Surg 1996;3:158–65.

[63] Hwang CS, Shau WY, Tegeler CH. Doppler velocity criteria based on receiver operating characteristic analysis for the detection of threshold carotid stenoses. J Neuroimaging 2002;12:124–30.

[64] Filis KA, Arko FR, Johnson BL, et al. Duplex ultrasound criteria for defining the severity of carotid stenosis. Ann Vasc Surg 2002;16:413–21.

ELSEVIER
SAUNDERS

SURGICAL
CLINICS OF
NORTH AMERICA

Surg Clin N Am 87 (2007) 995–1016

Current Trends in Managing Carotid Artery Disease

Kristen L. Biggs, MD*, Wesley S. Moore, MD

*UCLA Division of Vascular Surgery, 200 Medical Plaza,
Room 510-6, Box 956908, Los Angeles, CA 90095-6908, USA*

Indications for carotid endarterectomy based on Level I evidence (prospective randomized trials)

Symptomatic trials

North American Symptomatic Carotid Endarterectomy Trial

The North American Symptomatic Carotid Endarterectomy Trial (NAS-CET) was a multicenter prospective randomized controlled clinical trial designed to evaluate the benefit of carotid endarterectomy in reducing the risk of fatal and nonfatal stroke for patients who had experienced neurologic symptoms (prior transient ischemic attack [TIA] or mild stroke).

There were two main criteria for patient participation in the trial: (1) patients less than 80 years old must have experienced either a TIA or a minor, nondisabling stroke in the distribution of the study artery within the past 120 days; and (2) a selective carotid angiography performed within the past 120 days had to demonstrate at least a 30% stenosis of the study artery, which would be surgically accessible without significant tandem lesions or complete carotid occlusion. At the time of publication of the study design in 1991, a total of 1212 symptomatic patients had been randomized to either the surgical group, who would undergo carotid endarterectomy in addition to the best medical management, or the medical group, who would receive the best medical management alone [1]. Medical management consisted of drug therapy for hypertension and hyperlipidemia, risk factor modification, and antiplatelet therapy with 1300 mg/d of aspirin. For statistical analysis, the surgical and medical groups were further divided into

---

* Corresponding author.
E-mail address: kbiggs@mednet.ucla.edu (K.L. Biggs).

0039-6109/07/$ - see front matter © 2007 Elsevier Inc. All rights reserved.
doi:10.1016/j.suc.2007.07.005
surgical.theclinics.com

groups of moderate stenosis (30–69%) and high-grade stenosis (70–99%). End points of the NASCET were stroke and death.

In February 1991, the NASCET investigators issued a clinical alert because carotid endarterectomy was found to be highly beneficial for symptomatic patients with high-grade stenosis [2]. Within the high-grade stenosis group, 300 patients had been randomized to surgery, and 295 patients were to receive best medical management alone. Sixteen patients within the medical group (5.4%) crossed over and underwent carotid endarterectomy, but they were still considered to be part of the medical group because of the intent-to-treat design of the study. Although the 30-day perioperative stroke morbidity and mortality rate was higher in the surgical group (5%) than the rate over a similar period in the medical group (3%), the data at 18 months after the time of randomization were clearly in favor of carotid endarterectomy. Twenty-four percent of patients in the medical group experienced fatal or nonfatal ipsilateral stroke at 18 months, compared with only 7% of the patients in the surgical group, including perioperative events. This represented a highly significant 17% absolute reduction in the risk of fatal or nonfatal ipsilateral stroke for the surgical group ($P < .001$). When analyzing all strokes (ipsilateral, contralateral, vertebrobasilar, hemorrhagic, and so forth) and deaths in the high-grade stenosis group, again the data favored endarterectomy. Twelve percent of medical patients and only 5% of surgical patients experienced stroke in any distribution or death from any cause at 18 months after randomization ($P < .01$). Because these significant findings demonstrated the benefit of carotid endarterectomy for symptomatic patients with a high-grade stenosis, this arm of the study was halted. For patients with a moderate stenosis (30–69%), the trial continued, as the benefit of carotid endarterectomy was still uncertain [3].

The results in the moderate stenosis group were reported in 1998 [4]. In the group of patients with stenosis ranging from 30% to 69%, 1108 patients were randomized to carotid endarterectomy and 1118 received medical therapy alone. These groups were further subdivided according to degree of stenosis. Of the patients receiving surgical treatment, 430 had a stenosis of 50% to 69% and 678 had a stenosis of less than 50%. Similarly in the medical group, 428 had a stenosis of 50% to 69% and 690 had a stenosis of less than 50%. Again, the perioperative stroke and overall mortality rate was higher in the surgical group (6.7%) compared with the medical group (2.4%) at approximately 30 days after randomization. However, the 5-year rate of fatal and nonfatal stroke was 22.2% in the medical group and only 15.7% in the surgical group with 50% to 69% stenosis. Although this finding was statistically significant ($P = .045$), the long-term benefit of carotid endarterectomy in the 50% to 69% stenosis group was not as great as that seen in symptomatic patients with greater than 70% stenosis. Among symptomatic patients with less than 50% stenosis, no significant benefit was noted from carotid endarterectomy.

Medical Research Council European Carotid Surgery Trial

The Collaborative Group of the European Carotid Surgery Trial (ECST) concurrently enrolled symptomatic patients in a randomized controlled clinical trial to assess the risks and benefits of carotid endarterectomy in stroke prevention. The largest study to date, ECST randomized 3024 patients to either undergo carotid endarterectomy (n = 1811) or to avoid surgery for as long as possible (n = 1213) [5]. Although it was not strictly enforced by a protocol, patients in both groups were administered medical treatment, and the numbers of patients taking aspirin, antiplatelet medication, anticoagulants, and lipid-lowering drugs were similar in the two study groups. To qualify for the ECST, patients with symptoms (nondisabling ischemic stroke, TIA, or retinal infarction) during the previous 6 months had to undergo carotid angiography, and the treating physician had to be "substantially uncertain" as to whether endarterectomy was recommended after the angiogram was performed. Patients were subdivided into categories of disease by the percent of stenosis they demonstrated on angiography: mild (0%–29%), moderate (30%–69%), and severe (≥70%). After randomization to the surgery and no surgery groups, patients were followed from 1981 through 1994. Trial end points included 30-day perioperative stroke or death, any major stroke during follow-up, and death from any cause.

Before discussing the trial results, an important point should be acknowledged regarding the European method of determining percent of carotid stenosis by angiography. In the European method, the percent of carotid stenosis is calculated from the formula:

$$\%\text{Stenosis} = (1 - R/B) \times 100$$

where R is the minimal transverse diameter through the maximum point of stenosis, and B is the projected diameter of the carotid bulb. On angiography, only the contrast within the lumen is seen, and the vessel wall itself cannot be visualized. Thus, to determine the projected diameter of the carotid bulb, one must extrapolate lines drawn from the visible lumina of the common and internal carotid arteries. As expected, this method is not entirely reproducible between interpreters.

In North-American-based trials, such as the NASCET and the Veterans Administration Asymptomatic Trial, specific diameters are *measured* on angiography, and these values are used to calculate the percent of carotid stenosis:

$$\%\text{Stenosis} = (1 - R/D) \times 100$$

where R is as described above and D is the diameter of the normal internal carotid artery where the walls become parallel.

When comparing the two formulas, R is a constant value, and B will usually be a greater diameter than D. As a result, the European method not only lacks reproducibility but tends to overestimate the percent of carotid stenosis. A study conducted by Eliasziw and colleagues compared angiograms using the European and American methods (Table 1) [6].

The interim results for ECST patients with severe ($\geq 70\%$) and mild (0%–29%) stenosis were published in *The Lancet* in 1991 [7]. At that time, 778 patients were noted to have severe stenosis by angiography, 455 were randomized to undergo surgery, and the remainder continued medical management. Despite an initial 7.5% risk of stroke or death in the 30-day perioperative period, the patients with severe stenosis in the surgical group had an eightfold reduction in ipsilateral fatal and nonfatal ischemic strokes at 3 years. The risk was 1.1% in the surgical group and 8.4% in the medical group, and this difference was highly significant ($P < .0001$). It should be noted that the perioperative risk of stroke and death was higher at 7.5% in this study when compared with the 5.0% perioperative risk in NASCET. For 374 patients with mild stenosis, the risk of ischemic stroke at 3 years was negligible for all patients in the ECST, so any benefits of endarterectomy were outweighed by its perioperative risks.

The ECST's Collaborative Group reported their findings for 1599 patients with a moderate (30%–69%) stenosis in *The Lancet* in 1996 [8]. Of the 959 patients randomized to receive surgery within the moderate stenosis group, the 30-day perioperative risk of stroke and death was 7.9%. Once again, the perioperative risks outweighed the potential long-term benefits of carotid endarterectomy. The ECST recommended against surgery for symptomatic patients with up to a 69% stenosis, which would be classified as up to a 40% stenosis by the North American method and is consistent with the NASCET results.

Veterans Administration Symptomatic Trial

A third multicenter randomized prospective trial comparing carotid endarterectomy plus best medical therapy to medical management alone for symptomatic patients was the Veterans Administration (VA) Symptomatic Trial [9]. Between 1988 and 1991, 189 patients were enrolled at 16 participating Veterans Affairs medical centers. To qualify for enrollment, patients must have experienced symptoms of TIAs, transient monocular blindness, or mild stroke within the previous 120 days, and they must have had a greater than 50% stenosis of the carotid artery ipsilateral to

Table 1
Comparison of carotid stenosis estimated by European and North American methods

% Stenosis European	% Stenosis North American
60	18
70	40
80	61
90	80

the symptoms by angiography. Patients were randomized to undergo carotid endarterectomy (91 patients) or best medical management alone (98 patients). The study was halted after a mean follow-up of 11.9 months, in part because data from the earlier NASCET and ECST trials had already demonstrated the significant benefits of performing carotid endarterectomy on symptomatic patients with severe stenosis at the time this trial was getting under way. The results of the VA Symptomatic Trial at the 11.9-month follow-up were fully supportive of the NASCET and ECST findings. Of the medically managed patients, 19.4% experienced stroke or crescendo TIAs, but only 7.7% of the patients who underwent endarterectomy had this outcome. This represented an absolute risk reduction of 11.7% ($P = .011$) for the surgical group. An even greater 17.7% absolute risk reduction ($P = .004$) occurred in the subset of symptomatic patients with a stenosis greater than 70%.

Asymptomatic trials

Veterans Administration Asymptomatic Carotid Stenosis Study

The VA Asymptomatic Carotid Stenosis Study was a multicenter prospective randomized clinical trial initiated in 1983. The study was designed to determine the effect of carotid endarterectomy on the incidence of TIA, transient monocular blindness, and stroke for patients who had an asymptomatic hemodynamically significant stenosis of the carotid artery measuring 50% or more by angiography [10].

Eleven VA medical centers in the United States participated in this study, which enrolled 444 male patients. Patients were first screened for potential trial enrollment by ocular pneumoplethysmography (OPG) or optional B-mode duplex ultrasonography. Patients with positive OPG or duplex ultrasonography screening underwent conventional or digital subtraction angiography. Patients with a hemodynamically significant stenosis of 50% or more were considered for study participation. Patients were excluded from study participation if they had a previous stroke in the distribution of the study artery, previous endarterectomy with re-stenosis, or previous extracranial-to-intracranial bypass; were high surgical risk secondary to medical comorbidities; had a life expectancy of less than 5 years; were taking chronic anticoagulation or long-term high-dose aspirin therapy; or were intolerant of aspirin or noncompliant with medical therapy. They were then randomized to one of two treatment groups: carotid endarterectomy plus aspirin (the surgical group; 211 patients) or aspirin therapy alone (the medical group; 233 patients). Once randomized, therapy with aspirin 650 mg twice daily commenced. Patients randomized to the surgical group underwent carotid endarterectomy within 10 days of randomization. Study participants were followed for a mean of 47.9 months. End points of TIA, stroke, or stroke death were recorded. Crossovers from the medical to the surgical group were permitted if recommended by the coprincipal investigators.

Initial data analysis revealed a 30-day mortality of 1.9% (4/211) for the surgical group. All deaths were from myocardial infarction (MI). The incidence of postoperative stroke was 2.4% (5/211), and three of these strokes occurred as a result of angiography. Thus, the combined stroke and mortality rate within 30 days after randomization was 4.3% in the surgical group [11].

After the conclusion of the trial, 57 patients (24.5%) in the medical group sustained an ipsilateral or contralateral neurologic event (TIA, amaurosis fugax, stroke), compared with only 27 patients (12.8%) in the surgical group. This represented an absolute risk reduction of 11.6% (for the surgical group versus the medical group), which was statistically significant ($P < .002$). There were 65 ipsilateral neurologic events, 48 (20.6%) in the medical group, and 17 (8%) in the surgical group. For ipsilateral events, the absolute risk reduction was 12.6%, which was also statistically significant ($P < .001$). Thirty-two strokes occurred in the distribution of the study artery, 22 (9.4%) in the medical group and 10 (4.7%) in the surgery group. This difference was not statistically significant ($P < .06$), which may be related to the small sample size. There were no differences in the survival rates between the surgically and medically treated groups [12]. The overall conclusion of the study was that carotid endarterectomy, combined with optimal medical management, reduces the incidence of ipsilateral neurologic events in a selected group of male patients with asymptomatic, hemodynamically significant carotid stenosis.

Asymptomatic Carotid Atherosclerosis Study

Similar to the VA Asymptomatic Carotid Stenosis Trial, the Asymptomatic Carotid Atherosclerosis Study (ACAS) was initially designed to determine if carotid endarterectomy plus aspirin and risk-factor modification would reduce the incidence of ipsilateral TIA, amaurosis fugax, and retinal and cerebral infarction in patients with asymptomatic, hemodynamically significant carotid stenosis [13]. After criticism of the VA Asymptomatic trial, the end points were changed in March 1993 to cerebral infarction occurring in the distribution of the study artery or any stroke or death occurring in the perioperative period. TIA was no longer an end point. The ACAS, funded by the National Institute of Neurological Disorders and Stroke, is the largest prospective randomized multicenter trial of surgery for asymptomatic carotid stenosis to date.

Thirty-nine clinical sites across the United States and Canada enrolled a total of 1662 patients with asymptomatic carotid artery stenosis of 60% or greater between December 1987 and December 1993. Follow-up data were available on 1659 patients. Patients were eligible for study participation if an internal carotid artery stenosis of at least 60% was confirmed by two of three procedures. Qualifying procedures included OPG, Doppler sonography, and conventional or arterial digital subtraction angiography. Angiography was not required before randomization but was required before surgery in those so randomized. Therefore, any angiographic complications were charged against the surgery group, whether or not surgery was performed. Disease that constitutes a 60% stenosis by carotid duplex may not translate to a 60% stenosis by angiography, and it may not translate to an absolute 60% stenosis of the carotid artery (see later section, "Identification of The High Risk Plaque"). This must be taken into consideration when interpreting the results of the medically randomized group in ACAS.

The study participants were randomized to one of two groups: carotid endarterectomy plus aspirin and risk-factor modification (the surgical group; 825 patients) or aspirin therapy and risk factor modification alone (the medical group; 834 patients). Risk factor reduction consisted of counseling and intervention for hypertension, obesity, hyperlipidemia, diabetes mellitus, tobacco use, sedentary lifestyle, the use of estrogen compounds, and polycythemia. The dosage of aspirin administration was 325 mg/d. Those randomized to surgery underwent carotid angiography and carotid endarterectomy within 2 weeks of randomization. For quality control purposes, performance criteria were established to audit surgical results [14]. To participate in ACAS, a surgeon's operative experience had to include a minimum of 12 carotid endarterectomies per year. Upon review of the surgeon's last 50 endarterectomies, the neurologic morbidity and mortality rate must not exceed 3% for endarterectomies performed on asymptomatic patients and 5% for endarterectomies performed on symptomatic patients.

In September 1994, after a median follow-up of 2.7 years (4657 patient-years of observation), the ACAS trial was halted because carotid endarterectomy was found to be significantly better than medical management alone. A clinical advisory was issued, recommending that physicians participating in the study reevaluate patients in the medical group for the opportunity to undergo surgery [15]. The full report of the data was published in *JAMA* [16]. The risk of ipsilateral stroke and perioperative stroke and death for patients with asymptomatic carotid stenosis was 5.1% for patients in the surgical group, including the complications of angiography and perioperative events, compared with an 11.0% complication rate for patients in the medical group ($P = .004$). The study concluded that asymptomatic patients with a hemodynamically significant carotid stenosis would have a 5-year aggregate ipsilateral stroke risk reduction of 53% if carotid endarterectomy was performed by a surgeon with less than a 3% morbidity and mortality rate for the procedure.

The 30-day perioperative stroke morbidity and mortality rate for the surgical group of ACAS was 2.3% (19 events/825 patients). Only 724 of the 825 patients in the surgical group actually underwent carotid endarterectomy. Some of the strokes and deaths attributed to this group occurred before surgery, or as a result of angiography, but were included in the surgical group's data because of the intention-to-treat design of the study. The actual 30-day stroke rate for surgical patients after endarterectomy was 1.38%. Only one mortality occurred within 30 days of the 724 patients who underwent operations, yielding a 0.14% mortality rate. The low combined perioperative stroke and death incidence of 1.52% can be attributed in part to the stringent criteria used to select surgeons for participation in ACAS [17].

Asymptomatic Carotid Surgery Trial

The Asymptomatic Carotid Surgery Trial (ACST) was a large, European-based multicenter randomized controlled clinical trial designed to examine the effect of carotid endarterectomy on the end points of stroke and perioperative death for asymptomatic patients with substantial carotid narrowing. The original study design was published in the *European Journal of Vascular Surgery* in 1994, around the same time that results from the two aforementioned United States trials were available for review [18]. The ACST attempted to definitively assess the long-term effects of carotid endarterectomy on stroke risk for asymptomatic patients with significant carotid stenosis by enrolling an extremely large number of patients.

One hundred twenty-six hospitals in 30 countries participated in the ACST. Patients were eligible for the study if they demonstrated a greater-than-60% luminal diameter reduction of the carotid artery by duplex ultrasound and if this stenosis had not caused any neurologic symptoms, TIA, or stroke within the past 6 months. Carotid angiography was not an ACST requirement. Patients were excluded from study participation for reasons of previous ipsilateral carotid endarterectomy, prohibitive surgical risk, presence of a life-threatening condition other than carotid stenosis, or if the source of cerebral emboli were felt to be of cardiac rather than of carotid origin. A total of 3120 patients were enrolled in the trial between 1993 and 2003. Exactly half were randomized to undergo immediate carotid endarterectomy (the surgical group), and the other half were randomized to indefinite deferral of carotid endarterectomy (the nonsurgical group). All issues of medical management, including antiplatelet, antihypertensive, and lipid-lowering therapy, were left to the discretion of the physician. At the date of the last follow-up in 2002 to 2003, more than 90% of the patients were taking antiplatelet therapy, 81% were on antihypertensives, and 70% were on lipid-lowering medications. For quality control of the study, surgeons were considered eligible for participation only if their stroke morbidity and mortality did not exceed 6% of their most recent 50 endarterectomies performed on symptomatic patients. Study end points were perioperative stroke and death and non-perioperative stroke.

Results of the ACST were published in 2004 in *The Lancet* [19]. A total of 1650 endarterectomy procedures were performed in this trial, 1405 in the surgical group and 245 in the nonsurgical group. Collectively, the 30-day perioperative risk of stroke or death was 3.1%. When analyzing the 5-year risk of non-perioperative stroke, there was a statistically significant reduction in this risk for patients randomized to the surgical group. The actual risk was 3.8% for the surgical group and 10.9% for the nonsurgical group ($P<.0001$). In each group, half of the non-perioperative strokes were severely disabling or fatal. When including perioperative stroke and death in the analysis, the 5-year risk of stroke or perioperative death became 6.4% for the surgical group and 11.8% for the nonsurgical group. Again, half of the strokes in each group caused death or significant disability. After analyzing certain subgroups of gender, age, and percent carotid stenosis, the authors concluded that immediate carotid endarterectomy halved the net 5-year stroke and perioperative death risk from 12% to 6% for asymptomatic patients 75 years old or less with a diameter-reducing stenosis of 70% or greater as measured by duplex ultrasound.

Improving safety and durability of carotid endarterectomy

Intraoperative monitoring

Since carotid endarterectomy requires clamping of the internal carotid artery, the blood flow it provides to the ipsilateral cerebral hemisphere will be affected during the operation. Because adequate cerebral perfusion can be maintained from the contralateral carotid artery and the vertebral arteries via the Circle of Willis, clamping is usually of no significant consequence. Approximately 10% to 15% of the time, however, clamping will lead to symptomatic hemispheric cerebral ischemia, as determined from operations performed under local anesthesia [20–24]. Patients who have suffered prior cerebral infarction may be more sensitive to clamping due to pressure sensitivity for flow to the ischemic penumbra surrounding an infarct. The patients who become symptomatic with clamping benefit from placement of a silastic shunt to maintain prograde blood flow through the carotid artery during the operation. Because shunting can result in air or atheroma embolization, intimal dissection, creation of an intimal flap, or difficulty in visualizing the intimectomy end point, shunt placement has potential morbidity. Some surgeons advocate routine shunting, arguing that it can be performed with little morbidity in experienced hands and that it offers the patient the best protection from intraoperative cerebral ischemia [25]. Others use shunts more selectively, based on clinical observations or monitoring criteria. Still others do not shunt patients at all. Current practice guidelines support either routine shunting or selective shunting [26].

For carotid endarterectomy performed under local anesthesia, a neurologic deficit that becomes apparent with carotid clamping necessitates shunt placement. For patients under general anesthesia, internal carotid artery back-pressure, intraoperative electroencephalography (EEG), transcranial Doppler (TCD), or somatosensory-evoked potentials (SSEPs) can be used to determine whether to shunt. The technique of measuring carotid back-pressure was first described by Moore and colleagues [27,28]. A 22-gauge needle is connected to pressure tubing, which is joined to an arterial pressure transducer. After flushing the system with saline and zeroing it at the level of the carotid bifurcation, the needle is bent at a 45°angle and carefully inserted into the common carotid artery. The bend on the needle ensures that its distal tip is free within the arterial lumen and oriented in an axis parallel to blood flow. The common carotid artery proximal to the needle and the external carotid artery are clamped, and then the back-pressure is ascertained. The original criteria for mandatory shunting based on back-pressure included either a prior cerebral infarction ipsilateral to the operative artery (regardless of back-pressure) or no prior cerebral infarction but a back-pressure of 25 mm Hg or less. Currently, controversy exists as to which level of back-pressure mandates use of an internal shunt. Some surgeons have a lower threshold and report optimal benefit when shunting patients with back-pressures of up to 50 mm Hg [29].

When conducting EEG monitoring, multiple electrodes are affixed with conductive gel to the patient's scalp before surgery. A standard 16-lead configuration connected to the electrodes is used to measure voltage differences between parts of the brain. With this modality, brain activity can be monitored noninvasively and with high temporal resolution down to milliseconds. Different sinusoidal waves of various frequencies correlate with brain activity. Generally, higher frequencies (beta waves, ≥ 12 Hz) correspond to active thought, and lower frequencies (delta waves, ≤ 4 Hz) are associated with deep stages of sleep. EEG changes that denote cerebral ischemia include amplitude attenuation of higher frequencies by 50% or greater, an increase in delta wave activity, or a complete loss of EEG signals [25,30].

Two other intraoperative monitoring techniques, TCD and SSEPs, have been evaluated with mixed reviews in the literature. TCD uses a 2-MHz Doppler probe to noninvasively measure the blood velocity though the middle cerebral artery via a transtemporal approach [31]. A decrease in the middle cerebral arterial velocity by 60% to 70% has been used as a criterion for shunting. SSEPs, another type of intraoperative cerebral monitoring, record the electrical response to the mechanical stimulation of peripheral nerves. Unlike the EEG, which passively monitors cerebral electrical activity, SSEPs involve electrical stimulation of a peripheral nerve, such as the median nerve or the posterior tibial nerve. Electrodes placed on the scalp record the response to the stimulus. Criteria for shunting have included decreased amplitude or prolonged conduction time of the cortical SSEP. In a meta-analysis involving more than 3000 patients, no difference in intraoperative SSEP was found between patients who were shunted and those who were not shunted during carotid endarterectomy. The authors concluded that decreased or delayed cortical SSEPs could be used neither as a criterion for shunting, nor as a predictor of neurologic outcome after carotid endarterectomy [32].

Patch closure

Carotid endarterectomy can be performed in a variety of ways. Some surgeons favor eversion endarterectomy, which involves obliquely transecting the internal carotid artery at the level of the bulb, everting the artery to remove the plaque specimen, and subsequently rejoining the arterial segments with a circumferential suture line. Proponents of this technique argue that by creating an oblique anastomosis at the widest part of the carotid, re-stenosis rates are lower and use of a patch is unnecessary. Disadvantages of eversion endarterectomy include lack of plaque–end point visualization and difficulty in suturing around a shunt, if one is required. For these reasons, many surgeons prefer standard endarterectomy, creating a longitudinal arteriotomy that extends from the common onto the internal carotid artery beyond the level of disease. After the endarterectomy is complete, the arteriotomy can be closed primarily, but the literature now overwhelmingly supports patch angioplasty closure. The best patch material is still a matter of debate and surgeon preference. Patches can be made of autologous or synthetic substances, to include saphenous vein, cervical vein, bovine pericardium, polytetrafluoroethylene, and collagen-impregnated Dacron (Hemashield).

A meta-analysis comparing primary closure to carotid patch angioplasty reported the results of seven randomized controlled trials, representing a total of 1281 operations, in *The Journal of Vascular Surgery* in 2004 [33]. When examining the 30-day perioperative results, there was a statistically significant lower risk of ipsilateral stroke, any perioperative stroke, risk of stroke or death, return to the operating room, and acute arterial occlusion for the group undergoing patch angioplasty. Six of the seven trials reported follow-up results at a postoperative interval greater than or equal to 1 year. Again, a statistically significant lower risk of ipsilateral stroke, any stroke, combined stroke or death, and arterial occlusion or recurrent stenosis was noted in the patients who were given patch angioplasty.

These findings were supported by a recently published retrospective cohort study comparing primary closure (n = 233), patch angioplasty (n = 1377), and eversion endarterectomy (n = 362) in 1972 carotid endarterectomies [34]. Patients with primary closure had a 5.6% perioperative stroke risk, which was significantly greater ($P = .006$) than the risk with either patch angioplasty (2.2%) or eversion (2.5%). In addition, the risk of perioperative stroke or death was significantly higher in the primary closure group when compared with the other closure techniques (6.0% versus 2.5%, $P = .006$). The authors concluded that primary closure should be abandoned in favor of either standard endarterectomy with patch angioplasty or eversion endarterectomy.

Antiplatelet drugs

It has been long recognized that antiplatelet medical therapy interrupts the pathophysiology of atherosclerotic carotid disease. As evidenced by the different dosage of aspirin used in the randomized controlled clinical trials of the 1980s comparing carotid endarterectomy to best medical management, the optimal dosage of aspirin to prevent stroke has been controversial. Some investigators have hypothesized that after surgery, a high dosage of aspirin is necessary to prevent platelet aggregation at the site of the endarterectomy. Others have recommended a low dosage, suggesting that it was associated with a lower complication rate. The ASA and Carotid Endarterectomy (ACE) trial attempted to resolve this debate by investigating the effect of different dosages of aspirin on perioperative complication rates.

The ACE trial was an international multicenter controlled clinical trial that randomized 2849 patients scheduled to undergo carotid endarterectomy to different dosages of aspirin [35]. Most centers enrolled had also been participants in the NASCET. The patients were randomly assigned to 81 mg (n = 709), 325 mg (n = 708), 650 mg (n = 715), or 1300 mg (n = 717). Most patients had surgery within two days after starting aspirin therapy, and patients continued taking aspirin for 3 months after surgery. Study end points included all strokes, MIs, and deaths; all strokes and deaths; and ipsilateral strokes and deaths. Data were reported for end points occurring within 30 days, as well as 3 months, after surgery.

There were no significant differences in the outcomes for the 81 mg and 325 mg groups, or for the 650 mg and 1300 mg groups. Thus, the patients receiving the lower dosages were analyzed together as the low-dosage group, and those receiving the higher dosages were similarly combined into the high-dosage group. Because the antiplatelet effects of aspirin can persist for up to 1 week, an efficacy analysis was performed that excluded patients who had been taking high dosages of aspirin (650 mg and higher) before randomization in the trial. Also excluded were patients who received surgery within 1 day of randomization because they may not have had enough time for complete systemic circulation of the aspirin dose. In the efficacy analysis, 566 patients were in the low-dosage group, and 550 patients were in the high-dosage group. The combined rate of stroke, MI, and death was significantly lower in the low-dosage group (3.7%) than the high-dosage group (8.2%) at 30 days ($P = .002$). A significantly lower rate was also seen in the low-dosage group (4.2% compared with 10.0%, high-dosage group) at 3 months ($P = .0002$). The ACE trial concluded that patients taking a low dosage aspirin were less likely to suffer perioperative stroke, MI, and death than patients taking higher dosages. The American College of Chest Physicians strongly supported these findings and recommended with Grade IA evidence that patients begin preoperative therapy with low-dosage aspirin (81–325 mg) upon clinical presentation and continue medical therapy indefinitely after carotid endarterectomy [36,37].

Statins and beta blockers

A strong association has been identified between blood cholesterol levels and risk of coronary disease. To determine whether a similar association exists between low-density lipoprotein (LDL) cholesterol levels and risk of stroke, the Heart Protection Study (HPS) Collaborative Group randomized 20,536 patients to receive either 40 mg/d of simvastatin or placebo [38]. Of the study participants, 3280 patients had pre-existing cerebrovascular disease (nonhemorrhagic stroke occurring greater than 6 months prior, history of TIA, or history of carotid endarterectomy or angioplasty). The other 17,256 study participants had evidence of coronary disease, arterial occlusive disease, diabetes mellitus, or treated hypertension. They were considered to be at high risk for a major vascular event, defined as nonfatal MI or coronary death, stroke of any type, or need for a coronary or non-coronary revascularization procedure. LDL levels of all study participants were at least 3.5 mmol/L (135 mg/dL). After an induction phase involving 4 weeks of placebo followed by 4 to 6 weeks of 40 mg/d simvastatin, patients were then randomized to 5 years of treatment with simvastatin (n = 10,269) or placebo (n = 10,267).

When evaluating the entire patient database, there was a highly significant 25% reduction ($P < .0001$) in the first event rate of stroke for the patients taking simvastatin (n = 444, or 4.3%) compared with placebo (n = 585, or 5.7%). In addition, a significant 28% reduction in ischemic strokes ($P < .0001$) was also noted for the entire study population, favoring the patients randomized to simvastatin (n = 290, or 2.8%) instead of placebo (n = 409, or 4.0%). Analysis of the patient subgroup with pre-existing cerebrovascular disease showed no difference in the incidence of stroke for the simvastatin group (n = 169, or 10.3%) and the placebo group (n = 170, or 10.4%), although there was a nonsignificant trend toward fewer ischemic strokes for the simvastatin group. One possible explanation is that these patients may have had advanced carotid disease at the time of study enrollment, and simvastatin is unlikely to reduce the atherosclerotic plaque burden in the carotid artery.

Despite these findings, medical therapy with simvastatin or an equivalent lipid-lowering agent should still be recommended to patients with pre-existing cerebrovascular disease. The HPS Collaborative Group did find a highly significant 20% reduction ($P = .001$) in the combined rate of major vascular events (coronary events, strokes, and coronary and noncoronary revascularizations) in this patient subset taking simvastatin. The use of beta blockers has recently been advocated as a means of reducing the incidence of fatal and nonfatal MI in patients undergoing vascular surgery. Lindenauer and colleagues [39] performed a retrospective review of 663,635 patients in 329 hospitals between the years 2000 and 2001. In patients with no cardiac risk, there was no benefit in beta blockade. In patients with increasing cardiac risk, there was a statistically significant benefit in cardiac event reduction in favor of beta blockade. A review of available evidence to date was performed by Hackam and supports the use of beta blockers in patients at risk [40]. However, a prospective randomized trial reported by Yang and colleagues, which compared patients undergoing abdominal aortic surgery and lower extremity revascularization, failed to show a benefit in risk reduction for those patients on metoprolol when compared with placebo [41].

Identification of the high-risk plaque

Percent stenosis

The randomized controlled clinical trials of the late 1980s, which compared carotid endarterectomy to medical management alone, established the current practice guidelines for determining when to operate on symptomatic and asymptomatic patients based on percent stenosis. The NASCET trial clearly established that with each decile increase in percent stenosis, there was a corresponding increase in neurologic event rates in the medically randomized group. The inflection point at which the surgically managed group fared better than the medical group occurred at a 50% diameter-reducing stenosis, as measured using the North American method with contrast angiography. With each 10% increase in stenosis beyond 50%, there was a corresponding increase in benefit with carotid endarterectomy when compared with patients in the medical control arm of the trial. The effect of increasing percent stenosis was not as clear in asymptomatic patients. In the ACAS trial there was no apparent correlation between event rates and percent stenosis. However, the majority of the ACAS patients were in the 60% to 80% range, with relatively few patients having stenosis greater than 80%. Therefore, the failure to demonstrate a relationship between increasing percent stenosis and increasing neurologic event rates in ACAS may be a type 2 statistical error. This may also be the case in the ACST trial where there was a suggestion of correlation.

Ulceration

The relationship of plaque ulceration as an independent factor separate from percent stenosis was first documented by Moore and Hall [42,43]. The authors identified a group of patients experiencing focal TIAs in the absence of hemodynamically significant carotid stenosis, but with angiographically documented plaque ulceration. Carotid endarterectomy was successful in arresting these attacks. They went on to apply numeric characteristics to these ulcers and categorized them as small type A, medium type B, and large type C [44], making it possible to demonstrate that the presence of medium and large ulceration in asymptomatic plaques, when left untreated, had a 5% to 7% annual stroke rate [45,46]. The importance of plaque ulceration was further validated in the NASCET trial [47] and by a separate analysis of plaques removed from patients in the surgical arm of NASCET [48]. Further evidence of the importance of plaque ulceration and the genesis of cerebral emboli was shown by Valton and colleagues [49] using TCD and demonstrating a relationship between high-intensity signals and plaque ulceration.

Plaque composition

The Imaging in Carotid Angioplasties and Risk of Stoke registry was established to identify patients who might be at a higher or lower risk of periprocedural stroke during carotid angioplasty [50]. This multicenter international registry included 418 cases of carotid artery stenting. Preprocedurally, high-resolution B-mode ultrasound was used to image the carotid plaque. Images were then digitized, sent to a personal computer, and analyzed using Adobe Photoshop software [51]. The gray-scale median (GSM) of the carotid plaque, which is the median of the frequency distribution of the gray levels of the pixels in the plaque as compared with adventitia and blood, was then calculated. The GSM is a measure of plaque echolucency, and the authors arbitrarily established the value of 25 to discriminate between hypoechoic and hyperechoic plaques [52]. After patients underwent carotid angioplasty and stenting, outcomes were recorded. The overall rate of neurological complications was 3.6% and included 2.2% minor strokes and 1.4% major strokes. Of patients with GSM less than or equal to 25, 11 of 155 (7.1%) had strokes. Of patients with GSM greater than 25, 4 of 263 (1.5%) had strokes. This finding was statistically significant ($P = .005$). The authors concluded that patients with echolucent plaque (GSM $\leq$ 25), notably high in lipid and hemorrhagic content, were at increased risk of having a postprocedural stroke. Echolucent plaques have a significantly higher embolic potential when treated with angioplasty and stenting. Of interest, there was no correlation in this study between the degree of carotid stenosis and the GSM. Thus, plaque composition may be an independent characteristic of the high-risk plaque.

Identification of the high-risk patient

First introduced in the mid-1990s, the endovascular option of carotid angioplasty and stenting (CAS) has been evolving over the past decade. CAS in high-risk patients is currently approved only in the setting of clinical trials. CAS may offer a minimally invasive alternative for high-risk patients. Randomized controlled CAS trials have enrolled patients at high risk for open surgery with intent to eventually broaden the application of CAS to lower-risk patients if this technology is deemed not inferior to carotid endarterectomy.

The Stenting and Angioplasty with Protection in Patients at High Risk for Endarterectomy (SAPPHiRE) trial was the first to specifically enroll high-risk patients, defined as having (1) certain physiologic factors, including clinically significant cardiac disease (such as congestive heart failure, abnormal stress test, or need for open-heart surgery), severe pulmonary disease, or advanced age greater than 80 years, or (2) certain anatomic factors, including contralateral carotid occlusion, contralateral laryngeal nerve palsy, previous radical neck surgery, previous radiation therapy to the neck, or recurrent stenosis after endarterectomy [53]. Patients were required to have at least one high-risk factor to be eligible for participation in the SAPPHiRE trial. The results of this trial are described in the next section.

Carotid endarterectomy versus carotid angioplasty and stenting

Registries and historical comparison

At least two dozen case series, each involving more than 100 patients treated with CAS, have been published between 1996 and 2005 [54]. Overall 30-day stroke rates ranged from 1% to 8% in these series. Rates declined in later years, presumably due to increased experience and use of embolic protection devices (EPD). The average combined 30-day rate of stroke, MI, or death was 4% in these series.

Multiple industry-sponsored registries collected data on patients undergoing CAS. Although none is published in a peer-reviewed journal, their results have been presented at national meetings and are available on the Internet. The purpose of these registries, or single-arm uncontrolled trials, was to establish the safety of CAS and to gain approval for its use in randomized controlled clinical trials. Device safety was established by comparing the rate of adverse outcomes after stenting to historical controls of carotid endarterectomy and medically managed high-risk patients. The Acculink for Revascularization of Carotids in High Risk Patients registry quoted the historical rate of the 1-year composite primary end point (stroke, MI, or death at 30 days and ipsilateral stroke from 31 days to 1 year) to be as high as 14.5% for high-risk patients [55]. This historical risk may have been overestimated. The composite rate of stroke, MI, and death has been recently reported as 9.3% for symptomatic high-risk patients, and as low as 1.6% for asymptomatic high-risk patients, in a series of 323 patients who underwent carotid endarterectomy [56].

Approximately 10 CAS registries, each involving over 100 to almost 500 patients, have reported 30-day stroke rates ranging from 2 to 7% [54]. Combined stroke, MI, or death rates averaged 6% at 30 days. Of note, only a minority (27%) of patients treated with CAS in these registries had symptoms; the vast majority were asymptomatic from their carotid disease and therefore at the lowest risk for any intervention. Randomized controlled clinical trials are necessary to determine (1) whether the endarterectomy or the stented patient is at greater risk of having an adverse outcome, and (2) whether the expected risks are different for symptomatic and asymptomatic patients with carotid disease.

Data from CAS registries led to US Food and Drug Administration (FDA) approval of at least five stenting and EPD systems for use in randomized controlled clinical trials studying patients with either a greater-than-50% symptomatic or greater-than-80% asymptomatic carotid stenosis [57–61]. Some trials have targeted high-risk patients while others are presently enrolling average-risk patients.

Prospective randomized trials

Many prospective randomized trials comparing carotid artery stenting to endarterectomy have been published or are presently underway. To describe each in detail is beyond the scope of this review. This section outlines the conclusions of a few of the more recent trials.

The SAPPHiRE trial was designed to test the hypothesis that carotid artery stenting with an embolic protection device was a noninferior alternative to carotid endarterectomy in patients considered high-risk [53]. Patients were considered for study participation if they had (1) either a greater-than-50% symptomatic stenosis or a greater-than-80% asymptomatic stenosis of the carotid artery, and (2) at least one high-risk factor, such as clinically significant cardiac disease, severe pulmonary disease, contralateral carotid occlusion, contralateral laryngeal-nerve palsy, previous radical neck surgery, previous radiation therapy to the neck, recurrent stenosis after endarterectomy, or age greater than 80 years. Patients were randomized to CAS with a self-expanding nitinol stent and an EPD (n = 167), or to carotid endarterectomy (n = 167). The primary end point of the SAPPHiRE trial was the incidence of a major cardiovascular event at 1 year, defined as the combined rate of death, stroke, and MI occurring within 30 days and the rate of death or ipsilateral stroke occurring between 31 days and 1 year after the procedure. The primary end point occurred in 12.2% of the CAS patients and 20.1% of the endarterectomy patients. This outcome was statistically significant for noninferiority ($P = .004$) but not for superiority ($P = .053$). In other words, the SAPPHiRE trial concluded that in high medical- and anatomic-risk patients, CAS is a treatment alternative to endarterectomy with comparable risks of major cardiovascular events. The trial was terminated in 2002 because of a decline in patient enrollment.

The main criticism of the SAPPHiRE trial is that only 29.9% of patients randomized to CAS and 27.7% of patients randomized to endarterectomy had a stenosis that was symptomatic. Most of the patients enrolled in this trial had asymptomatic stenoses, which are less likely to result in stroke than symptomatic stenoses. The "high-risk" patients who were treated with open surgery had increased risks of MI compared with those who underwent stenting both at 30 days (6.6% carotid endarterectomy [CEA] versus 1.9% CAS, $P = .04$) and at 1 year (8.1% CEA versus 2.5% CAS, $P = .03$). Whether the physiologic stresses induced by general anesthesia contributed to an increased risk of MI for endarterectomy patients was not commented on in the SAPPHiRE results. Increased risk of MI may have accounted for the overall increased cardiovascular event rate for the patients randomized to open surgery. When the results were analyzed with conventional end points (stroke or death at 30 days plus ipsilateral stroke or death from neurologic causes within 31 days to 1 year), there was essentially no difference between the two groups (5.5% for CAS versus 8.4% for CEA, $P = .36$).

The Carotid Revascularization using Endarterectomy or Stenting Systems (CaRESS) trial questioned if CAS with EPD was comparable to carotid endarterectomy in both symptomatic and asymptomatic patients [62]. Of significant note, this trial was nonrandomized, with treatment modality determined by physician and patient preference. Patients with a greater-than-50% symptomatic or greater-than-75% asymptomatic stenosis were eligible for study participation, and presence of a high risk factor was not required. Although approximately 85% of the patients were considered to be high-risk by the study investigators (120 of the 143 CAS patients and 220 of the 254 endarterectomy patients), most were asymptomatic (68%), similar to the SAPPHiRE trial. No statistically significant difference was observed in the baseline characteristics of the CAS and endarterectomy groups.

The CaRESS trial reported lower rates of adverse outcomes than those reported in the SAPPHiRE trial. The combined event rate of death, stroke, and MI was 2.1% for CAS and 4.4% for endarterectomy ($P = .241$) at 30 days, and 10.9% for CAS and 14.3% for endarterectomy ($P = .288$) at 1 year. Because patients were not randomized to a treatment arm in the CaRESS trial, these lower morbidity and mortality rates were likely a product of careful patient selection. The investigators concluded that the 30-day and 1-year risk of death, stroke, or MI was equivalent for patients with symptomatic and asymptomatic carotid stenosis undergoing CAS or CEA.

In 2004 a German trial was announced which would investigate if the two modalities were indeed equivalent in the treatment of severe symptomatic carotid stenosis [63]. Patients had to have symptoms of a TIA or stroke in the prior 180 days and an ipsilateral carotid stenosis of greater than 50% by NASCET criteria to participate in the Stent-Supported Percutaneous Angioplasty of the Carotid Artery versus Endarterectomy (SPACE) trial. The primary end point was ipsilateral ischemic stroke or death within 30 days after the procedure. Twelve hundred patients were randomized to the treatment arms. The primary end point occurred in 6.84% of the 605 CAS patients and in 6.34% of the 595 CEA patients [64]. The one-sided P value for noninferiority was 0.09; thus, the SPACE trial failed to prove noninferiority for CAS compared with endarterectomy for the periprocedural complication rate. The investigators concluded that widespread use of CAS was not justified and that more data was needed for long-term comparison of CAS to endarterectomy.

A French study was enrolling patients at the same time as the SPACE trial. The Endarterectomy Versus Angioplasty in Patients with Symptomatic Severe Carotid Stenosis (EVA-3S) trial enrolled patients who had had a TIA or stroke in the prior 4 months and at least a 60% stenosis by the NASCET criteria [65]. Patients were randomized to CAS, either with or without an EPD, or endarterectomy, and the primary end point investigated was any stroke or death occurring within 30 days of the procedure. On January 30, 2003, the safety committee of EVA-3S recommended stopping unprotected CAS [66]. At that time, approximately 80 patients had been randomized to CAS, and the 30-day rate of stroke was 3.9 times higher in the group without EPD (4 strokes in 15 patients) than the group with EPD (5 strokes in 58 patients). The trial continued until September 2005, when it was stopped prematurely because of reasons of safety and futility [67]. Of the 527 patients enrolled, the primary outcome was reached by 9.6% of the CAS group and only 3.9% of endarterectomy patients ($P = .01$). Significantly higher rates of stroke and death were seen at 6 months in the stenting group as well (11.7% CAS with EPD versus 6.1% CEA, $P = .02$). Although the EVA-3S investigators defended their process of selecting interventional physicians, stating that it did not adversely affect the stroke rate, the question remains whether the poorer outcomes among the CAS group occurred secondary to the inexperience of the interventionalists. The interventional physician had to have performed at least 12 carotid stenting procedures or at least 35 stenting procedures in the supra-aortic trunks, of which five were carotid stents, to qualify. Centers that filled all study requirements but lacked a qualifying interventional physician could participate under the supervision of an "experienced tutor" until the local interventionalist met the criteria. The NASCET and ACAS trials enforced technical standards that minimized the morbidity and mortality attributable to the surgeon. If similarly higher standards were required to perform CAS, perhaps the stroke and death rates would be lower for the patients receiving this intervention.

Approved indications for carotid angioplasty and stenting

The only approved indication for CAS at the present time is a symptomatic patient who, in the opinion of a surgeon, is at high risk for carotid endarterectomy. Otherwise, CAS use is only approved for patients participating in an FDA-approved clinical trial. The largest trial for both symptomatic and asymptomatic high-risk patients is the Carotid Revascularization Endarterectomy versus Stent Trial (CREST) trial. This study is continuing to enroll patients and has not yet reached an end point.

References

[1] North American Symptomatic Carotid Endarterectomy Trial (NASCET) Steering Committee. North American Symptomatic Carotid Endarterectomy Trial. Methods, patient characteristics, and progress. Stroke 1991;22:711–20.

[2] North American Symptomatic Carotid Endarterectomy Trial (NASCET) investigators: clinical alert: benefit of carotid endarterectomy for patients with high-grade stenosis of the internal carotid artery. Stroke 1991;22:816–7.

[3] North American Symptomatic Carotid Endarterectomy Trial Collaborators: beneficial effect of carotid endarterectomy in symptomatic patients with high-grade carotid stenosis. N Engl J Med 1991;325:445–53.

[4] Barnett HJM, Taylor DW, Eliasziw M, et al. Benefit of carotid endarterectomy in patients with symptomatic moderate or severe stenosis. N Engl J Med 1998;339:1415–25.

[5] European Carotid Surgery Trialists' Collaborative Group. Randomised trial of endarterectomy for recently symptomatic carotid stenosis: final results of the MRC European Carotid Surgery Trial (ECST). Lancet 1998;351:1379–87.

[6] Eliasziw M, Smith RF, Singh N, et al. Further comments on the measurements of carotid stenosis from angiograms. Stroke 1994;25:2445–9.

[7] European Carotid Surgery Trialists' Collaborative Group. MRC European Carotid Surgery Trial: interim results for symptomatic patients with severe (70–99%) or with mild (0–29%) carotid stenosis. Lancet 1991;337:1235–43.

[8] European Carotid Surgery Trialists' Collaborative Group. Endarterectomy for moderate symptomatic carotid stenosis: interim results from the MRC European Carotid Surgery Trial. Lancet 1996;347:1591–3.

[9] Mayberg MR, Wilson SE, Yatsu F, et al. Carotid endarterectomy and prevention of cerebral ischemia in symptomatic carotid stenosis. JAMA 1991;266:3289–94.

[10] Veterans Administration: a Veterans Administration cooperative study: role of carotid endarterectomy in asymptomatic carotid stenosis. Stroke 1986;17:534–9.

[11] Towne JB, Weiss DG, Hobson RW. First phase report of cooperative Veterans Administration asymptomatic carotid stenosis study—operative morbidity and mortality. J Vasc Surg 1990;11:252–9.

[12] Hobson RW, Weiss DG, Fields WS, et al. Efficacy of carotid endarterectomy for asymptomatic carotid stenosis. N Engl J Med 1993;328:221–7.

[13] Asymptomatic Carotid Artery Stenosis Group: study design for randomized prospective trial of carotid endarterectomy for asymptomatic atherosclerosis. Stroke 1989;20:844–9.

[14] Moore WS, Vescera CL, Robertson JT, et al. Selection process for surgeons in the Asymptomatic Carotid Atherosclerosis Study. Stroke 1991;22:1353–7.

[15] Clinical advisory: carotid endarterectomy for patients with asymptomatic internal carotid artery stenosis. Stroke 1994;25:2523–4.

[16] Executive Committee for the Asymptomatic Carotid Atherosclerosis Study: endarterectomy for asymptomatic carotid artery stenosis. JAMA 1995;273:1421–8.

[17] Moore WS, Young B, Baker WH, et al. Surgical results: a justification of the surgeon selection process for the ACAS Trial. J Vasc Surg 1996;23:323–8.

[18] Halliday AW, Thomas D, Mansfield A. The Asymptomatic Carotid Surgery Trial (ACST): rationale and design. Eur J Vasc Surg 1994;8:703–10.

[19] Halliday A, Mansfield A, Marro J, et al. Prevention of disabling and fatal strokes by successful carotid endarterectomy in patients without recent neurological symptoms: randomized controlled trial. Lancet 2004;363:1491–502.

[20] Evans WE, Hayes JP, Waltke EA, et al. Optimal cerebral monitoring during carotid endarterectomy; neurologic response under local anesthesia. J Vasc Surg 1985;2:775–7.

[21] Rockman CB, Riles TS, Gold M, et al. A comparison of regional and general anesthesia in patients undergoing carotid endarterectomy. J Vasc Surg 1996;24:946–56.

[22] Stroughton J, Nath RL, Abbott WM. Comparison of simultaneous electroencephalographic and mental status monitoring during carotid endarterectomy with regional anesthesia. J Vasc Surg 1998;28:1014–23.

[23] Calligaro KD, Dougherty MJ. Correlation of carotid artery stump pressure and neurological changes during 474 carotid endarterectomies performed in awake patients. J Vasc Surg 2005; 42:684–9.

[24] Hans SS, Jareunpoon O. Prospective evaluation of electroencephalography, carotid artery stump pressure, and neurologic changes during 314 consecutive carotid endarterectomies performed in awake patients. J Vasc Surg 2007;45:511–5.

[25] Roseborough GS. Pro: routine shunting is the optimal management of the patient undergoing carotid endarterectomy. J Cardiothorac Vasc Anesth 2004;18:375–80.

[26] Bond R, Rerkasem K, Rothwell PM. Routine or selective carotid artery shunting for carotid endarterectomy (and different methods of monitoring in selective shunting). Cochrane Database of Syst Rev 2002;CD000190.

[27] Moore WS, Hall AD. Carotid artery back pressure: a test of cerebral tolerance to temporary carotid occlusion. Arch Surg 1969;99:702–10.

[28] Moore WS, Yee JM, Hall AD. Collateral cerebral blood pressure. An index of tolerance to temporary carotid occlusion. Arch Surg 1973;106:521–3.

[29] Baker WH, Littooy FN, Hayes AC, et al. Carotid endarterectomy without a shunt: the control series. J Vasc Surg 1984;1:50–6.

[30] Blume WT, Ferguson GG, McNeil DK. Significance of EEG changes at carotid endarterectomy. Stroke 1986;17:891–7.

[31] Schneider PA, Rossman ME, Torem S, et al. Transcranial Doppler in the management of extracranial cerebrovascular disease: implications in diagnosis and monitoring. J Vasc Surg 1988;7:223–31.

[32] Wober C, Zeitlhofer J, Asenbaum S, et al. Monitoring of median nerve somatosensory evoked potentials in carotid surgery. J Clin Neurophysiol 1998;15:429–38.

[33] Bond R, Rerkasem K, Naylor AR, et al. Systematic review of randomized controlled trials of patch angioplasty versus primary closure and different types of patch materials during carotid endarterectomy. J Vasc Surg 2004;40:1126–35.

[34] Rockman CB, Halm EA, Wang JJ, et al. Primary closure of the carotid artery is associated with poorer outcomes during carotid endarterectomy. J Vasc Surg 2005;42:870–7.

[35] Taylor DW, Barnett HJM, Haynes RB, et al. Low-dose and high-dose acetylsalicylic acid for patients undergoing carotid endarterectomy: a randomized controlled trial. Lancet 1999; 353:2179–84.

[36] Clagett GP, Sobel M, Jackson MR, et al. Antithrombotic therapy in peripheral arterial occlusive disease: the Seventh ACCP Conference on Antithrombotic and Thrombolytic Therapy. Chest 2004;126:609S–26S.

[37] Albers GW, Amernco P, Easton JD, et al. Antithrombotic and thrombolytic therapy for ischemic stroke: the seventh ACCP Conference on antithrombotic and thrombolytic therapy. Chest 2004;126:483S–512S.

[38] Heart Protection Study Collaborative Group. Effects of cholesterol-lowering with simvastatin on stroke and other major vascular events in 20,536 people with cerebrovascular disease or other high-risk conditions. Lancet 2004;363:757–67.

[39] Lindenauer PK, Pekow P, Wang K, et al. Perioperative beta-blocker therapy and mortality after major noncardiac surgery. N Engl J Med 2005;353:349–61.

[40] Hackam DG. Perioperative beta-blocker therapy in vascular surgery: clinical update. J Vasc Surg 2006;43:632–4.

[41] Yang H, Raymer K, Butler R, et al. The effects of perioperative beta-blockade: results of the Metoprolol after Vascular Surgery (MaVS) study, a randomized controlled trial. Am Heart J 2006;152:983–90.

[42] Moore WS, Hall AD. Ulcerated atheroma of the carotid artery—a cause of transient cerebral ischemia. Am J Surg 1968;116:237–42.

[43] Moore WS, Hall AD. Importance of emboli from carotid bifurcation in pathogenesis of cerebral ischemic attacks. Arch Surg 1970;101:708–16.

[44] Maddison FE, Moore WS. Ulcerated atheroma of the carotid artery: arteriographic appearance. Am J Roentgenol 1969;107:530–4.

[45] Moore WS, Boren C, Malone JM, et al. Natural history of nonstenotic asymptomatic ulcerative lesions of the carotid artery. Arch Surg 1978;113:1352–9.

[46] Dixon S, Pais SO, Raviola C, et al. Natural history of nonstenotic asymptomatic ulcerative lesions of the carotid artery: a further analysis. Arch Surg 1982;117:1493–8.

[47] Eliasziw M, Streifler JY, Spence JD, et al. Prognosis for patients following a transient ischemic attack with and without a cerebral infarction on brain CT. North American Symptomatic Carotid Endarterectomy Trial (NASCET) Group. Neurology 1995;45: 428–31.

[48] Fisher M, Paganini-Hill A, Martin A, et al. Carotid plaque pathology: thrombosis, ulceration, and stroke pathogenesis. Stroke 2005;36:253–7.

[49] Valton L, Larrue V, Arrue P, et al. Asymptomatic cerebral embolic signals in patients with carotid stenosis. Correlation with appearance of plaque ulceration on angiography. Stroke 1995;26:813–5.

[50] Biasi GM, Ferrari SA, Nicolaides AN, et al. The ICAROS registry of carotid artery stenting. Imaging in Carotid Angioplasties and Risk of Stroke. J Endovasc Ther 2001;8:46–52.

[51] Sabetai MM, Tegos TJ, Nicholaides AN, et al. Reproducibility of computer-quantified carotid plaque echogenicity: can we overcome the subjectivity? Stroke 2000;31:2189–96.

[52] Biasi GM, Froio A, Diethrich EB, et al. Carotid plaque echolucency increases the risk of stroke in carotid stenting: the Imaging in Carotid Angioplasty and Risk of Stroke (ICAROS) Study. Circulation 2004;110:756–62.

[53] Yadav JS, Wholey MH, Kuntz RE, et al. Protected carotid-artery stenting versus endarterectomy in high-risk patients. N Engl J Med 2004;351:1493–501.

[54] Goodney PP, Schermerhorn ML, Powell RJ. Current status of carotid artery stenting. J Vasc Surg 2006;43:406–11.

[55] Available at: http://www.strokecenter.org/trials/TrialDetail.aspx?tid=100. Accessed April 20, 2007.

[56] Mozes G, Sullivan TM, Torres-Russotto DR, et al. Carotid endarterectomy in SAPPHiRE-eligible high-risk patients: Implications for selecting patients for carotid angioplasty and stenting. J Vasc Surg 2004;39:958–66.

[57] Available at: http://www.fda.gov/cdrh/mda/docs/p040012.html. Accessed April 20, 2007.

[58] Available at: http://www.fda.gov/cdrh/mda/docs/p040038.html. Accessed April 20, 2007.

[59] Available at: http://www.fda.gov/cdrh/mda/docs/p030047.html. Accessed April 20, 2007.

[60] Available at: http://www.fda.gov/cdrh/mda/docs/p050025.html. Accessed April 20, 2007.

[61] Available at: http://www.fda.gov/cdrh/mda/docs/p060001.html. Accessed April 20, 2007.

[62] CaRESS Steering Committee. Carotid Revascularization Using Endarterectomy or Stenting Systems (CaRESS) phase I clinical trial: 1-year results. J Vasc Surg 2005;42:213–9.

[63] Ringleb PA, Kunze A, Allenberg JR, et al. The stent-supported percutaneous angioplasty of the carotid artery vs. endarterectomy trial. Cerebrovasc Dis 2004;18:66–8.

[64] The SPACE Collaborative Group. 30-day results from the SPACE trial of stent-protected angioplasty versus carotid endarterectomy in symptomatic patients: a randomised non-inferiority trial. Lancet 2006;368:1239–47.

[65] EVA-3S Investigators. Endarterectomy vs. angioplasty in patients with symptomatic severe carotid stenosis (EVA-3S) Trial. Cerebrovasc Dis 2004;18:62–5.

[66] EVA-3S Investigators. Carotid angioplasty and stenting with and without cerebral protection: clinical alert from the endarterectomy versus angioplasty in patients with symptomatic severe carotid stenosis (EVA-3S) Trial. Stroke 2004;35:e18–21.

[67] Mas JL, Chatellier G, Beyssen B, et al. Endarterectomy versus stenting in patients with symptomatic severe carotid stenosis. N Engl J Med 2006;355:1660–71.

ELSEVIER
SAUNDERS

SURGICAL
CLINICS OF
NORTH AMERICA

Surg Clin N Am 87 (2007) 1017–1033

Current Management of Infrarenal Abdominal Aortic Aneurysms

Jonathan L. Eliason, MD[a],*, W. Darrin Clouse, MD[b,c]

[a]Section of Vascular Surgery, Department of Surgery, The University of Michigan Health System, CVC 5463, 1500 E. Medical Center Drive, SPC 5867, Ann Arbor, MI 48109-5867, USA
[b]Division of Vascular Surgery Wilford Hall Medical Center, 2200 Bergquist Drive, Suite 1, Lackland AFB, San Antonio, TX 78236, USA
[c]Uniformed Services University of the Health Sciences, 4301 Jones Bridge Road, Bethesda, MD 20814, USA

The management of infrarenal abdominal aortic aneurysms (IAAAs) changed considerably 16 years ago when Juan Parodi ushered in the concept of endovascular aneurysm repair (EVAR) [1]. The subsequent EVAR era has been far from static, however, with many technological advances and multiple generations of aortic stent-graft devices being used. In this rapidly changing environment, the determination of the optimal management of patients with aneurysmal disease can be difficult. The goal of this article is to provide the best level of evidence within the contemporary literature to answer two simple questions: when should an IAAA be repaired? and what method of repair should be used? The management of ruptured abdominal aortic aneurysms (AAAs) and approaches to repair of complex aortic aneurysms are outlined in subsequent articles within this issue.

Although it seems straightforward, the question of "when," or at what size, an IAAA should be repaired is complicated. Patient comorbidities, gender, chosen method of repair, and a host of other variables may alter the management approach. Two randomized controlled clinical trials have helped considerably to provide a framework for answering this question. The UK Small Aneurysm Trial and the subsequent Aneurysm Detection and Management (ADAM) Trial both compared open surgical repair with aneurysm surveillance for aneurysm sizes in the 4.0- to 5.5-cm range [2–5]. Each of these studies demonstrated no benefit in overall mortality for surgical repair of these small aneurysms. Many surgeons, therefore, limited elective aneurysm repair to asymptomatic patients with aneurysm sizes

---

* Corresponding author.
E-mail address: jonaelia@med.umich.edu (J.L. Eliason).

0039-6109/07/$ - see front matter © 2007 Elsevier Inc. All rights reserved.
doi:10.1016/j.suc.2007.08.002

of 5.5 cm or greater. However, both studies were encumbered by a large number of crossovers from the observation arms to the surgical arms owing to patients' IAAAs becoming symptomatic or expanding to 5.5 cm or greater. Indeed, a mean 8-year follow-up to the UK Small Aneurysm Trial in 2002 showed that nearly three-quarters of trial participants under surveillance had crossed over to surgery [3]. Despite the high crossover rate, both studies concluded that early surgery for IAAAs measuring 4.0 to 5.5 cm did not produce a long-term survival advantage, but that most patients will ultimately come to need surgical repair (Table 1).

The waters were again muddied with an ever-growing number of single- and multicenter experiences suggesting that EVAR offered a substantial improvement in length of hospital stay, morbidity, and even mortality, over open repair [6–8]. Several randomized controlled clinical trials (RCTs) were subsequently conducted in Europe in an attempt to prospectively evaluate these potential advantages. The first was the Dutch Randomized Endovascular Aneurysm Management (DREAM) Trial [9,10]. Patients with asymptomatic IAAAs greater or equal to 5.0 cm and considered suitable candidates for open or endovascular repair were randomized to either technique. This study suggested a 30-day benefit in mortality favoring EVAR (1.2% EVAR versus 4.6% open repair), with a risk ratio for open repair of 3.9 (95% confidence interval, 0.9–32.9; $P = .10$). The implied mortality advantage for EVAR was lost, however, at the 2-year study endpoint.

The second and third RCTs were from the United Kingdom and were labeled EVAR trial 1 (EVAR 1) and EVAR trial 2 (EVAR 2) [11,12]. EVAR 1 compared EVAR with open repair in patients with suitable EVAR anatomy and aneurysm size of 5.5 cm or greater. EVAR 2 compared EVAR with no treatment in patients with aneurysm size of 5.5 cm or greater who were deemed unfit for open repair. EVAR 1 was similar to the DREAM Trial in its demonstration of an early perioperative mortality benefit for EVAR (1.7% EVAR versus 4.7% odds ratio [OR]), with an adjusted odds ratio 0.37 (95% confidence interval, 0.17–0.83; $P = .016$), although all-cause mortality at the 4-year study endpoint showed no survival advantage for EVAR over open repair. In EVAR 2, 4-year follow-up revealed that, when compared with no intervention, EVAR in patients unfit for open repair did not improve patient survival. The post hoc analyses and discussion regarding these studies are beyond the scope of this article. Suffice it to say that issues such as long treatment delays, a high number of patient crossovers, and patients in EVAR 2 actually undergoing open repair made the application of these trials to everyday practice patterns difficult.

More recent data used the National Surgical Quality Improvement Program (NSQIP) database to compare open aneurysm repair with EVAR in the high-risk population [13]. This highly validated and clinically relevant database used prospectively entered data from the 123 participating centers in The Department of Veteran Affairs system for retrospective review. The high-risk criteria included age greater than 60; American Society of

Table 1
Randomized controlled trials comparing surgery to surveillance of small aneurysms

| Trial | Patient number randomized | Aneurysm size at randomization (cm) | Follow-up duration | 30-day operative mortality OR[a] group (%) | All-cause final mortality (%) | | Number (%) of surveillance patients who underwent surgical repair during follow-up |
					OR[a]	Obs.[b]	
ADAM[c]	1136	4.0–5.4 cm	4.9 years (mean)	11 (2.1)	143 (25.1)	122 (21.5)	349 (61.6)
United Kingdom Small Aneurysm Trial	1090	4.0–5.5 cm	10 years (at minimum)	(5.8)	362 (63.9)	352 (67.3)	401 (76.1)

[a] Surgery group.
[b] Surveillance group.
[c] Aneurysm Detection and Management trial.

Anesthesiology classification 3 or 4; and the comorbidity variables of history of cardiac, respiratory, or hepatic disease, cardiac revascularization, renal insufficiency, and low serum albumin level. The all-cause 30-day mortality (3.4% versus 5.2%, $P = .047$) and morbidity (16.2% versus 31.0%, $P < .0001$) were both statistically lower for EVAR, and the mortality benefit for EVAR persisted through the 1-year study duration (9.5% versus 12.4%, $P = .038$). Although this study was not of prospective randomized controlled clinical design, the NSQIP's robust clinical information-facilitating risk-stratified comparisons, as well as the study's relatively large enrollment, make the persistent 1-year mortality advantage of EVAR over open repair an important finding.

Although most studies since the UK Small Aneurysm and the ADAM trials have focused on aneurysm sizes of 5.5 cm or greater, some nonrandomized studies have shown superior results using EVAR in smaller aneurysms [14]. Retrospective analysis of the large European Collaborators on Stent/graft Techniques for aortic Aneurysm Repair database revealed that EVAR for aneurysms with diameters between 4.0 and 5.4 cm had lower Type I endoleak rates and improved cumulative freedom from aneurysm-related death than two comparison groups with aneurysm diameters of 5.5 to 6.4 cm, and 6.5 cm or greater [15]. The small aneurysm advantage with EVAR is thought to be due to less aortic tortuosity and a lower incidence of iliac aneurysmal disease, leading to more precise endograft placement and a better seal both proximally and distally. Some practitioners have therefore argued that it is this patient population that should be targeted for EVAR. Level 1 evidence is currently lacking, however. The Positive Impact of EndoVascular Options for Treating Aneurysms EarLy (PIVOTAL) and Comparison of surveillance versus Aortic Endografting for Small Aneurysm Repair (CEASAR) trials were initiated to provide such evidence [16]. Both are device specific, but are randomizing patients with smaller aneurysms to EVAR or observation. Until these studies are concluded and the data analyzed, the optimal management of aneurysms with a diameter less than 5.5 cm will likely remain in question.

Synthesizing these data, some general guidelines can be made about the "when" to fix an IAAA. Aneurysm size of 5.5 cm or greater appears to be an appropriate threshold to consider aneurysm repair in most patients. Repair can be considered at smaller diameters for asymptomatic patients with rapid growth, female gender [17,18], and a strong family history [19,20], as well as less common situations outlined by the subcommittee of the Joint Council of the American Association for Vascular Surgery and Society for Vascular surgery [21]. Patient preference for endovascular repair of aneurysm size of less than 5.5 cm may also be an important consideration as public awareness of shorter hospital stays and lower perioperative morbidity and mortality rates associated with EVAR continues to increase. Although strong arguments can be made for both open repair and EVAR, at this point a patient-specific approach should be used when considering what type of repair to perform. Morbidity, mortality, cost, durability, freedom from re-intervention, patient comorbidities, and patient preference should all be considered when deciding which repair to use. Once a decision is made to treat an IAAA, the technical aspects of the chosen method of repair will need to be considered. The following sections provide an overview of these technical aspects for both open and endovascular aneurysm repair.

Open repair

Retroperitoneal and transperitoneal approaches

Remarkably, the described principles of extraperitoneal surgical exposure of the aortoiliac segments date back to 1796. It is fascinating that although the first successful infrarenal aortic aneurysm reconstruction by Dubost and colleagues was performed via a retroperitoneal (RP) approach, use of this tool remained quiescent until Charles Rob re-popularized its use in 1963 [22,23]. Since then, the benefits and drawbacks of the RP exposure compared with transperitoneal exposure have been scrutinized extensively. Certain patient-specific physiologic and anatomic considerations are important, and may predict technical benefits of one exposure over another. However, the cumulative result of these appraisals is that one type of open repair is not obviously superior to the other. In the view of the present authors, it is now obsolete to debate the issue, as both randomized and uncontrolled studies show that both exposures have well-recognized merits [24,25]. Aortic surgeons should be trained in both exposures and often find each approach useful and effective.

Retroperitoneal approach

The RP approach may be preferable in those with renal ectopia, inflammatory aneurysms, prior abdominal surgery, or in the obese. Here, the term *retroperitoneal* is reserved for incisions no higher than the 11th rib where the peritoneum is not entered. Incisions in the 10th interspace or above are considered *thoracoabdominal*, irrespective of peritoneal entry. Chief considerations are the level of the incision and whether the left kidney is to be elevated medially or left in situ. The patient is placed on an air-vacuum beanbag in a right lateral decubitus position. The left arm is rotated onto the right with a 60° rotation of the torso, and the hips and lower extremities are rotated back as close as possible to horizontal. The iliac crests should be placed at the level of the operating table break with the table flexed to maximally open the flank. For infrarenal aneurysms with an infrarenal cross-clamp, the incision is started at the tip of the 12th rib and extended inferomedially to the semilunar line of the rectus abdominus muscle. This may be extended inferiorly to assist pelvic dissection of the iliac arteries. The authors avoid dividing the rectus. For suprarenal or visceral segment cross-clamps the incision may be placed in the 9th or 10th interspace, and for full supraceliac exposure, the 8th or 9th interspace is used. The left pleura is usually entered on these more superior exposures, and partial diaphragmatic division may be necessary.

The peritoneal sac is swept anteromedially, defining the RP space. Small vessels to the musculature of the flank are encountered and easily ligated. This is continued until the dissection has been performed over the proximal aorta, aneurysm, and iliac arteries as necessary. The left ureter is identified and swept up in the peritoneal sac. Care must be taken to mobilize it well in the pelvis. The authors divide the posterior fold of Gerota's fascia and continue this inferiorly to leave a soft tissue layer on the posterior muscles (quadratus lumborum and iliopsoas) to avoid injuring lumbosacral plexus nerve branches. For aneurysmal disease, a retrorenal plane is preferred except in instances of retroaortic left renal vein and the need to access the renovisceral segment for occlusive disease, in which case the kidney is left down. Care must be taken not to create a left renal artery traction injury with renal elevation. The inferior mesenteric artery can be ligated external to the aneurysm sac to facilitate full inferior exposure. Specific identification and ligation of the left renolumbar vein must be achieved. Identification of this vein and its hemiazygos connections is imperative, as injury can result in significant hemorrhage. For higher cross-clamp sites, division of the left crus over the aorta facilitates dissection. Aortic dissection and control may be circumferential, but this is based on surgeon preference. The aid of self-retaining retraction is crucial; the authors use the Omni-tract (Omni-Tract Surgical, St. Paul, MN). Right iliac control may require use of an intraluminal balloon catheter. Once the aortoiliac segments are properly exposed (Fig. 1), the conduct of operation is similar to that of the subsequently outlined transperitoneal approach.

Transperitoneal approach to the aorta

For the purposes of this section, a transperitoneal approach to the aorta consists of a midline approach. Other transperitoneal incisions have been

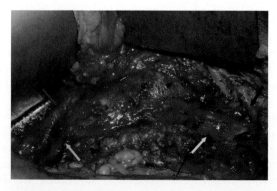

Fig. 1. Standard infrarenal RP AAA. Left renal artery (*black arrow*); aortic neck (*white arrow*); left ureteric fold in pelvis (*blue arrow*); aortic bifurcation (*yellow arrow*).

described for dealing with abdominal aortic branch artery disease, such as transverse incisions or bilateral subcostal incisions. However, the vast majority of transperitoneal incisions for infrarenal aortic aneurysmal disease are in the midline.

A generous midline skin incision is made first and the fascia divided along the linea alba. Once safe entry into the peritoneum is made, the contents of the abdomen are inspected for cancers or other unexpected abnormalities. After the abdominal contents have been surveyed, the small bowel is eviscerated to the right side of the abdomen, providing exposure of the infrarenal aortic space and easy palpation of the aortic aneurysm. With the transverse colon reflected superiorly, the RP tissue is divided longitudinally. Included in this portion of the exposure is the careful division of the ligament of Treitz and mobilization of the proximal jejunum. Near the level of the ligament of Treitz, and contained within the RP tissue, the inferior mesenteric vein and associated lymphatic channels course gradually from the patient's left to cross over the aorta as it ascends to join the splenic vein. Secure ligation and division of this vein and the lymphatic channels are typically necessary for exposure of the infrarenal aortic neck. Placement of an Omni Tract self-retaining retractor is prudent at this point, as formal dissection around the aorta is now undertaken.

Dissection and exposure of the anterior surface of the aorta can be undertaken with scissors or electrocautery. It is helpful to keep the dissection just to the right of the midline of the aneurysm to avoid injury to the inferior mesenteric artery. The dissection should proceed cephalad up to, and including, the left renal vein (Fig. 2). It is rarely necessary to divide the left renal vein for repair of an infrarenal aneurysm, but full mobilization of the vein is recommended. With ligation and division of the lumbar, adrenal, and gonadal venous tributaries, the vein can be encircled with a vessel loop to facilitate clamp placement during repair. If a decision is made to divide the left renal vein to facilitate exposure, the venous branches should be left intact with division of the vein nearer the vena cava. This allows at least some venous drainage for the left kidney should re-anastomosis of the left renal vein be precluded. With the left renal vein fully mobilized, the infrarenal neck of the aneurysm can be dissected free, and the proximal renal arteries exposed as needed. If insufficient infrarenal neck for clamping is encountered and the anatomy of the renal artery origins is suitable, it may be possible to position the clamp above one renal artery and below the other, thus maintaining antegrade flow to one kidney while the proximal anastomosis is performed. If the renal artery origins preclude this type of clamp placement, a suprarenal or supraceliac clamp will be required. A supraceliac exposure will not be detailed in this description, as it is infrequently necessary for repair of the IAAA.

Distal dissection of the aorta and its branches should be undertaken along the right common iliac artery preferentially. The tissues can then be reflected toward the left side to expose the left iliac artery. This method of

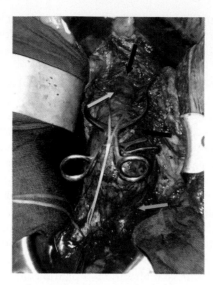

Fig. 2. Standard infremesocolic transperitoneal aortic aneurysm exposure. Renal arteries (*black arrow*); aortic neck (*white arrow*); ligated inferior mesenteric artery (*blue arrow*); aortic bifurcation (*yellow arrow*).

dissection helps to maintain the sympathetic fibers in an attempt to avoid the notable complication of retrograde ejaculation. If the aneurysmal disease includes the common iliac arteries, dissection can proceed caudally, keeping in mind that the ureters will cross the iliac vessels near their bifurcations. Once adequate exposure has been obtained, surgeon's preference will then dictate the size and type of graft used for repair. The patient is then fully heparinized, iliac clamps are applied first, followed by placement of the proximal clamp. The aneurysm is then opened longitudinally, any existing thrombus and debris are removed, and back-bleeding lumbar arteries are oversewn. The inferior mesenteric artery (IMA) should be assessed. If no bleeding or pulsatile bleeding is noted from the IMA, ligation of this vessel is appropriate. If only a trickle of back-bleeding is noted, a temporary clamp should be applied in consideration of re-implantation onto the aortic graft.

The graft is sutured in place proximally with a permanent suture. Once the anastomosis is complete, an atraumatic vascular clamp should be applied to the graft, the proximal clamp slowly released, and the proximal anastomosis assessed for suture line bleeding. Once hemostasis is assured, the graft can be cut to length and attention turned toward the distal anastomoses. Before completing the distal suture line(s), retrograde bleeding from the iliacs should be undertaken, followed by a flush of antegrade flow through the graft. Flow should be restored to the lower extremities one side at a time to limit hemodynamic instability. Reversal of heparin with protamine sulfate, if necessary, is appropriate once femoral pulses and distal perfusion to the feet are assessed and found to be adequate.

The aneurysm sac is then plicated around the newly placed graft with a running suture, followed by careful closure of the retroperitoneum with a separate running suture.

Endovascular aneurysm repair

Technical aspects of endovascular repair

Since the procedure's inception in 1991, the complexities and nuances of placing an endograft in an abdominal aortic aneurysm have continued to mature. However, if one breaks down EVAR into four basic components, its intricacies are more easily appreciated. These components include (1) iliofemoral access, (2) main body deployment and positioning, and (3) iliac limb deployment. All three funnel into the fourth and final consideration: device selection. Each component is critical to proper placement of the graft and achievement of adequate wall apposition, attachment site seal, and exclusion of the sac from the systemic circulation (Fig. 3A–C). Failure or insecurity in any of these procedural aspects may result in continued systemic flow within the aneurysm sac, or endoleak (Fig. 4) [26].

Procedural planning therefore becomes the most critical aspect of EVAR. Given today's highly resolute, multichannel, multislice CT with volumetric reconstruction, pre-procedural imaging before EVAR is frequently limited to CT. This reserves aortography and selective arteriography for either pre-procedural adjunctive interventions, or the occasional need when aortoiliac topography remains unclear and suitability for EVAR requires further inquiry. MRI can also be performed using gadolinium and a breath-hold technique. It can facilitate reasonably accurate measurements of aneurysm diameter and stenoses in the branch arteries. Unfortunately, it cannot accurately delineate calcified aortic plaque, an important component to consider in procedural planning.

Device selection

At present, four - devices approved by the US Food and Drug Administration for endovascular repair of IAAAs are being marketed. Each device has a slightly different design and attributes, making device selection critical (Table 2). Frequently, device selection is based on the anatomic characteristics of the aneurysm that are of the most concern and the graft that ostensibly best addresses these issues. Furthermore, as these aneurysm-specific considerations strongly influence EVAR outcomes, the Ad Hoc Committee for Standardized Reporting Practices of the Society for Vascular Surgery formally identified and graded each morphologic aspect of AAAs in 2002 [27,28]. This communication serves as a benchmark with which to grade and score the anatomic risks associated with EVAR that can lead to access failure, endograft limb thrombosis, distal embolism, endoleak, and deployment failure.

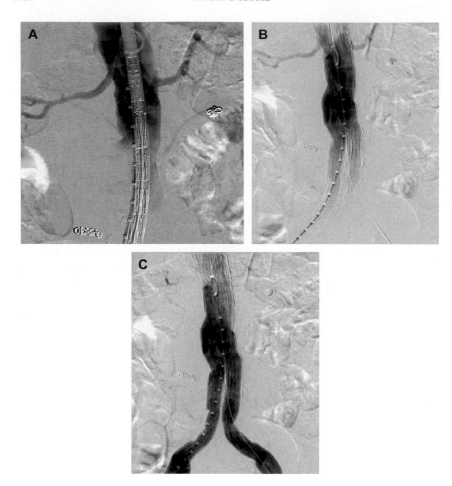

Fig. 3. (*A*) Aortogram marking renal artery location before proximal endograft deployment. (*B*) Early completion aortogram revealing normal renal artery opacification and proper endograft sealing with suprarenal fixation. (*C*) Midcompletion aortogram revealing normal flow through the endograft and preserved pelvic circulation.

Iliofemoral access

The procedure begins with preparation and procurement of sites for graft delivery. Iliac artery size, tortuosity, calcification, thrombus, and length of graft sealing are key matters here. Currently, standard access is via open bilateral control of the proximal common femoral arteries. However, concern regarding these access sites may lead one to perform an open exposure higher in the iliac system, usually via a RP approach. Either direct arterial puncture or a graft conduit may then be used. Another option in those with challenging unilateral iliofemoral anatomy is placement of an aortouniiliac main endograft with contralateral iliac artery adjunctive occlusion and

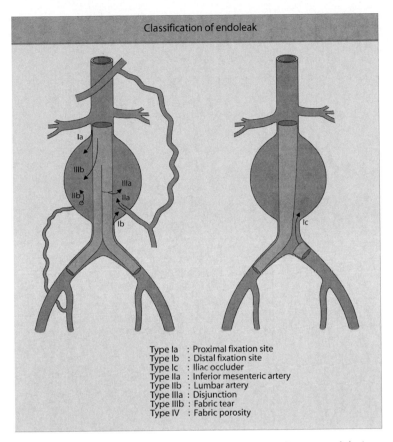

Classification of endoleak

Type Ia   : Proximal fixation site
Type Ib   : Distal fixation site
Type Ic   : Iliac occluder
Type IIa : Inferior mesenteric artery
Type IIb : Lumbar artery
Type IIIa : Disjunction
Type IIIb : Fabric tear
Type IV   : Fabric porosity

Fig. 4. Classification of endoleak by morphologic etiology. Not shown is endoleak type V or endotension. This represents continued sac pressurization in the absence of radiographically demonstrated sac flow. (*From* van Sambeek MRHM, van Dijk LC, Hendriks JM. Abdominal aneurysms–EVAR. In: Hallett Jr JW, Mills JL, Earchshaw JJ, et al, editors. Comprehensive vascular and endovascular surgery. Philadelphia: Mosby; 2004. p. 409–24; with permission.)

femoro-femoral bypass to achieve sac isolation. This technique has been shown to be a durable alternative for those who have complex iliac scenarios [29]. Conversely, if the anatomy of the iliofemoral systems is appropriate, some now are advocating either a unilateral or a totally percutaneous approach, with excellent results [30,31]. Regardless, properly chosen techniques facilitate successful endograft placement based on accurate assessment of patient-specific iliofemoral access. Large series of EVAR emphasize the impact of the iliac arteries to EVAR success, as the use of additional iliac graft limb extensions appears to be an important cause for procedural failure and subsequent secondary intervention [32].

Iliofemoral size is also important, as delivery systems for the currently approved devices range from 18 to 22 Fr. Although material engineering is continually improving the delivery platforms in terms of strength, profile,

Table 2
U.S. Food and Drug Administration-approved infrarenal aortic stent-graft devices

Device	Stent material	Graft material	Main body diameter (mm)	Main body delivery size (Fr)	Iliac limb diameter (mm)	Graft construction	Fixation
Cook Zenith	Stainless steel	Woven polyester	22–36	18–22	8–24	Modular	Self-expanding stents and active suprarenal hooks
Endologix Powerlink	Cobalt-chromium alloy	ePTFE	25–28	21	16–20	Unibody	Self-expansion
Gore Excluder	Nitinol	ePTFE	23–28.5	18	12–20	Modular	Self-expansion and active barbs in neck
Medtronic AneuRx AAA Advantage	Nitinol	Woven polyester	20–28	21	12–24	Modular	Self-expansion

Main body and iliac extension devices available for all grafts. Aorto-uni-iliac converter grafts available for Cook Zenith and Endologix Powerlink. Contralateral occlusion devices available from Cook Zenith.
Abbreviation: ePTFE, expanded polytetrafluoroethylene.

and trackability, the compliance and straightness of the iliofemoral system remain fundamental in endograft access. Adjuncts such as angioplasty and stenting may be used to aid in providing appropriate arterial access diameters. A major point of stress in standard EVAR access occurs at the iliac bifurcation, and in a significant proportion of cases the external iliac artery origin is the site of diminutive iliac size. Tortuosity of the iliac vessels may also be a limiting factor. Calcification and thrombus also play a significant role in both the possibility for vessel injury and risk of thromboembolic events. In relatively healthy vessels with little calcification or thrombus, tortuosity may be overcome by stiff guide wires and available large-diameter delivery sheaths.

Although there are no clear absolute thresholds for any of these features that contraindicate EVAR, some general recommendations can be made. All iliac angulations should be considered in three dimensions. Angulations of 90° or more in contiguous iliofemoral segments should be viewed with caution. Calcification of greater than or equal to 50% of the artery circumference may severely limit vessel compliance, and thrombus burden of 25% to 50% of the lumen or more increases thromboembolic risk. Access site selection involves evaluation of both iliac systems to decide on the side of main body delivery as well as the side for contralateral graft delivery. Finally, the importance of the length of seal within the iliacs produced by graft placement is now appreciated more clearly than when endografting was in its initial stages. The seating of the graft limbs inferiorly appears to play a significant role in endograft structural integrity, influencing not only the potential for type IB endoleaks, but also the risk of distal graft migration [33]. It is generally held that an iliac seal zone of at least 15 to 20 mm is ideal.

Main body deployment and positioning

Deployment of the endograft's main body is perhaps the most critical aspect in terms of selection for EVAR suitability. Unfavorable neck morphology has been the most common cause of denial for EVAR as difficulties with seal in the aneurysm neck lead to persistent in-line systemic flow (type IA endoleak) and procedural failure. Although delivery platforms differ and techniques are unique to each of the approved devices, universal comments can be made regarding aneurysm neck features important for success. Similar to the distal iliac arteries, these features include the length of the neck, calcification, thrombus burden, and angulation. These features impact the length of graft seal necessary to provide adequate fixation. A neck length of 10 mm or less is concerning, whereas 25 mm or more is ideal. Neck morphology is also significant, with reverse conical tapering of more than 20% raising concern for temporal enlargement, decreasing seal and ultimate graft migration. Calcification of more than 50% of the neck circumference may lead to poorer graft seating and increased failure. Circumferential calcium should be viewed as having a high potential for fixation failure. Similarly, a thrombus burden of 50% or more of the neck lumen greatly increases the potential for thromboembolic events and seal failures. Ideal features of an aortic neck for endografting include minimal calcium, no thrombus burden, and a lengthy seal area.

Regarding neck angulation, the currently approved devices' instructions for use recommend the angle created by the aortic center line between the distal neck and the aortic bifurcation and the center line from the level of the renal arteries to the distal neck be no more than 45° to–60°. During EVAR, it is important to place the image intensifier in a plane orthogonal to the anterior–posterior surface of the aortic neck and the axis of the renal artery origins. This allows for the most precise view for device deployment. An accurate estimation of this angle is attainable using the reconstructed CT, and should be a consistent method of preoperative image planning.

Use of active fixation with barbs or hooks to attach the graft to the aortic wall appears to be helpful in stabilizing and seating the endograft proximally. Bare suprarenal fixation is also used, and has been associated with very low migration rates in mid- and long-term follow-up [34,35]. Yet, more recent communications have emphasized that proximal fixation may be less important than iliac limb fixation as close as possible to the iliac bifurcation [31]. The four endografts currently marketed in the United States use self-expanding stent technology and the proximal graft must be oversized 10% to 20%. This is potentially problematic, as oversizing has been implicated in continued neck enlargement and graft failure [36]. Currently, in the United States, certain approved devices will allow endovascular treatment of neck diameters of 34 mm or less. When a poor aortic neck seal is encountered, endovascular methods available to treat this problem include balloon angioplasty, endograft cuff extensions, and bare Palmaz stenting. More complex and involved open or hybrid procedures, such as plication, buttressing, and renovisceral debranching with extension, have been described and are also used.

Another important consideration is how the device will sit in the aortoiliac segment to facilitate contralateral graft limb cannulation. This is important, as most currently approved devices require accessing the endograft from the contralateral side using guide-wire techniques. Further, a judgment must be made whether to place the graft in a straight bifurcated or crossed iliac limb configuration. This latter configuration may be used in instances where there is desire to shorten overall graft length 5 to10 mm, such as in hypogastric preservation, or to simplify contralateral cannulation. Although the importance of type II endoleak on aneurysm-related outcomes continues to be debated, there may be a place for either augmented surveillance or pre-EVAR embolization of larger inferior mesenteric, lumbar, and accessory renal arteries in certain instances [37]. The number of patent branch vessels and size over 4 mm may increase the overall prospect of type II leak [28].

Iliac limb deployment

Proper overlap of all modular components is necessary to reduce risk of seal disruption (type IIIA endoleak). In general, as long as the main body's flow divider level is maintained, the more overlap the better, and it appears overlap lengths of less than 2 cm are at highest risk of temporal modular disruption. Achieving adequate overlap, therefore, may require iliac extension in some cases. Imaging with orthogonal views of the iliac system, particularly the common iliac and its bifurcation, aids in iliac limb deployment. Distal flaring of the iliac graft modules through the use of either aortic cuffs or the newer generation enlarging tapered extensions may also be useful in creating adequate seating and seal. Discrimination in their use must be used. Unless the patient is clearly in need of an endovascular solution, the authors try not to maintain systemic continuity of iliac segments larger than 25 mm. Iliac endograft components used in the seal zone should be 1 to 2 mm larger than the native arteries as self-expansion is used for fixation. When active occlusion techniques are used due to adverse iliac anatomy, one internal iliac artery should be preserved if at all possible. Sacrifice of both hypogastrics may lead to unrecoverable complications owing to pelvic ischemia or debilitating buttock claudication. Moreover, a significant proportion of those with one remaining hypogastric will have buttock claudication [38].

Summary

Advances in both EVAR technology and the understanding of how it is best implemented continue to progress. Consistent data revealing short-term advantages in morbidity and mortality make EVAR a very appealing option for practitioners and patients. However, mid- and long-term data proving an all-cause mortality benefit are lacking. A maximum transverse measurement of greater than 5.5 cm is still a reasonable threshold to recommend repair in most patients with asymptomatic IAAAs; repair at smaller diameters may be recommended for women and other select cases. Open repair has proven durability, and should be strongly considered in younger and lower-risk patients. Nevertheless, the decision as to whether open repair or EVAR is the best option for each individual should be made on the basis of the specific patient.

References

[1] Parodi JC, Palmaz JC, Barone HD. Transfemoral intraluminal graft implantation for abdominal aortic aneurysms. Ann Vasc Surg 1991;5:491–9.

[2] The United Kingdom Small Aneurysm Trial Participants. Mortality results for randomized controlled trial of early elective surgery or ultrasonographic surveillance for small abdominal aortic aneurysms. Lancet 1998;352:1649–55.

[3] The United Kingdom Small Aneurysm Trial Participants. Long-term outcomes of immediate repair compared with surveillance of small abdominal aortic aneurysms. N Engl J Med 2002;346:1445–52.

[4] The United Kingdom Small Aneurysm Trial Participants. Final 12-year follow-up of surgery versus surveillance in the UK Small Aneurysm Trial. Br J Surg 2007;94:702–8.

[5] Lederle FA, Wilson SE, Johnson GR, et al. Immediate repair compared with surveillance of small abdominal aortic aneurysms. N Engl J Med 2002;346:1437–44.

[6] Matsamura JS, Brewster DC, Makaroun MS, et al. A multicenter controlled clinical trial of open versus endovascular treatment of abdominal aortic aneurysm. J Vasc Surg 2003;37: 262–71.

[7] May J, White GH, Waugh R, et al. Improved survival after endoluminal repair with second-generation prostheses compared with open repair in the treatment of abdominal aortic aneurysms: a 5-year concurrent comparison using life table method. J Vasc Surg 2001;33:21–6.

[8] Zarins CK, White RA, Schwarten D, et al. AneuRx stent graft versus open surgical repair of abdominal aortic aneurysms: multicenter prospective clinical trial. J Vasc Surg 1999;29: 292–308.

[9] Prinssen M, Lerhoeven ELG, Buth J, et al. A randomized trial comparing conventional and endovascular repair of abdominal aortic aneurysms. N Engl J Med 2004;351:1607–18.

[10] Blankensteijn JD, de Jong SE, Prinssen M, et al. Two-year outcomes after conventional or endovascular repair of abdominal aortic aneurysms. N Engl J Med 2005;352:2398–405.

[11] EVAR Trial Participants. Endovascular aneurysm repair versus open repair in patients with abdominal aortic aneurysm (EVAR trial 1): randomised controlled trial. Lancet 2005;365: 2179–86.

[12] EVAR Trial Participants. Endovascular aneurysm repair and outcome in patients unfit for open repair of abdominal aortic aneurysm (EVAR trial 2): randomised controlled trial. Lancet 2005;365:2187–92.

[13] Bush RL, Johnson ML, Hedayati N, et al. Performance of endovascular aortic aneurysm repair in high-risk patients: results from the Veterans Affairs National Surgical Quality Improvement Program. J Vasc Surg 2007;45:227–34.

[14] Ouriel K, Srivastava SD, Sarac TP, et al. Disparate outcome after endovascular treatment of small versus large abdominal aortic aneurysm. J Vasc Surg 2003;37:1206–12.

[15] Peppelenbosch N, Buth J, Harris PL, et al. Diameter of abdominal aortic aneurysm and outcome of endovascular aneurysm repair: does size matter? A report from Eurostar. J Vasc Surg 2004;39:288–97.

[16] Cao P, CAESAR Trial Collaborators. Comparison of surveillance vs Aortic Endografting for Small Aneurysm Repair (CAESAR) trial: study design and progress. Eur J Vasc Endovasc Surg 2005;30:245–51.

[17] Brown LC, Powel JT. Risk factors for rupture in patients kept under ultrasound surveillance. The UK Small Aneurysm Trial Participants. Ann Surg 1999;230:289–97.

[18] Heikkinen M, Salenius J-P, Auvinen MD. Ruptured abdominal aortic aneurysm in a well-defined geographical area. J Vasc Surg 2002;36:291–6.

[19] Darling RC III, Brewster DC, Darling RC, et al. Are familial abdominal aortic aneurysms different? J Vasc Surg 1989;10:39–43.

[20] Verloes A, Sakalihasan N, Koulischer L, et al. Aneurysms of the abdominal aorta: familial and genetic aspects in three hundred thirteen pedigrees. J Vasc Surg 1995;21:646–55.

[21] Brewster DC, Cronenwett JL, Hallett JW Jr, et al. Guidelines for the treatment of abdominal aortic aneurysms. Report of a subcommittee of the Joint Council of the American Association for Vascular Surgery and Society for Vascular Surgery. J Vasc Surg 2003;37:1106–17.

[22] Dubost C, Allary M, Oeconomos N. Resection of an aneurysm of the abdominal aorta: reestablishment of the continuity by preserved human arterial graft, with results after five months. Arch Surg 1952;64:405–8.

[23] Rob C. Extraperitoneal approach to the abdominal aorta. Surgery 1963;53:87–9.

[24] Cambria RP, Brewster DC, Abbott WM, et al. Transperitoneal versus retroperitoneal approach for aortic reconstruction: a randomized prospective study. J Vasc Surg 1990;11: 314–25.

[25] Sicard GA, Reilly JM, Rubin BG, et al. Transabdominal versus retroperitoneal incision for abdominal aortic surgery; report of a prospective randomized trial. J Vasc Surg 1995;21: 174–83.

[26] van Sambeek MRHM, van Dijk LC, Hendriks JM, et al. Abdominal Aneurysms-EVAR. In: Hallett JW Jr, Mills JL, Earnshaw JJ, editors. Comprehensive vascular and endovascular surgery. Philadelphia: Mosby; 2004. p. 409–24.

[27] Chaikof EL, Blankensteijn JD, Harris PL, et al. Reporting standards for endovascular aortic aneurysm repair. J Vasc Surg 2002;35:1048–60.

[28] Chaikof EL, Fillinger MF, Matsumura JS, et al. Identifying and grading factors that modify the outcome of endovascular aortic aneurysm repair. J Vasc Surg 2002;35:1061–6.

[29] Clouse WD, Brewster DC, Marone LK, et al. EVT/Guidant Investigators. Durability of aortouniiliac endografting with femorofemoral crossover: 4-year experience with evt/guidant trials. J Vasc Surg 2003;37:1142–9.

[30] Starnes BW, Anderson CA, Ronsivalle JA, et al. Totally percutaneous aortic aneurysm repair: experience and prudence. J Vasc Surg 2006;43:270–6.

[31] Lee WA, Brown MP, Nelson PR, et al. Total percutaneous access for endovascular aortic aneurysm repair ("Preclose" technique). J Vasc Surg 2007;45:1095–101.

[32] Hobo R, Laheij RJF, Buth J, et al. The influence of aortic cuffs and iliac limb extensions on the outcome of endovascular abdominal aortic aneurysm repair. J Vasc Surg 2007;45:79–85.

[33] Benharash P, Lee JT, Abilez OJ, et al. Iliac fixation inhibits migration of both suprarenal and infrarenal aortic endografts. J Vasc Surg 2007;45:250–7.

[34] Tonnessen BH, Sternbergh WC III, Money SR. Mid- and long-term device migration after endovascular abdominal aortic aneurysm repair: a comparison of AneuRx and Zenith endografts. J Vasc Surg 2005;42:392–401.

[35] Talent AAA Retrospective Longterm Study Group. Long-term outcome after Talent endograft implantation for aneurysms of the abdominal aorta: a multicenter retrospective study. J Vasc Surg 2006;43:277–84.

[36] Tonnessen BH, Sternbergh C, Money SR. Late problems at the proximal aortic neck: migration and dilation. Semin Vasc Surg 2004;17:288–93.

[37] Sheehan MK, Hagino RT, Canby E, et al. Type II endoleaks after abdominal aortic aneurysm stent grafting with systematic mesenteric and lumbar coil embolization. Ann Vasc Surg 2006;20:458-63.

[38] Lee WA, Nelson PR, Berceli SA, et al. Outcome after hypogastric bypass and embolization during endovascular aneurysm repair. J Vasc Surg 2006;45:1162–9.

ELSEVIER
SAUNDERS

SURGICAL
CLINICS OF
NORTH AMERICA

Surg Clin N Am 87 (2007) 1035–1045

Ruptured Abdominal Aortic Aneurysms: Remote Aortic Occlusion for the General Surgeon

CPT Zachary M. Arthurs, MD[a],*,
CPT Vance Y. Sohn, MD[a],
Benjamin W. Starnes, MD, FACS[b]

[a]Department of Surgery, Madigan Army Medical Center, Fitzsimmons Drive,
Building 9040, Tacoma, WA 98431, USA
[b]Division of Vascular Surgery, University of Washington, Harborview Medical Center,
325 Ninth Avenue, Seattle, WA 98104, USA

When Parodi and colleagues [1] implanted the first endograft to treat an infrarenal abdominal aortic aneurysm (AAA) in 1991, they forever changed the treatment of aortic aneurysmal disease. This technology has reduced the mortality risk compared with open repair, and it has eliminated the associated morbidity of an abdominal operation in high-risk patients [2–5]. Similarly, whereas open surgery has remained the primary therapy for ruptured abdominal aortic aneurysms (RAAA), it is nonetheless associated with significant morbidity and mortality ranging from 30% to 80% [6]. Despite technological advances and advances in critical care, the actual surgical approach and resultant mortality has only marginally changed over the last 50 years [7,8].

The success of endovascular aneurysm repair (EVAR) for elective aneurysms has been slow to transition into the treatment of emergent aneurysmal disease. There are several obstacles preventing this from occurring, ranging from institutional limitations, imaging, graft availability, and availability of an endovascular surgeon. Although not all vascular surgeons and general surgeons are capable of performing EVAR, there are basic endovascular techniques that can be useful for standard open repair.

During the Korean War, Lieutenant Colonel Hughes [9] introduced the technique of remote aortic occlusion by placement of transfemoral Foley catheters in three injured soldiers who presented in hemorrhagic shock from penetrating truncal trauma. He used this technique as compassionate

* Corresponding author.
E-mail address: arthursz@mac.com (Z.M. Arthurs).

0039-6109/07/$ - see front matter © 2007 Elsevier Inc. All rights reserved.
doi:10.1016/j.suc.2007.07.002   *surgical.theclinics.com*

use and noted all three patients to temporarily experience hemodynamic improvement. A decade later, Hesse and Kletschka [10] used intralumenal aortic occlusion specifically for ruptured abdominal aneurysms in 1961. Their technique involved placing a Foley catheter through the aneurysmal rent in the aorta and guiding it into the thoracic aorta. If the aneurysm was not easily defined, the balloon was placed through an arteriotomy placed in the common iliac artery. Within the past 2 decades, endovascular procedures have become commonplace in the United States, and vascular surgeons are using remote aortic occlusion to manage RAAAs [11–13].

This article addresses the challenges associated with performing endovascular procedures in an after-hours environment, the preoperative preparation of patients who have RAAAs, and the technique of remote aortic occlusion.

Remote aortic occlusion for ruptured abdominal aortic aneurysms

Institutional preparation

When a patient presents to the emergency room with a presumed RAAA, the institution must have a predetermined algorithm to rapidly assess the patient, prepare the operative suite, obtain axial imaging, and transport the patient to the operative suite. At the authors' institution, endovascular training is provided on an annual basis to the house officers, surgical staff, and operating room technicians to rehearse the prepared algorithm for RAAAs. Mehta and colleagues [14] found that mock preparation for emergent ruptured aneurysms highlighted the importance of early diagnosis and institutional readiness. Additionally, rehearsing the emergent algorithm with each elective aneurysm prepared the anesthesiologists, operating room staff, and radiographic technicians for emergent cases.

In order to use endovascular techniques, the institution must have an available fluoroscopic C-arm and operative imaging table. In addition, there must be a basic set of endovascular supplies readily available for the surgeon. The scrub technicians and circulating nurses must also have familiarity with access needles, wires, sheaths, and contrast agents. Whereas most general surgeons have had experience with intraoperative cholangiograms, few have used intraoperative vascular imaging in their practice. The majority of general surgeons are extremely comfortable with gaining access in the groin using Seldinger's technique, however. Having a team with basic endovascular knowledge is imperative for using this technique for emergent cases.

Preoperative management

Once the patient is identified as having an RAAA, the patient's clinical status dictates the urgency of treatment. The ideal perfusion pressure has brought about much debate with regards to resuscitation of patients who have RAAAs. The majority of research in this area has focused on hypotensive (systolic blood pressure <90 mmHg) trauma patients suffering from hemorrhagic shock, and a consensus suggests that delayed resuscitation until hemorrhage is controlled improves survival and reduces postoperative morbidity, primarily multisystem organ failure [15,16]. This literature has been applied to RAAAs, and although there are multiple animal studies in this arena, no prospective studies have been performed in patients who have RAAAs [17]. Increasing the patient's systolic blood pressure could exacerbate ongoing hemorrhage or convert a contained rupture to free rupture. If the patient is mentating, resuscitation (crystalloid and blood products) should be reserved until the aortic occlusion balloon (AOB) is secured.

If a vascular surgeon is available for potential endovascular repair of an RAAA, a preoperative CT scan will be valuable for endograft sizing. Transferring a patient who has an RAAA to the CT scanner contradicts general surgical training principles, and can be viewed as a deplorable decision; however, Lloyd and colleagues [18] performed a time-to-death analysis of patients who presented with RAAAs and were not able to undergo repair secondary to malignancies or secondary to comorbidities that precluded open repair. The median time from onset of symptoms to admission was 2.5 hours, and death occurred in 12.5% within 2 hours of admission (4.5 hours from onset of symptoms); the remainder died after 2 hours. The median time-to-death in this study was 16 hours and 38 minutes [18]. This study illustrates the feasibility of obtaining preoperative axial imaging. Most CT scanners can perform 2 to 3 mm collimation imaging of the aorta in 5 to 10 minutes en route to the operative suite. If the decision is made to defer preoperative axial imaging, intraoperative sizing of the aneurysm can be performed with aortography and intravascular ultrasound should a vascular surgeon be available.

Once the decision is made to repair the aneurysm, the patient should proceed to the operative suite, and it is imperative that the patient be placed on an imaging table. Having the imaging table and C-arm available in the assigned operative suite must be part of the operative personnel's checklist. Before induction of anesthesia, central access and arterial monitoring should be obtained. Blood products for massive resuscitation should be in the operative suite. A Foley catheter should be placed, and then the patient should be prepared and draped. At this time, the surgical team can place the AOB before induction of general endotracheal anesthesia. If an endovascular approach is going to be attempted, regional anesthesia or even local anesthesia can be used based on the hemodynamic status of the patient. Box 1 lists the basic inventory that should be readily available when placing AOBs.

Technique

Access to the common femoral artery

With the patient prepped and draped, the operator should use a standard access needle that will accept a 0.035" wire. The authors prefer the groin

---

Box 1. Basic inventory necessary for aortic occlusion balloon placement

- Fluoroscopic C-arm and imaging table.
- Access needle
- 30 cc aspiration syringe
- 6 Fr sheath and 11 Fr sheath
- 150 cm, 0.035″ Bentson wire
- 150 cm, 0.035″ Glide wire
- 150 cm, 0.035″ Amplatz wire
- 125 cm, 33 mm AOB
- 65 cm Kumpe catheter
- 65 cm, 11 Fr sheath
- Bottle of contrast (Visipaque, GE Healthcare, Waukesha, Wisconsin)

---

because of the straightforward percutaneous approach, and the right side keeps the surgeon on the opposite side of the table as the C-arm. Utilizing Seldinger's technique, the vessel is accessed, ideally over the medial third of the femoral head. Most of these patients do not have palpable groin pulses; therefore the surgeon must rely on anatomic landmarks, image guidance, or a cutdown procedure. The authors' standard approach is to place a Kelly clamp inline with the proposed access site, and then check our planned site with fluoroscopic imaging. The tip of the Kelly clamp is then adjusted such that the tip is overlying the common femoral artery just over the medial third of the femoral head. Often the calcifications in the vessel wall can be visualized on fluoroscopic images. Once the vessel is marked, we attempt access.

Another modality that is readily accessible in the operative suite is duplex ultrasound. If access is difficult, an ultrasound probe can be brought onto the field to aid in the identification of the common femoral artery. Once differentiated from the vein by its lateral location and noncompressibility, the common femoral artery can be mapped caudally until identification of the profunda femoris artery, with access obtained just cranial to the profunda takeoff. Access is obtained with the duplex image in an axial view, and the access needle placed at a 45° angle to the ultrasound probe. As the needle is advanced, the path of the needle can be visualized under ultrasound by separation of the tissue planes. Ultrasound-guided access of the femoral vessels has yielded excellent success and deferred the need for cutdown in the authors' practice. Finally, if all attempts at percutaneous access fail, a femoral cutdown can be performed in less than three minutes under local anesthesia, still avoiding induction of general anesthesia. Patients in profound shock require no local anesthesia for access, be it percutaneous or open.

Once adequate flash is obtained from the access needle, The authors first pass a Bentson wire (Cook Medical, Bloomington, Indiana) into the common femoral artery, and if the wire does not easily pass, we then use a hydrophilic glide wire. If this fails, we redirect the access needle and repeat the steps. Once the wire easily passes into the artery, a 6 Fr sheath is placed in the groin, which is just an initial step to serially dilate the vessel to our working sheath, the 11 Fr sheath. After the sheath has been flushed, we then replace the 6 Fr sheath with an 11 Fr sheath. At this point, the operator has a working system from the right groin that can accept a 33 mm AOB.

Selecting the supraceliac aorta

At this point the Bentson wire should be followed under fluoroscopic guidance through the iliac vessels and into the aneurysm sac. Fig. 1 illustrates the proceeding steps. The wire should be advanced under direct fluoroscopic imaging into the supraceliac aorta. If the wire advances easily into the thoracic aorta, it has already bridged the RAAA, but not uncommonly, the wire will coil in the redundant and tortuous aneurysmal sac (see Fig. 1A).

At this point, a selective catheter is required to direct the wire into the supraceliac aorta. The authors' catheter of choice is the Kumpe catheter

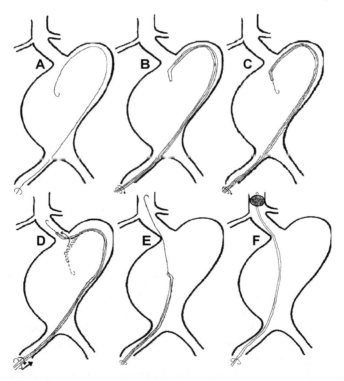

Fig. 1. Illustration of aortic balloon placement. (*A*) Placement of the access wire. (*B*) Using a Kumpe catheter to select the proximal aorta. (*C*) Positioning the tip of the Kumpe catheter just beyond the proximal aorta. (*D*) Retracting the catheter, applying torque to the catheter, and advancing the Bentson wire. (*E*) Purchasing hold in the supraceliac aorta and retracting the Kumpe catheter. (*F*) Advancing the AOB into position.

(Cook Medical), which has a hockey-stick bend at the tip. This catheter is advanced over the Bentson wired through our working sheath (11 Fr sheath), and then advanced over the tip of the wire (see Fig. 1B). When selecting vessels, the selective catheter and wire should never be pushed into the orifice; instead, the catheter should be advanced beyond the orifice with the floppy tip of the Bentson wire just beyond the end of the Kumpe catheter (see Fig. 1C). From this vantage point, counterclockwise torque is applied to the Kumpe catheter in the right groin while slowly withdrawing the catheter and watching the catheter under fluoroscopic imaging. The wire can then be advanced into the supraceliac aorta (see Fig. 1D). Once the wire is in the thoracic aorta, the redundant loop in the aortic sac will snap into a straight line across the aneurysm (see Fig. 1E).

Placement of the aortic occlusion balloon

Once the wire is secured in the thoracic aorta, the Kumpe catheter can be withdrawn over the wire, and the 33 mm AOB can be advanced over the wire into a supraceliac position (see Fig. 1F). With the balloon in position, the authors shoot a hand-injected aortogram through the central channel of the AOB to confirm its position. In addition, we test the balloon by inflation with contrast and saline mixed 50/50. The compliant characteristic of the AOB allows conformation to the wall of the fairly noncompliant aorta. Therefore, the balloon will initially appear spherical, but once it accommodates the endoluminal surface of the aorta, it will expand by elongating along the walls of the aorta (Fig. 2).

The occlusion balloon is injected under fluoroscopy, and once the balloon profiles the aorta, the location of the balloon is secured in the right groin by the assistant. In addition, the volume of contrast required to achieve a change in balloon profile, and hence occlusion is recorded (Fig. 3). At this time, the balloon is deflated, and anesthesia can start resuscitation (crystalloid and blood products) and prepare for induction.

Perform the open repair

The AOB is reserved only for periods of hemodynamic instability. With induction of anesthesia or upon opening the abdominal fascia, the patient may require interval inflation of the AOB and continued resuscitation from the anesthesia provider. Having proximal control secured allows the surgeon a relatively bloodless field to dissect the infrarenal neck of the RAAA (Fig. 4). Once the infrarenal neck is isolated, a vascular clamp can replace the AOB; the balloon is simply retracted into the aneurysm sac before clamp application.

Once the balloon has been inflated and deflated, it is more difficult to retract through an 11 Fr sheath; therefore, once the aneurysm sac is opened, the authors cut the balloon tip off the catheter and retract the system through the groin. The standard open repair of an AAA ensues.

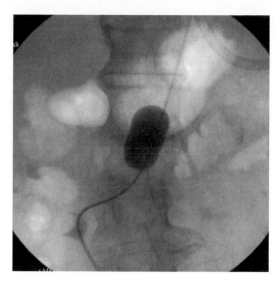

Fig. 2. Test inflation of the AOB. The balloon has opposed the aortic wall and started to elongate with continued inflation. Note the wire inferior to balloon buckling against the cranial to caudal pressure.

Discussion

Although an AOB can be placed in less than 5 minutes in experienced hands, technical difficulties can occur with any of the above steps. Most general surgeons are comfortable with obtaining access in the groin, and depending on their comfort with ultrasound, ultrasound-guided access is an alternative. If percutaneous attempts fail, general surgeons can perform a rapid cutdown at the groin and access the common femoral vessel.

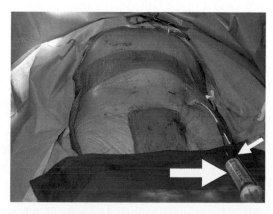

Fig. 3. The AOB is secured at the groin. The contrast (*large white arrow*) has been marked from test occlusion, and the wire (*small white arrow*) remains in place throughout the procedure. This particular patient had a prior right groin exploration; therefore, the AOB was placed from the left groin.

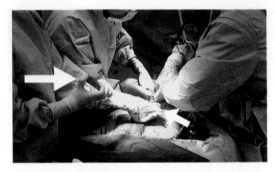

Fig. 4. Remote AOB for proximal control. The assistant inflates the AOB (*large white arrow*) and secures the position (*small white arrow*) while the open operation ensues. This patient experienced free rupture of the aneurysm, prompting inflation of the AOB for proximal control.

General surgeons are probably least familiar with selecting the supraceliac aorta using a directional catheter (ie, the Kumpe). For endovascular surgeons, this is a very common maneuver, and is performed at the beginning of every elective endovascular aneurysm repair. The authors recommend using this opportunity under elective circumstances to gain experience with handling wires in the aneurysm sac and selecting the supraceliac aorta before attempting this technique in the emergent setting.

Once proximal placement is confirmed, the assistant must secure the AOB at the groin or the patient's pressure will force the balloon caudally into the aneurysm sac. When the test occlusion is performed under fluoroscopy, the force on the balloon can be felt by the assistant securing the catheter. If the patient's aortic pressure is greater than the columnar strength of the catheter system, the wire and balloon will start to buckle. This can be seen ion Fig. 2 just caudal to the balloon. To increase the columnar support of the system, the Bentson wire can be replaced with an Amplatz wire (Cook Medical), which is more rigid. If this fails to secure the balloon in place, then the AOB can be removed, and a 65 cm 11 or 12 Fr sheath can be placed over the Amplatz wire into the supraceliac aorta. The AOB can then be passed through the sheath so that the balloon extends just beyond the tip of the sheath. When the balloon is inflated, the sheath will wedge against the caudal aspect of the balloon and prevent migration. Veith and colleagues [23] have described this modification as an adjunct to EVAR for RAAAs. Typically, an Amplatz wire has enough columnar support to hold the balloon in position; therefore, the authors only place the 65 cm, 11 Fr sheath if it fails to secure the balloon.

Some authors have used a transbrachial approach for placement of the AOB [11,12,20,21]. The primary reported benefit of this approach is lack of balloon migration into the aneurysm sac. The transbrachial approach, initially used when the surgeon planned to repair the RAAA with an endograft, allowed both groins still available for graft insertion. The disadvantage of this technique is the required cutdown procedure over the brachial artery near the median nerve and the placement of a very large sheath relative to the normal size of the brachial artery. Additionally, using the right brachial artery places the patient at risk for cerebral embolization as the innominate and left common carotid arteries are crossed. Utilizing the left arm will place the operators in a difficult location between the patient and the C-arm. In addition, the stiffness associated with the AOB and sheaths make them difficult to navigate through the arch into the descending thoracic aorta. Relative risk of ischemic complications to the hand is also a concern.

For these reasons, the authors feel that the femoral approach is superior. Dr. Veith and colleagues [22] have reported the largest experience treating RAAAs with EVAR; their group uses a transfemoral AOB and then places the endograft from the contralateral groin [23]. If a transfemoral AOB is placed as a temporizing measure until the vascular surgeon arrives, it does not hinder the placement of an endograft.

The risks associated with AOB placement include a time delay such that the patient experiences a poor outcome. Those patients that survive through transport to the hospital typically have a contained rupture that is dependent on the retroperitoneal hematoma and tone of the abdominal wall musculature. Based on Lloyd and colleagues' [18] time-to-death analysis, most patients have 2.5 hours after being admitted to the hospital before free rupture. The authors feel that the benefits of securing the proximal aorta before anesthetic induction and release of the tamponade effect of the abdominal wall far outweigh the risks of a relatively small time delay.

Manipulating wires and catheters within the aneurysm sac could potentially convert a contained rupture to free rupture. The authors have not experienced this complication, nor has it been reported in the literature. Surgeons have used AOBs for penetrating truncal trauma and experienced the balloon exiting the injury site in the aorta [19]. If this were to occur during placement, we feel that it would be recognized by using fluoroscopic guidance.

The most devastating complication of occluding the aorta is spinal cord, visceral, and lower extremity ischemia. The balloon is only inflated if the patient's hemodynamic status demands proximal control. Based on the patient's underlying vascular disease, collateral flow, and moribund state, the ischemia time is variable. Intermittent periods of aortic occlusion are better tolerated than prolonged occlusion [19]; therefore, the authors limit periods of occlusion to 10 minutes with variable periods of reperfusion. This complication is inherent in all types of proximal control, and the AOB could theoretically reduce periods of hypotension.

At the authors' institution, we have adopted the approach of placing a transfemoral AOB before resuscitation, induction of anesthesia, and exclusion of the RAAA. The availability of commercial endografts and surgeons trained in the art of endovascular technique is such that each patient is considered for endovascular repair. The utility of remote aortic occlusion has served as an invaluable adjunct to our experience of open RAAA repair, and we feel that this is a useful adjunct for the general surgeon faced with an RAAA.

Summary

Although the treatment and mortality for RAAAs has changed very little in the last 50 years, the elective repair of abdominal aortic aneurysms has dramatically changed because of endovascular technology. EVAR for RAAAs has been limited to relatively few centers, but remote endovascular occlusion of the aorta is a technique that can be used by both vascular and general surgeons alike. Preoperative placement of a remote AOB from the groin is a rapid and effective method of obtaining proximal control and has the potential to improve the morbidity and mortality in this moribund population of patients.

References

[1] Parodi JC, Palmaz JC, Barone HD. Transfemoral intraluminal graft implantation for abdominal aortic aneurysms. Ann Vasc Surg 1991;5(6):491–9.

[2] EVAR Trial Participants. Endovascular aneurysm repair and outcome in patients unfit for open repair of abdominal aortic aneurysm (EVAR trial 2): randomised controlled trial. Lancet 2005; 365(9478):2187–92.

[3] EVAR Trial Participants. Endovascular aneurysm repair versus open repair in patients with abdominal aortic aneurysm (EVAR trial 1): randomised controlled trial. Lancet 2005; 365(9478):2179–86.

[4] Blankensteijn JD, de Jong SE, Prinssen M, et al. Two-year outcomes after conventional or endovascular repair of abdominal aortic aneurysms. N Engl J Med 2005;352(23): 2398–405.

[5] Prinssen M, Verhoeven EL, Buth J, et al. A randomized trial comparing conventional and endovascular repair of abdominal aortic aneurysms. N Engl J Med 2004;351(16):1607–18.

[6] Harris LM, Faggioli GL, Fiedler R, et al. Ruptured abdominal aortic aneurysms: factors affecting mortality rates. J Vasc Surg 1991;14(6):812–8 [discussion: 819–20].

[7] Bown MJ, Sutton AJ, Bell PR, et al. A meta-analysis of 50 years of ruptured abdominal aortic aneurysm repair. Br J Surg 2002;89(6):714–30.

[8] Gerbode F, Parsons H, Da Costa IA. The surgical treatment of abdominal aortic aneurysms; report of a case treated by resection of the aneurysm with restoration of the aorta by homograft. Stanford Med Bull 1953;11(3):179–82.

[9] Hughes CW. Use of an intra-aortic balloon catheter tamponade for controlling intra-abdominal hemorrhage in man. Surgery 1954;36(1):65–8.

[10] Hesse FG, Kletschka HD. Rupture of abdominal aortic aneurysm: control of hemorrhage by intraluminal balloon tamponade. Ann Surg 1962;155:320–2.

[11] Greenberg RK, Srivastava SD, Ouriel K, et al. An endoluminal method of hemorrhage control and repair of ruptured abdominal aortic aneurysms. J Endovasc Ther 2000;7(1):1–7.

[12] Veith FJ, Ohki T, Lipsitz EC, et al. Endovascular grafts and other catheter-directed techniques in the management of ruptured abdominal aortic aneurysms. Semin Vasc Surg 2003;16(4):326–31.

[13] Arthurs Z, Starnes B, See C, et al. Clamp before you cut: proximal control of ruptured abdominal aortic aneurysms using endovascular balloon occlusion—case reports. Vasc Endovascular Surg 2006;40(2):149–55.

[14] Mehta M, Taggert J, Darling RC 3rd, et al. Establishing a protocol for endovascular treatment of ruptured abdominal aortic aneurysms: outcomes of a prospective analysis. J Vasc Surg 2006;44(1):1–8 [discussion: 8].

[15] Martin RR, Bickell WH, Pepe PE, et al. Prospective evaluation of preoperative fluid resuscitation in hypotensive patients with penetrating truncal injury: a preliminary report. J Trauma 1992;33(3):354–61 [discussion: 361–2].

[16] Bickell WH, Wall MJ Jr, Pepe PE, et al. Immediate versus delayed fluid resuscitation for hypotensive patients with penetrating torso injuries. N Engl J Med 1994;331(17):1105–9.

[17] Roberts K, Revell M, Youssef H, et al. Hypotensive resuscitation in patients with ruptured abdominal aortic aneurysm. Eur J Vasc Endovasc Surg 2006;31(4):339–44.

[18] Lloyd GM, Bown MJ, Norwood MG, et al. Feasibility of preoperative computer tomography in patients with ruptured abdominal aortic aneurysm: a time-to-death study in patients without operation. J Vasc Surg 2004;39(4):788–91.

[19] Gupta BK, Khaneja SC, Flores L, et al. The role of intra-aortic balloon occlusion in penetrating abdominal trauma. J Trauma 1989;29(6):861–5.

[20] Veith FJ, Ohki T. Endovascular approaches to ruptured infrarenal aorto-iliac aneurysms. J Cardiovasc Surg (Torino) 2002;43(3):369–78.

[21] Matsuda H, Tanaka Y, Hino Y, et al. Transbrachial arterial insertion of aortic occlusion balloon catheter in patients with shock from ruptured abdominal aortic aneurysm. J Vasc Surg 2003;38(6):1293–6

[22] Veith FJ, Ohki T, Lipsitz EC, et al. Treatment of ruptured abdominal aneurysms with stent grafts: a new gold standard? Semin Vasc Surg 2003;16(2):171–5.

[23] Malina M, Veith F, Ivancev K, et al. Balloon occlusion of the aorta during endovascular repair of ruptured abdominal aortic aneurysm. J Endovasc Ther 2005;12(5):556–9.

ELSEVIER
SAUNDERS

Surg Clin N Am 87 (2007) 1047–1086

SURGICAL
CLINICS OF
NORTH AMERICA

Descending Thoracic Aortic Dissections

Riyad Karmy-Jones, MD[a],*, Alan Simeone, MD[a],
Mark Meissner, MD[b], Brian Granvall, MPH, PA-C[a],
Stephen Nicholls, MD[a]

[a]Divisions of Thoracic and Vascular Surgery, Heart and Vascular Institute,
Southwest Washington Medical Center, P.O. Box 1600 Vancouver,
WA 98668, USA
[b]Department of Surgery, Division of Vascular Surgery, University of Washington School
of Medicine, Seattle, WA 98195, USA

Acute aortic dissection has been estimated to affect 14 to 20 million individuals globally per annum [1–3]. Alternatively, it has been described as having an incidence of 2.9/100,000/y [4]. Dissections predominantly affect males (male/female ratio 5:1). Two thirds involve the ascending aorta (proximal), with a peak incidence for proximal dissections being 50 to 60 years of age and for distal dissections, 60 to 70 years [2,3,5,6]. Ascending aortic dissection is usually managed as a surgical emergency, because of the risk for rupture, and is a distinct topic that is not addressed in this article.

In general, acute uncomplicated distal dissections are best treated with medical therapy, with attention to blood pressure and rate control. The in-hospital mortality with medical therapy is approximately 10%, and this is considered the standard of care [2,6]. If patients present with or develop acute complications (such as rupture, major branch vessel occlusion, or mesenteric ischemia) that require operative intervention, then mortality increases to approximately one in three [6]. In addition, although the data are not entirely clear, predicting which patients may go on to develop more chronic complications (such as aneurysmal changes) is uncertain. Finally, the definition of "failure of medical therapy," which often relies on persistent pain, can be difficult.

The risk for operation may be increased because of advanced age, extent of aortic disease, presence of connective tissue disorders, or visceral or cerebral ischemia. Endovascular approaches, including fenestration, visceral

* Corresponding author.
E-mail address: rkarmyjo@swmedctr.com (R. Karmy-Jones).

0039-6109/07/$ - see front matter © 2007 Elsevier Inc. All rights reserved.
doi:10.1016/j.suc.2007.08.003
surgical.theclinics.com

stenting, and more recently endovascular stent grafting, have offered a method of improving patient physiology before surgery or definitive treatment, avoiding the need for surgical reconstruction. Even in the setting of proximal dissection, stenting or fenestration to restore perfusion to critical branch vessels before operative repair may be appropriate [7]. The role of interventional approaches remains ill defined, primarily because of uncertainty about how durable these procedures are and what the risk/benefit ratio is, depending on the clinical scenario. Some centers propose using endovascular approaches only in the presence of defined complications, whereas others believe they may be appropriate even in uncomplicated dissections to avoid the development of late complications [8]. To define the role of medical, surgical, or interventional approaches, a review of pathophysiology, classification, natural history, relevant anatomy, and current technologies with outcomes must be performed. Ultimately, however, this is an area that continues to evolve, and as such each case needs to be evaluated by an individual surgeon based on the exact clinical scenario, recognizing that often there are multiple options with no clear-cut best approach.

Pathophysiology

The principle pathologic mechanism of aortic dissection is a tear in the aortic intima, usually transverse but not completely circumferential, which results in separation between the intimal and medial layers of the aortic wall. Although this usually occurs in pathologic settings (connective tissue disease, atherosclerotic ulcer, and so forth) it can occur in histologically normal aortas also. The most common underlying risk factors for distal dissection are hypertension in conjunction with advanced age [4,9]. Connective tissue disorders, including Marfan and Ehlers-Danlos syndromes and the broad-spectrum condition of cystic medial necrosis, result in medial degeneration. Marfan syndrome has been found to be responsible for 6% to 12% of all distal aortic dissections, and has been linked to mutations in fibrillin-1 [10,11]. Aortic ulcers have also been described as a cause in "normal" aortas [9]. Pregnancy, particularly if associated with pre-eclampsia, has been implicated possibly because of progesterone-mediated weakening of the aortic wall [12]. Acute hypertensive crises caused by cocaine ingestion have been documented [13]. Weight-lifting has also been associated with acute dissection, although predominantly involving the ascending aorta [14]. Trauma rarely results in true dissection, and if it does it should be considered a different entity because the management is based on different urgency and timing. Coarctation can be complicated by dissection, particularly in pregnancy. Loeys-Dietz, an inheritable connective tissue disorder attributed to mutations in the gene for either transforming growth factor β type I or II receptors, has been relatively recently recognized as having a marked propensity toward rupture or dissection at early ages with smaller aortic

diameters [15,16]. Finally, dissection can be iatrogenic and caused by operative or catheter treatments in areas removed from the thoracic aorta [17].

Taking all dissections into account, the primary tear occurs in the ascending aorta in 65%, arch in 10%, descending aorta in 20%, and abdominal
aorta in 5% [6]. There are usually multiple secondary fenestrations, often
at the origin of branch vessels (intercostal and visceral). In many instances
the distal auto-fenestrations do not completely decompress the false lumen.
There is thus a pressure gradient that promotes false lumen distension, promoting aneurysmal dilatation. The increased thrombogenicity of the false
lumen can lead to distal false lumen thrombosis further increasing the propensity for aneurysm formation [18].

The dissection proceeds for variable distances distally and on occasion in
a retrograde fashion, following a spiral path [19]. The false channel tends to
occupy the left lateral/inferior portion of the aorta as it propagates distally;
the left renal artery arises from the false lumen in 25% of cases. At the aortic
bifurcation the dissection proceeds bilaterally in many cases and often ends
at the iliac bifurcations, although there is a tendency for the false lumen to
expand particularly on the left, resulting in limb ischemia [10]. As it proceeds, the intimal flap is torn away from branch vessels, resulting in multiple
spontaneous fenestrations [2]. Critical obstruction may result from one of
three mechanisms, all of which may occur simultaneously. In dynamic obstruction, the septum may prolapse across the origin of the vessel, impinging
flow although the vessel remains anatomically intact. Static obstruction results from the dissection plane entering the ostia of the vessel with subsequent narrowing or distal thrombosis. As the false lumen dilates, the true
lumen is compressed, and this can lead to critical limitation of vessels that
arise from the true lumen. Because the distal fenestrations are smaller
than the entry tear, the false lumen tends to be over-pressurized leading
to gradual dilation while at the same time further compromising the diameter of the true lumen [20,21].

Classification

In 1965 DeBakey and colleagues [22] proposed an anatomic classification
that is based on the origin and the extent of the dissection (Table 1). Dailey
and associates proposed a method based on the inherent different outcomes
and operative issues that combined ascending aortic dissections, regardless
of origin, as Stanford type A (DeBakey types I and II) and those that originate in and are limited to the descending thoracic aorta (with or without
abdominal aortic involvement, DeBakey types IIIa and IIIb) as Stanford
type B [23]. It is important to recognize the small number of cases in which
the primary tear occurs in the descending aorta or arch, but which lead to
retrograde dissection involving arch or ascending aorta. DeBakey types I
and II and Stanford A are often grouped together as proximal dissections,
whereas the remainder are considered distal.

Table 1
The DeBakey classification

Type	Origin of dissection	Extent of dissection
I	Ascending aorta	Through arch, extending into thoracic or abdominal aorta
II	Ascending aorta	Limited to ascending aorta (up to innominate origin)
III	Descending aorta	Limited to descending aorta, IIIa; involves descending and portions of abdominal aorta, IIIb

A nonanatomic classification is acute versus chronic. If the dissection is diagnosed within 2 weeks of onset of symptoms, it is considered acute. Particularly with ascending aortic dissections, complications, such as rupture, are more likely to occur without prompt medical management, and in the case of ascending dissection, operation. As discussed later, whether distal dissections are acute or chronic has major implications in determining whether endovascular or operative approaches should be undertaken. In brief, operative results are improved if distal dissections can be repaired during the chronic phase [24]. On the other hand, the behavior of endovascular stents seems to be more predictable if performed during the acute phase.

Presentation

The classic presenting symptom of aortic dissection is abrupt onset of chest pain [6,25]. With distal dissections the pain is located in the back and characterized in half of cases as tearing but in two thirds additionally as sharp and in approximately one fifth as migratory [6]. In 43% of cases the pain primarily involved or included the abdominal area, raising suspicion of mesenteric ischemia [6]. Unfortunately, if the nature and quality of the pain is not specifically sought after, the initial differential does not include dissection in as many as 85% of cases, leading to significant delay in starting treatment [4,26]. Syncope was much more commonly associated with dissections involving the ascending aorta or retrograde arch involvement [6]. Presentation with paralysis is reported to occur in 2% to 8% of patients who had distal dissection, and hypertension is much more common than hypotension ($>70\%$ versus $<5\%$, respectively) [2,3,5,27]. Indeed, hypertension that is difficult to control or refractory to medical management is present in nearly two thirds of patients [28]. Approximately 14% of patients who have dissections involving the distal aorta present with femoral pulse deficits [2]. Although as many as one third of patients may spontaneously resolve lower extremity pulse deficits, a significant number require intervention, and even more critically, this finding suggests an extensive dissection that should prompt evaluation of possible renal and visceral compromise

[29]. Data from the International Registry of Aortic Dissection (IRAD) suggested that absence of pain, presence of hypotension, and branch vessel involvement were significantly associated with increased risk for death [30].

Simple initial screening tests, such as plain chest radiography and ECG, are of limited value. The initial chest radiograph may suggest mediastinal widening but considering all cases of dissection is normal in 12% of cases [6]. The ECG is normal in one third of cases, but the presence of severe chest pain and normal ECG should suggest the diagnosis of dissection, particularly distal dissection [6].

The primary diagnostic tool has become CT angiography (CTA) using thin (1.5 mm) slices and encompassing the entire aorta, through the iliac and femoral vessels [2]. CTA can define true lumen and branch vessel compromise, identify which lumen is the predominant source of perfusion to specific branch vessels, and be used to plan treatment. Three-dimensional reconstruction can be readily performed permitting increased accuracy. Intravascular ultrasound can be used to help differentiate the diagnosis if intramural hematoma is suspected and can also accurately define the physiology of branch malperfusion [21,31]. Magnetic resonance angiography (MRA) has also been used in cases of contrast allergy or renal insufficiency, although recently there has been concern that in this latter situation the gadolinium contrast agent should also be limited. Transesophageal echocardiography is somewhat less attractive in the setting of type B dissection compared with type A because portions of the arch may be obscured, but distal dissection and in some cases celiac or superior mesenteric artery compromise can be confirmed [2,32].

Natural history/medical management

The mortality associated with acute uncomplicated distal aortic dissection managed medically is as low as 10.7%. This figure increases to 31% (or higher) if complications arise that require surgical intervention, particularly during the acute phase [6,24].

Estrera and colleagues [27] followed 159 consecutive patients, admitted between January 2001 and April 2006, who had acute type B dissection, all initially managed medically. Median time to obtain a systolic blood pressure less than 140 mm Hg and to control primary pain was 48 hours. The overall hospital mortality was 8.8%, but in the 23 (14.5%) patients who required an intervention, there were four (17%) deaths compared with mortality of 7.7% if medical management was maintained. These four deaths occurred among the 8 patients who presented with or developed rupture. Complicated dissection, defined as rupture or malperfusion (cerebral, visceral, spinal, or limb) was present in nearly half of patients, and the mortality was significantly greater (18%) compared with uncomplicated dissection (1.2%). Neurologic complications included stroke (5%), intracranial hemorrhage (2%), and paraplegia (8%). Of the patients who had paraplegia two thirds resolved within 24 hours. Frank intestinal or hepatic ischemia occurred in 8.6% and acute renal failure in 20%, of whom two thirds required dialysis. Three (1.9%) patients required open cardiac repair because of retrograde dissection.

An intriguing aspect of this report was the observation that limb, spinal, and visceral malperfusion could in a significant number of cases spontaneously resolve. At the same time it took on average 48 hours to obtain symptomatic relief and blood pressure control. Our own observations suggest that in some instances dropping the blood pressure may aggravate renal or visceral malperfusion or lead to confusion suggesting cerebral hypoperfusion. Deciding when to intervene on any given case may not be straightforward and may require multiple physical, laboratory, and radiographic examinations over the initial 24- to 48-hour period.

A Swedish study of 66 patients who had uncomplicated dissection treated medically had an actuarial survival rate at 5 years of 82% and at 10 years of 69%. Freedom from dissection-related death at 5 years was 85% and at 10 years was 82% [33]. In addition, quality of life was not appreciably affected when patients could be maintained on medical management [34].

A simple summary of these findings would include the following observations: In the acute setting, uncomplicated type B dissection is best managed medically, with acute mortality less than 10% and complication rate 5% to 20% [35,36]. The rationale is that medical therapy, although not necessarily proved to be better than surgical therapy, is at least as good as surgical therapy [37,38]. A report from the IRAD database analyzing outcomes of acute type B dissection in 242 patients who survived initial hospitalization showed 3-year survival for medical therapy to be 77.6% ± 6.6%, surgical repair 82.8% ± 18.9%, and endovascular therapy 76.2% ± 25.2%, respectively [39].

As many as half of all patients develop or present with complications requiring intervention and have a marked increase in mortality. The leading complication is malperfusion, followed by a smaller incidence of acute rupture. A complication-specific treatment plan is recommended, with malperfusion issues currently being addressed predominantly by endovascular stent grafting, branch artery stenting, or fenestration [10,40]. There is a growing body of data that supports the notion that in the acute, complicated setting, endovascular approaches, if feasible, are associated with lower paralysis, pain, blood loss, length of stay, and probably mortality, compared with open repair [41].

Patients who survive the initial episode remain at risk for the development of aneurysm or further dissection, particularly if the false lumen remains patent [42,43]. As many as 50% of patients who have distal dissection who are managed medically progress to aneurysm formation or death within 4 years of their initial presentation [6,9,41,42,44]. Dialetto and colleagues [45] found that 28.5% of uncomplicated type B dissections managed medically progressed to aneurysmal dilatation at a mean of 18.1 ± 16.9 months. Patients who had patent false lumens or in whom the distal aortic diameter is greater than 40 mm (or 45 mm in some series) are at particular risk [35,46–48]. Bernard and associates [43] described actuarial survival rates with distal dissection as 76% at 1 year, 72% at 2 years, and 46% at 10 years, with survival being significantly affected by age greater than 70 years or patent false lumen.

Whether or not earlier intervention (either open surgical or endovascular repair) in asymptomatic patients at higher risk is justified still awaits clarification but is the subject of ongoing trials [49]. For example, Roseborough and colleagues [50] estimated that 37% of patients might benefit acutely from prophylactic stent grafts, and a further 13% might benefit in avoiding chronic complications.

Indications for intervention

There are four indications for acute intervention: rupture, aortic expansion (> 5.0 cm), critical vessel malperfusion, and intractable pain. Many authors argue that an aortic diameter in the involved segment of greater than 40 or 45 mm is a reasonable indication for intervention, at least with stent grafts, because of the risk for later aneurysmal development, progressive dissection, or death [8,36,41,51]. Intractable hypertension has been also used as an indication, although as discussed earlier this is hard to define because it may take as long as 48 hours to achieve ideal pressure control [41]. Retrograde dissection usually involves ascending or proximal arch and requires operative intervention. In the acute setting with type B dissection the leading risk factor for mortality is malperfusion [27]. As discussed earlier, it may not be immediately apparent that intervention is required. Intractable pain may be more of an issue for the nervous surgeon than the patient, and the definition varies. The predominant principle is that intervention is reserved for specific complications, the primary therapy initially being medical. The use of endovascular stent grafts in particular in uncomplicated acute type B dissections should be restricted to investigational trials [52]. Although there are emerging data that stabilizing the aorta in patients at higher risk (patent false lumen, aortic diameter > 40 mm) who are asymptomatic may reduce the risk for late rupture, further studies are needed before this can be accepted universally [53].

In the chronic setting, indications advocated for intervention, at least for endovascular techniques, have included aortic diameters greater than 50 mm (or 55 mm) or growth of greater than 5 mm over a 6-month period [41,51]. Others argue that 6.5 cm should be the indication [40,54]. New onset of back pain or other acute symptoms is another indication [41]. Distal false lumen thrombosis with persistent large proximal entry may promote expansion of the thoracic component (Fig. 1).

Malperfusion syndromes represent a complex of physiologic and anatomic changes. Dynamic obstruction implies that either the septum has prolapsed over the vessel origin or that the true lumen is compressed to a degree

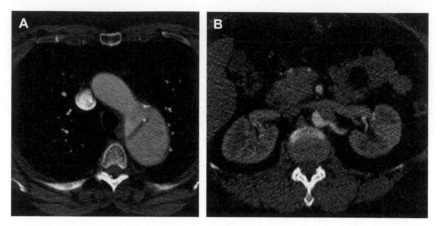

Fig. 1. Patient who has a chronic dissection with the primary entry site 1-cm distal to the origin of the left subclavian artery. There has been expansion of the total thoracic aortic diameter, with persistent filling from the proximal entry site (A) but minimal distal decompression of the false lumen because of thrombosis (B).

that it can no longer provide adequate perfusion. In static obstruction, thrombosis within the false lumen or branch vessel coupled with varying degrees of dissection into the vessel results in an anatomic limitation to flow [20]. The former, which may be responsible for as much as 80% of malperfusion syndrome, is more recently being managed with endovascular stenting, with fenestration or stenting being reserved for second-line therapy in most cases [20,52,55,56]. This practice represents a significant change, because until the turn of the century, fenestration or branch limb stenting was the primary therapy for dissection complicated by malperfusion syndromes [3]. Significant static obstruction requires stenting or operative bypass. Both forms of malperfusion may coexist. If fenestration is needed, intravascular ultrasound facilitates the procedure [57].

One contraindication to endovascular approaches seems to be defined connective tissue disorders, particularly Marfan syndrome. Although endovascular stents have been used in Marfan cases in the setting of aneurysmal disease, most centers are concerned that with the current technology available, there is too high a risk for creating retrograde dissection or acute or delayed perforation [54,58–60]. This concept is particularly relevant when considering that centers with extensive experience have excellent results with operative intervention. Coselli and LeMaire [61] reported on 50 patients who had Marfan syndrome who underwent operative repair of thoracoabdominal aneurysms, 41 of whom had chronic dissection. The 30-day survival was 96% and postoperative lower extremity neurologic injury was only 4%. In the settings of connective tissue disorders, at least currently, endovascular stent grafts are reserved for patients who have associated risk factors that would complicate operative repair.

Operative repair of type B dissection

In contrast to the primacy of open surgical therapy for dissection involving the ascending aorta, the role of open surgery in type B aortic dissection has for years been less well-defined. Enthusiasm for surgical approaches to descending dissection has had peaks and valleys, and with a few notable exceptions, most centers have adopted a protocol of intensive anti-impulse therapy for acute type B dissection [62–64]. Surgical treatment has for the most part been reserved for complicated acute dissection along with symptomatic or expanding aneurysmal degeneration of chronic dissection [24,65–68].

In 1935 the first report of a fenestration procedure for dissection-induced malperfusion was published by Gurin and colleagues [69]. DeBakey and colleagues [22] in 1965 were the first to advocate an aggressive operative approach to descending aortic dissection, citing an operative mortality of 25%, which compared favorably to a group of nonoperatively treated patients who had 90% mortality at one year. Their results and patient population were not easily reproduced, and data began to accrue supporting the nonoperative management of uncomplicated cases. Wheat and colleagues [62–64] showed that with aggressive antihypertensive therapy early mortality could be reduced to 16%, and most centers adopted the policy of medical treatment of uncomplicated dissection. Surgical intervention was reserved for patients who had rupture, intractable pain, visceral or peripheral malperfusion, progression of dissection, uncorrectable hypertension, or aneurysm [24,65–68].

Controversy persisted, however, spurred by reports from the group at Stanford and others showing equivalent early results with medical and surgical treatment of selected patients who had uncomplicated dissection [23,24,65,70,71]. Although most groups have continued to use a complication-specific approach to surgical intervention, impressive improvements in operative outcomes over the last 20 years have made aggressive surgically based care more attractive, particularly in selected uncomplicated patients [6,27,30,33,40,66,68,72,73].

The standard central aortic operative approach has involved a left posterolateral thoracotomy through the fourth or fifth interspace. If more distal exposure is needed, a more caudal thoracotomy or thoracoabdominal incision, either trans- or retroperitoneal, is created. The principle in acute dissection is to replace as short a segment of the aorta as possible encompassing the most significantly diseased region, preferably including the intimal tear. Proximal and distal anastomoses are performed where the aortic diameter is normal or at least close to normal, usually the proximal third of the thoracic aorta. By controlling the proximal intimal injury and reconstructing the layers of the aorta distally, most malperfusion issues resolve. In the acute setting, buttressing the anastomosis with Teflon helps protect the proximal portion from tearing, and distally this can be used to help exclude the false lumen. Biologic glues have also been used to reinforce the anastomosis and promote false lumen closure [74,75]. Alternatively, particularly in chronic dissections, the septum can be excised or fenestrated. Although this allows for resection of the portion of the aorta at risk for rupture and for perfusion into the false lumen if there is concern that critical branch vessels may be affected by exclusion, it does mean that the distal false lumen may go on to aneurysmal degeneration over the period of follow-up. Persistent malperfusion is addressed by percutaneous fenestration, bypass, or rarely thromboexclusion [40]. The Stanford group has shown that direct central aortic reconstruction is associated with improved results compared with local vascular bypass or reconstruction [76,77].

For chronic dissection with aneurysmal degeneration the approach is by necessity tailored to the anatomy, and limited aortic replacement is often not an option. The natural history of these enlarged aortas, which are correctly termed pseudoaneurysms because the dissection process by definition splits the wall in a subintimal plane, is difficult to predict. Some reports indicate that they behave analogously to degenerative thoracic aortic aneurysms [6,40,66,68,78]. Conversely, some reports suggest that they behave much more virulently, particularly if there is flow documented in the false lumen [79,80]. Regardless, at a diameter of 6 cm, or any size if symptomatic or if a connective tissue disorder exists, or if serial imaging suggests a significant interval increase in size has occurred, the aorta should be replaced. Traditionally the approach involved a sequential "clamp and sew" technique, with reimplantation of visceral vessels and intercostal arteries as Carrel patches. Operative mortality varied from around 15% to 70%, depending on acuity, comorbidity, and center. The incidence of the most dread morbidity, paraplegia, ranged from around 10% to 30%, again depending on anatomic extent, acuity, comorbidity, and center. The passage of time has brought dramatic improvements in diagnostic capability, anesthetic, and perioperative critical care, all of which have had a positive effect on outcome [81]. Operative technique has likewise matured. Perfusion adjuncts such as standard venoarterial and left heart bypass have been associated with reduced mortality and paraplegia rates, particularly when used with moderate hypothermia [82–87]. The addition of deep hypothermic circulatory arrest is associated with further reductions in mortality and paraplegia [88–95]. An intervention specifically directed at maximizing spinal cord perfusion, lumbar cerebrospinal fluid (CSF) drainage, has been adopted as an essential adjunct by most thoracic aortic surgeons [85,86,96–98]. This technique has also been shown to be an important treatment of delayed postoperative paraplegia and paraplegia associated with endovascular aortic stent grafting [99,100].

Operative management of intercostal arteries is another potentially revolutionary area; standard belief held that reimplantation of as many intercostal arteries as was feasible was essential to minimize paraplegia risk. Surprisingly, aggressive imaging to identify and ensure subsequent reimplantation of tributaries of the artery of Adamkiewicz [101] has not been shown to prevent paraplegia. There are data that suggest that reimplantation may often be unnecessary, and that a new paradigm for spinal cord perfusion may be warranted [102–105]. Along these lines, there is support for the use of intraoperative evaluation of motor and sensory evoked potentials to help guide operative conduct [106–109].

Although many groups believe that complications of type B dissection are best treated by aortic reconstruction, the role of primary open procedures for visceral, renal, and limb ischemia is unclear. This consideration is particularly true now for two reasons: the improvement in outcomes for open aortic surgery, and probably more importantly, the explosion and rapid advancement of percutaneous endovascular techniques. Open aortic fenestration, branch vessel bypass, and extra anatomic bypass have been reasonable techniques in selected instances, and their early outcomes were certainly better than what could have been be achieved with medical therapy alone. An additional technique, thromboexclusion of the proximal thoracic aorta by placement of an ascending to descending conduit, can be useful in select cases of acute dissection [40,68]. It is estimated that malperfusion occurs in 10% to 75% of cases and is associated with mortality of up to 60% to 80% [5,56,110–114]. Surgical fenestration has been found to decrease early mortality to around 20% to 40% [110–113]. The critical drawback of primary fenestration or bypass is that the central pathology—the diseased aorta—is not addressed. In addition, the conditions for which they are used have been shown to be markers for increased severity of aortic damage. Finally, visceral ischemia is a grave prognostic indicator, and renal ischemia is extraordinarily time-sensitive and can be difficult to diagnose early.

Endovascular management

The recognized difficulties in operative management of acute dissections have led to an increased interest in endovascular approaches, including stent grafting. The enthusiasm was stimulated by the Stanford group's initial report in 1999 [115]. It has been further invigorated by encouraging data in the atherosclerotic aneurysm population, particularly with reduced incidence of spinal cord injury, although how well this translates to the dissection population is still open to question [116].

A survey of eight centers performing endovascular stent procedures for thoracic aortic pathologies was performed collecting data on 1180 patients who underwent interventions between June 2003 and June 2004 [117]. The bulk of cases (64.2%) were performed for degenerative aneurysms of the descending thoracic aorta. Nearly 20% were performed for distal dissections or variants, however. The authors commented that except for chronic dissection, endovascular treatment was at least equivalent to, or better than, conventional approaches (Table 2) [117].

The primary goal of endovascular stent grafting in the setting of a type B dissection is to occlude the primary and proximal entry site. It has been argued that aortic pressure and perfusion becomes preferentially diverted to

Table 2
Incidence of endovascular stent graft management of acute aortic syndromes

Pathology	Total cases (%)	30-day mortality (%)
Acute dissection	7.8	9.9
Intramural hematoma with ulcer	2.2	7.2
Giant penetrating ulcer	1.0	0
Chronic dissection	8.4	3.3

the false lumen, which expands, becomes aneurysmal, and compresses the true lumen (Fig. 2). This compression can lead to inadequate perfusion of vessels arising from the true lumen or compression of visceral, spinal, and limb vessels because of dynamic compromise [2,46]. Malperfusion is the most common form of complication arising from type B dissection requiring intervention [2]. The anticipated result of covering the primary entry site is that with pressurized flow being redirected through the true lumen, the false lumen collapses and ideally thrombosis occurs (Fig. 3). If the septum is pliable, with the false lumen depressurized, it shifts back toward the false lumen. Vessels arising from the false lumen are perfused through auto-fenestrations in the septum (Fig. 4).

These assumptions give rise to various questions in any given case and are the subject of ongoing research. The first question is, what is the proper sizing of the endograft? Oversizing can result in increased risk for rupture, creating retrograde dissection, cutting through the septum distally with resultant vigorous retrograde perfusion. In the setting of malperfusion, how reliably can one predict successful reperfusion? If there is thickening of the septum or thrombus in the false lumen, a particular concern with

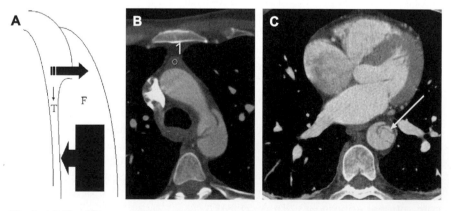

Fig. 2. (A) The thinner-walled false lumen (F) is pressurized, resulting in expansion of the false lumen with compression of the true (T). (B) Patient who has acute dissection with proximal entry site who presents with abdominal pain, acidosis, and developing renal insufficiency. (C) Distally, the true lumen (arrow) is nearly completely obliterated.

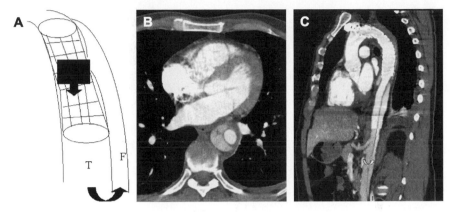

Fig. 3. (*A*) As cardiac output is redirected into the true (T) lumen, the false (F) is depressurized and the septum shifts back toward the false. Distal fenestrations may still permit filling of the false lumen. (*B*) Same patient as in Fig. 2, post–endovascular stent. The true lumen has expanded, although there is still false lumen filling, and the patient's mesenteric and renal ischemia completely resolved. (*C*) Sagittal reconstruction of the same patient illustrating how the stent graft has redirected the cardiac output into the true lumen. There is still distal retrograde filling of the false lumen. The false lumen along the treated area has thrombosed. At 1-year follow-up the anatomy has remained stable, but this patient might be considered acutely or subsequently for extension (possibly bare metal) to assist remodeling of the untreated aorta.

chronic dissection, compression or complete distal collapse of the endograft may occur (Fig. 5) [118]. How much of the descending aorta should be covered to promote false lumen compression and thrombosis? The greater the length of descending aorta completely excluded, presumably the greater the risk for spinal cord ischemia [103,119]. Will distal components that

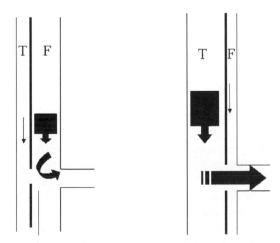

Fig. 4. Branch vessels arising from the false (F) lumen have usually an auto-fenestration where the septum has torn away from their origin. Once a more proximal stent graft occludes the primary entry site, in the acute setting, the septum shifts back toward the false lumen and perfusion is restored from the true (T) lumen through the fenestration.

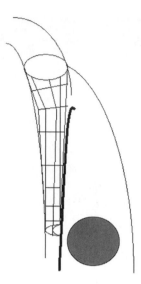

Fig. 5. Endograft placed in a chronic dissection. The thick, less-pliable septum may resist move-ment or distal thrombosis leading to distal compression or collapse of the endograft.

are bare metal be an adequate compromise? Proximal fixation is also an is-sue. Can proximal bare stent components provide more reliable fixation with short landing zones or is there an increased risk for rupture or retro-grade dissection?

Unlike the setting of atherosclerotic aneurysmal disease, in which it is rec-ommended that an oversizing of 10% to 20% of the proposed landing zones be used, in acute dissection anecdotally many centers believe that 10% to 15% of the normal aorta at the landing zone be used. This practice is to avoid the risk for creating a new dissection. At the time of deployment, ide-ally no ballooning is performed or, if deemed necessary because of signifi-cant proximal endoleak, very gentle ballooning at most [120].

Most, but not all, entry sites are in the region of the origin of the left sub-clavian artery [36]. In most cases the most proximal normal aorta is in proxim-ity to the origin of the left subclavian artery. To achieve a proximal landing zone of 1 cm in length, and one that does not result in deployment into the an-gle of the descending aorta with resultant lack of apposition, in a significant number of cases (25% or more) it is necessary to cover the origin of the left sub-clavian artery [41,121]. If the retrograde component of the dissection involves only a portion of the artery's origin, it may be reasonable to try to land across the origin, although one must be prepared to extend the endograft.

In most acute cases, endovascular occlusion of the primary entry site suc-cessfully resolves malperfusion syndromes (>90% of cases) with the need for additional stenting, bypass, or fenestration reduced to less than 10% of cases [36,41,55,120,122]. Intravascular ultrasound or manometry can help predict the degree to which dynamic or static compromise is present.

A bulge toward the true lumen at the origin of the vessel in question implies a significant dynamic component [21]. Fenestration can be used as an adjunct to endovascular stenting if needed [20]. Persistent iliac occlusion can be managed by further stenting or femoral–femoral bypass [123].

Eliminating the false lumen in the chronic setting is more difficult to predict. Although persistent proximal filling of a chronically dilated false lumen with distal thrombosis seems to be an ideal indication and has a high success rate, how the distal portion of the graft will behave is difficult to anticipate. If the septum is too thick or the false lumen filled with noncompressible thrombus, the distal graft may collapse [124]. At least in our experience, one method of assessing this is to perform intravascular ultrasound. If the septum moves, we have more confidence that the graft will deploy in a reasonable fashion. At the time of deployment we cautiously hand-inflate an angioplasty balloon to document whether or not the septum is pliable.

Clinical experience with endovascular stent grafting in the management of type B dissection

Before considering some of the larger trials of endovascular stent graft management of type B dissections, it must be remembered that these trials vary in patient population, acuity, presentation, and indications. Furthermore, few compare medical versus surgical management outcomes head-to-head.

Shimono and Shimpo [125] reported on 60 patients (19 chronic, 27 complicated acute, 14 uncomplicated acute) who underwent endovascular repair. Hospital mortality was 4.9% among the acute cases and 0 among the chronic, and actuarial survival among acute cases at 5 years was 90%.

Resch and colleagues [51] described the outcomes of 129 patients (49 chronic) who underwent endovascular repair. Indications in the acute population included rupture (20), end-organ ischemia (28), true-lumen compression without clinical signs of end-organ ischemia, persistent pain or hypertension (5), acute aortic dilatation (4), and intramural hematoma (10). Indications in the chronic population included diameter greater than 5.5 cm, growth greater than 5 mm over 6 months, and in 6 cases symptomatic or rupturing thoracic aneurysms. Perioperative mortality was 18% among the acute cases and 4% among the chronic. Overall stroke occurred in 8% and spinal cord injury in 6%.

Guo and colleagues [126] reported on 178 cases (76 acute, 19 type A), in which visceral and/or great vessel bypass was performed simultaneously in 10 cases. The left subclavian origin was covered without bypass in 36 cases. Thirty-day mortality was 3.4% and at 1 month the endoleak rate was 6.4% (compared with 12.9% acutely); there was no spinal cord injury and blood loss averaged 140 mL.

Eggebrecht and colleagues [49] reported the results of a meta-analysis of 39 studies totaling 609 patients. Studies that reported three or more cases or retrograde endovascular repair of type B dissections were included. Procedural success rate was 98.2% ± 0.5%, major complication rate 11.1% ± 1.4% (stroke 1.9% ± 0.6%, paraplegia 0.8% ± 0.4%) and 30-day mortality was 5.3% ± 0.9% (21.7% ± 2.8% acute versus 9.1% ± 2.3% chronic, $P = .005$). Kaplan-Meyer analysis yielded overall survival rates of 89.9% ± 1.7% at 1 year and 88.8% ± 1.9% at 2 years. The authors note that these results compare favorably with surgical repair, especially in the setting of complicated acute dissection, but that further studies are needed to clarify the benefit of this approach compared with medical management in uncomplicated cases.

Leurs and colleagues [58] presented a combined report from the EUROSTAR and United Kingdom Thoracic Endograft registries. One hundred thirty-one patients underwent endografting, 57% for complications of dissection and the remainder being asymptomatic. Primary success rate was 89%, 30-day mortality overall was 6.5% (12% if emergent), and paraplegia occurred in 0.8%. Overall 1-year survival of the 67 who had follow-up was 90%.

Xu and colleagues [127] reviewed 63 patients who presented with acute type B dissection and were managed with endovascular stents, 59 after 2 weeks of medical therapy. The primary entry site was completely sealed at the initial procedure in 95% of cases, 30-day mortality was 3.2%, retrograde dissection occurred in 3.2%, and the false lumen was completely thrombosed in the thoracic aorta at 1 year in 98%. Follow-up averaged 11.7 ± 10.6 months, during which time 3 (4.8%) died. In one case death was procedural (retrograde dissection). Kaplan-Meier–derived survival at 4 years was estimated to be 89.4%.

As noted, despite encouraging results, there is some debate as to whether stent grafts should be used in the setting of chronic dissection in patients who are operative candidates [49,128,129]. It has been argued that the problem in chronic dissection is false lumen dilation, and because of the multiple fenestrations, in many cases the false lumen continues to be perfused leading to persistent risk for expansion or rupture [130]. There are data that support the endovascular approach in high-risk patients. Czerny and associates [131] reported on six patients who underwent endograft procedures for chronic type B dissection complicated by aneurysmal growth. In four cases proximal extrathoracic debranching was required to obtain a suitable landing zone. At a mean of 16 months' follow-up, five patients exhibited thrombosis of the false lumen with shrinkage of the aneurysm and one patient had a persistent proximal endoleak.

The INSTEAD trial (INvestigation of STEnt grafts in patients with type B Aortic Dissection) is a prospective trial designed to compare outcomes of patients randomized to either stent graft or best medical management. Inclusion criteria include age greater than 18 years, uncomplicated type B dissection, and lack of spontaneous thrombosis in the false lumen 14 days after the index event. In designing the trial a retrospective analysis of 80 patients treated endovascularly by the lead author were compared with 80 patients treated medically. Two-year survival in the endovascular group was 94.9% and in the medical group, 67.5% [132]. These results, when published, will provide clarity in deciding when patients with chronic dissections may truly benefit from an endovascular approach.

Stent graft design

Various endovascular stent grafts have been used to manage type B dissection (Table 3). The three with which the authors have some personal experience and that are more readily available in North America are described in Tables 4 to 6 (Figs. 6–8). These devices have several inherent advantages and disadvantages that require individual experience so that the surgeon can feel comfortable in choosing which device would fit an individual case, much as with any operative case. Endografts can come with uncovered proximal or distal portions, or both. The argument for an uncovered proximal extension is that it permits covering across the origin of the left subclavian vessel without occlusion [36,122]. Distal uncovered grafts offer the opportunity to cover visceral vessels to achieve fixation without malperfusion [55]. Although gaining increasing support, we personally have been concerned about using bare metal stents routinely because of the possibility of cutting through the septum and causing a significant new entry site that could lead to complications [2,55]. Despite this concern, there is a growing body of data to support this approach to remodeling the aorta [132,133].

Three grafts, which have tended to be used more commonly in North America, are described in more detail. The Gore-TAG (W.L. Gore & Associates, Flagstaff, Arizona, USA) is constructed from ePTFE, wrapped in self-expanding nitinol stents that have a sutureless attachment. There is a radiopaque band at each end, with 0.5-cm proximal and distal extension flares covered to assist in wall apposition (see Fig. 6). These flares can be placed partially across an orifice without occluding the orifice. The device is introduced through a 30-cm sheath, the outer diameter varying depending on the diameter of the graft. The delivery catheter is fairly flexible and 100 cm in

Table 3
Brand names of thoracic endografts used in North America and Europe

Type	Company
Gore TAG	W.L. Gore & Associates, Flagstaff, AZ
Gore Excluder	
Medtronic Talent	Medtronic, Minneapolis, MN
Medtronic Valiant	
Cook-Zenith TX2	Cook, Bloomington, IN
Bolton Relay	Bolton Medical, Sunrise, FL
Endomed	Endomed, Phoenix, AZ
Jotec Evita	Jotec, Hechingen, Germany

Table 4
Characteristics of the Thoracic Aortic Graft

Stent diameter (mm)	Length (cm)	Landing zone inner diameter (mm)	Introducer size (French)	Access vessel diameter (mm)
26	10	23	20	7.6
28	10	24–26	20	7.6
	15			
31	10	26–29	22	8.3
	15			
	20			
34	10	29–32	22	8.3
	15			
	20			
37	10	32–34	24	9.1
	15			
	20			
40	10	34–37	24	9.1
	15			
	20			

length (see Table 4). The device is released by pulling a rip-cord that unlaces the constraining system with rapid (less than 1 second) release starting in the center. This central deployment prevents a "wind sock" effect and there is rarely any need to critically lower blood pressure during deployment to beyond normal ranges to prevent distal migration. When advancing the catheter there can be built up tension, and the device should be advanced just beyond the proposed landing zone and then brought back into the proper alignment just before deployment. One characteristic of the TAG device is that it rarely if ever jumps forward. Rather, it may drop a millimeter or two back (distally). In appropriately sized patients, the TAG offers an exceptionally good approach because of its flexibility and rapid deployment characteristics.

The Cook-Zenith TX2 (Cook, Bloomington, Indiana, USA) is made of woven polyester fabric over stainless steel Z-stents. The TX2 has a proximal form, which has no bare stents but does have 5-mm long barbs. The distal component does have a bare metal distal segment (see Fig. 7). The proximal device can be uniform or tapered. The diameters range from 28 to 42 mm (in 2-mm increments) and the lengths vary from 120 to 216 mm. The tapered form narrows at the third Z-stent and the distal diameter is 4 mm less than the proximal (see Table 5). The sheaths are precurved and 75 cm long. A 20-French sheath (OD 23 Fr) is used for 28- to 34-mm stents, and a 22-French sheath (OD 25 Fr) for 38- to 42-mm endografts. Although it would be rare to need it in the trauma setting, the TX2 is designed with a distal component to allow modification of the distal portion of the graft to fit the anatomic requirements of the distal landing zone. This portion has an uncovered

Table 5
Characteristics of the Cook-Zenith TX2 proximal component

Non-tapered

Diameter (mm)	Length (mm)	Introducer sheath (French-internal diameter)
28	120	20
	140	
	200	
30	120	20
	140	
	200	
32	120	20
	140	
	200	
34	127	20
	152	
	202	
36	127	22
	152	
	202	
38	127	22
	152	
	202	
40	108	22
	135	
	162	
	216	
42	108	22
	135	
	162	
	216	

Tapered

Proximal diameter (mm)	Distal diameter (mm)	Length (mm)	Introducer sheath (French-ID)
32	28	160	20
		200	
20	20	157	20
		197	
36	32	157	22
		197	
38	34	152	22
		202	
40	36	158	22
		208	
42	38	158	22
		208	

bare area. The device is unsheathed, but three trigger wires continue to constrain the device, reducing any wind sock effect, and allowing final careful positioning before complete release.

The Medtronic Talent Thoracic graft has recently been released in Europe in a modified form, the Valiant (Medtronic, Santa Rosa, California,

Table 6
Characteristics of the Talent-Valiant graft

Straight section

Proximal end	Distal end	Proximal diameter (mm)	Covered length (cm)	Catheter size (French)
FreeFlo	Closed web	24, 26, 28, 30, 32	100, 150	22
FreeFlo	Closed web	30, 32	200	22
FreeFlo	Closed web	34, 36, 38, 40	100, 150, 200	24
FreeFlo	Closed web	42, 44, 46	100, 150, 200	25
Closed web	Closed web	24, 26, 28, 30, 32	100, 150	22
Closed web	Closed web	30, 32	200	22
Closed web	Closed web	34, 36, 38, 40	100, 150, 200	24
Closed web	Closed web	42, 44, 46	100, 150, 200	25
Closed web	Bare spring	24, 26, 28, 30, 32	100	22
Closed web	Bare spring	34, 36, 38, 40	100	24
Closed web	Bare spring	42, 44, 46	100	25
Tapered Section (distal diameter is 4 mm less than proximal)				
Closed web	Closed web	28, 30, 32	150	22
Closed web	Closed web	34, 36, 38, 40	150	24
Closed web	Closed web	42, 44, 46	150	25

USA). The Valiant differs in that although it is still made of a low-profile polyester monofilament material, the nitinol stents are on the outside with two proximal configurations, one covered and the other with 12-mm flexible bare stents to allow adaptation to the aortic curvature and greater fixation. In addition, there has been improved conformability of the distal end, which may be covered or have a bare extension also (FreeFlo) (see Fig. 8, Table 6). The Medtronic company tends to recommend the FreeFlo model over the

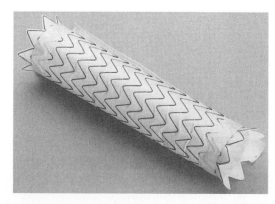

Fig. 6. The Gore Thoracic Aortic Graft (TAG). (*Courtesy of* W.L. Gore & Associates, Flagstaff, AZ; with permission.)

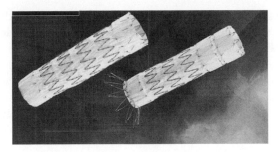

Fig. 7. The Cook-Zenith TX2 Graft with proximal and distal components. (*Courtesy of* Cook, Inc., Bloomington, IN; with permission.)

covered proximal stent because the experience, at least with nontraumatic aortic pathology, is that the increased flexibility allows the uncovered portion to conform well with the aorta, leading to better fixation. Like the Cook-TX2, the Valiant comes in both a proximal and distal (if needed) component, although with short lesions the proximal component alone is often sufficient. Both come in straight or tapered versions. The delivery system involves an unsheathing maneuver. The device allows retraction and repositioning to permit exact placement. The Talent does come in a slightly smaller model than the Valiant, 22 mm, which may be useful in aortas with diameters of 18 to 19 mm.

The endovascular procedure

Although probably more comfortable to perform under general anesthesia, especially if very precise imaging is required, endovascular stent grafting for type B dissection has been performed under spinal, epidural, or even local anesthesia [41].

Vascular access can be a major issue. Occasionally a completely percutaneous approach can be used, but this requires confidence in the integrity of the femoral artery, and our bias has been to use this method less frequently than in the setting of atherosclerotic aneurysms. An iliac conduit may be

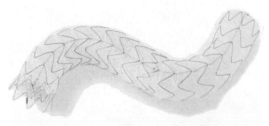

Fig. 8. The Medtronic Valiant Thoracic Stent Graft with proximal and distal components together. (*Courtesy of* Medtronic, Santa Rosa, CA; with permission.)

required if the femoral-external iliac arteries are too small or diseased to permit passing the sheaths or device. If at the close of the case this remains a concern, rather than closing the conduit as a patch it can be converted to an iliofemoral bypass that permits repeat intervention if required [55]. Dias and colleagues [120] found that 6 of 31 patients required operative repair (5 femoral, 1 iliac graft) after the procedure. In general, vascular access–related complications occur in the 2% range, but can be as much as 10% to 15% if there is extensive calcification or tortuosity of the particular vessel [134].

However one achieves access of the vasculature, negotiating the true lumen can be difficult. Slowly advancing the catheter with serial contrast injections can help assure that the false lumen has not inadvertently been entered. One approach is to pass a wire from the right arm, and snare it at the groin [36,120].

Other authors have championed passing a catheter by way of the left brachial, which serves to mark the left subclavian origin, permits stenting of this if needed, and allows imaging to be performed pre- and post-deployment without the need for multiple exchanges from the groin or a bilateral groin approach [8,35,133].

Intravascular ultrasound is an invaluable tool in this setting. It permits confirmation that the wire along which the device will track is in the true lumen completely, confirms measurements of the aorta, and adds comfort that there is no occult more proximal entry site. After deployment intravascular ultrasound gives a good assessment as to the degree of false versus true lumen perfusion and the restoration of flow to compromised branch vessels, and in ideal circumstances demonstrates a shift of the septum back toward the false lumen, confirming depressurization (Fig. 9) [41,133–135].

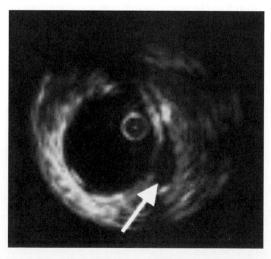

Fig. 9. Intravascular ultrasound documenting the primary proximal entry site.

Complications

Retrograde dissection

Retrograde dissection, converting a type B case into an acute type A, has been described with virtually all devices, although initially there was a sense that bare metal proximal extension had a higher risk for this [55,120, 136–139]. The reported incidence, in larger series of dissection cases, is roughly 0.5% to 3%, but has been reported in as many as 10% [36,41,125,127,140,141]. In addition, because most dissections require extension into the arch to achieve proximal coverage, one must be concerned that a stiff wire can lead to new proximal intimal tears [124]. The cause has been variously attributed to excessive oversizing (using criteria for atherosclerotic aneurysmal disease), vigorous ballooning, inadequate apposition against the inner curve of the arch with resultant trauma, or attempting to land proximally in an area with dissection or other trauma to a fragile endothelium [120]. Guide-wire manipulation can also create a proximal tear leading to an arch/ascending dissection [142]. This dissection usually occurs immediately, but on rare occasion can develop in a delayed fashion [122,127]. As with all acute type A dissections, in most cases immediate conversion to open repair is used.

Persistent filling of the false lumen

If the primary goal of endovascular treatment is to occlude the proximalmost entry site to promote false lumen thrombosis, clearly persistent perfusion of the false lumen should be a concern, particularly if the false lumen exhibits expansion during followup [122]. In 80% to 90% of cases the false lumen thromboses along the length of the endograft, whereas in the distal uncovered thoracic aorta it remains patent in 50% to 60%, and at the level of the celiac artery perhaps only one in five achieve thrombosis [36,51]. Persistent false lumen perfusion from distal sites can lead to growth over time and pose a risk for rupture (see Fig. 3C) [8,41]. This risk is probably greater if the false lumen perfused is in the thoracic component, and is one argument for covering the entire descending thoracic aorta [8]. Nienaber and colleagues described secondary extension with bare metal stents distally to successfully promote false lumen thrombosis, although others have worried about the possibility of the distal bare portion creating a new, large distal entry site if it tears through the septum [120,133]. Mossop and colleagues [143] reported 25 cases in which distal bare stenting of the thoracoabdominal aorta in the setting of persistent false lumen perfusion resulted in 100% 2.5-year survival, thrombosis of the entire false lumen resulted in 85% 2.5-year survival, and reparative remodeling in all cases. Nevertheless, not all persistent false lumen filling from distal entry sites requires early intervention. Song and associates [41] found that at less than 1 month, complete thrombosis along the treated area was 60%, but by 12 months this had increased to 88%. Schoder and colleagues [36] noted that one third of patients who acutely had persistent false lumen filling within the thoracic aorta developed evidence of false lumen dilation at 2-year follow-up. Just over half of those who had filling at the celiac level had documented increase at that level. Resch and colleagues [51] found that in the acute setting 12% of cases with persistent perfusion evidenced an increase in diameter during follow-up. In the chronic setting, 23% of those who had persistent perfusion of the false lumen had demonstrable growth. Persistent perfusion of the false lumen may be more of a risk in the setting of chronic type B dissections, owing to stiffness of the septum and multiple distal fenestrations [124,131].

In summary, it seems that persistent distal perfusion of the false lumen, when the primary entry site has been documented to have been excluded, does not necessarily require immediate further intervention. If follow-up imaging demonstrates shrinking of the false lumen, no intervention is required. If follow-up imaging documents growth of the false lumen, consideration to further intervention, either by graft extension (probably with bare metal stents) or operation should be considered. If the false lumen diameter does not change, then continued close observation with serial imaging is reasonable. Planning extensive coverage of the entire thoracic aorta with bare metal extension may reduce the risk for this while also reducing the risk for paralysis (Fig. 10).

This plan presupposes that the source of the persistent filling is distal entry sites. In a small number of cases the persistent perfusion may arise from retrograde flow from the left subclavian artery [36,51]. If this is believed to

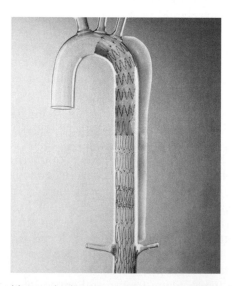

Fig. 10. An endograft with extensive bare metal distal coverage that may promote further false lumen thrombosis and aortic remodeling at markedly reduced risk for spinal cord injury. (*Courtesy of* Cook, Inc., Bloomington, IN; with permission.)

be the case either coil occlusion or ligation with or without subclavian bypass is required [8,36].

Arm ischemia

In several cases complete coverage of the origin of the left subclavian artery may be required to assure an adequate landing zone, either because of the extent of dissection or to avoid landing the graft in the curve of the aorta and thus having inadequate apposition along the inner wall [121]. Most, but not all, investigators have noted that clinically significant arm ischemia is an uncommon occurrence when this is required [8,36,41,55,139]. If it does occur, it can usually be electively managed with carotid-subclavian bypass. Other methods that have been described include using bare metal proximal extension, preprocedure carotid subclavian bypass, or deployment of a stent into the origin at the time of endovascular procedure [8,36,134].

Stroke

Cerebrovascular complications have been referred to as the Achilles heel of thoracic aortic stenting, and occur more frequently than spinal cord injury [49]. In the report by Resch and colleagues [51], strokes occurred in 9 of 80 acute and 2 of 49 chronic cases treated endovascularly. The cause of stroke falls into two broad categories. The first relates to embolic phenomena caused by wire or catheter manipulation through a diseased arch [8,144]. Embolic events may be detected if transcranial Doppler is used during the procedure [144]. The second is occlusion of a critical left vertebral artery resulting in a posterior circulation stroke. Song and colleagues [41] noted an incidence of such stroke in 2 of 11 patients in whom the origin of the left subclavian was completely covered as opposed to 1 in 31 in which it was not. Options in elective cases in which it is believed that to achieve adequate seal the left subclavian must be covered include preprocedure carotid-subclavian bypass or transposition in all cases, or to assess the posterior circulation using CT or intra-arterial or MRA [8,36,134,145]. Alternatively, test occlusion of the left subclavian while monitoring basilar flow with transcranial Doppler ultrasound can permit a more selective approach.

Paralysis

One of the primary advantages that an endovascular approach seems to have over open repair is a lower incidence of paralysis [55]. It has been argued that endovascular approaches are not associated with variations of pressure or risk for emboli as may be present with open repair. In open repair, there may be an increased risk for a steal phenomenon, either because of decreased perfusion of important collaterals, back bleeding from uncontrolled intercostals, or increased shunting if nitroprusside is used [103]. In addition, postoperatively, because one is not so concerned about suture lines in a tenuous aorta, a more liberal approach to blood pressure control can be instituted. Endograft procedures can nevertheless cover a significant portion of the thoracic aorta, presumably increasing the risk for cord ischemia. Recognizing that collateral supply (such as from the hypogastric and subclavian arteries) can provide critical collateral perfusion may modify the endovascular strategy [103].

In general, in dissection cases (acute and chronic) the reported incidence of spinal cord injury is approximately 0% to 6% [41,51,55,58,134]. Risk factors have included: prior abdominal aortic aneurysm repair; hypogastric disease; coverage of more than 20 cm of thoracic aorta; or complete coverage, including the left subclavian or coverage below T8 [41,51,55,58,134,144]. Some centers argue that if a dominant artery of Adamkiewicz can be identified, and if open surgery would result in preservation of this, then open repair might be favored over endovascular approaches [146]. Alternatively, if segmental collateral supply can be documented (using, for example, preoperative MRA), the risk for paralysis by covering an artery of Adamkiewicz is reduced [119]. The use of lumbar drains in higher-risk cases (aiming, for example, to keep the CSF pressure ≤ 10–14 mm Hg) does seem to provide additional protection [8,51,104,120,134]. The use of steroids before cross-clamping still has significant support and may have a role to play during endovascular procedures deemed to be at higher risk [103]. It has been argued that sensory or motor evoked potentials should be monitored so that spinal cord ischemia can be detected immediately, permitting early institution of therapy to raise mean arterial pressure, rather than waiting for the patient to recover from anesthesia, and allowing more selective use of spinal drainage [99,103,119,136]. Our bias has been to have a low threshold for prophylactic drainage because we have found that after heparin and emergence from anesthesia there tends to be a delay in getting the drainage instituted. If neurologic injury has occurred, CSF drainage, elevation of systemic pressure with volume or vasopressors, and possibly steroids have been shown to correct or reduce spinal cord injury in as many as half of all cases [8,99,134,147]. Finally, the use of endografts with bare metal distal extension, or deploying bare metal extensions on follow-up if needed, has been proposed as a method of achieving greater thoracic coverage at a lower risk for paralysis [51,132,133].

Endoleak

Overall endoleaks are less common in dissection cases than aneurysmal disease, being reported at 6% or less [126]. True type I endoleak (either proximal or distal forms) is uncommon in dissection cases [51,134]. In up to one third of cases, small, late-appearing proximal endoleaks have sealed at follow-up studies [126,134]. If proximal type I endoleaks are noted at the time of the procedure, and are early-appearing and large, options can include careful ballooning of the proximal graft (staying within the graft material and being gentle to reduce the risk for creating a retrograde dissection) or, if possible, extending the graft proximally [139]. This procedure can be done with a covered graft but some have, at least anecdotally, used bare metal stents to gently expand and fix the device.

Type II endoleaks arising from retrograde subclavian flow have been discussed. Occasionally, persistent intercostal back-flow can cause a type II endoleak [118]. In the absence of dilation of the involved segment, it is probably safe to follow these cases. Should dilation occur, consideration to CT-guided injection, angiogram to look for collaterals that might be embolized, or open repair might have to be considered.

Junctional (type III) endoleaks occur when attempting to cover a longer segment of aorta that has tortuosity. These are usually treated by ballooning or deploying a further endograft across the site of the leak [41].

Type IV endoleak implies a graft failure and the treatment can include re-endografting or primary surgical repair depending on the circumstances.

Type V endoleak represents endotension without any evidence of leak [148]. This type is manifested by persistent growth of an aneurysm and is presumably more an issue with atherosclerotic aneurysmal disease. These can be treated by repeat endografting.

Migration or proximal endograft collapse

Migration should be a relatively rare complication in dissection because in most cases the distal true lumen is actually relatively small. Although attempting to size the endograft at about 10% of the normal aortic diameter proximally, undersizing can lead to large endoleak and the risk for migration, which, depending on the patient's age and risk factors, may be managed by open repair or extending proximally. On the other hand, particularly with currently available thoracic devices, landing in aortas with diameters less than 23 mm can lead to collapse even with minimal oversizing [149]. Similarly, proximal collapse is less often reported but can occur if there is significant lack of apposition along the inner aortic curve in patients who have excellent cardiac output, a consequence in many cases of trying to land across the curve of the aorta (the "gray zone" or "no-man's-land") [150].

Related conditions

Intramural hematoma (IMH) and penetrating aortic (or atheromatous) ulcer (PAU) complete, with dissection, the triad of acute aortic syndromes [151–153]. There are some distinct differences between IMH and PAU, however, notably that (1) PAU tends to occur more often in older patients who have extensive calcification, and (2) whereas PAU can be associated with dissection, either often exists alone [151,154]. Although PAU and IMH probably share cellular processes (such as apoptosis with medial degeneration), PAU can be considered a disease of the intima and IMH (even though often associated with PAU) is a disease of the media [155–160]. Compared with dissection, PAU and IMH tend to occur in patients who have larger aortic diameters and there is an increased incidence of abdominal aortic aneurysm (42% with PAU, 30% with IMH in the Yale series) [159]. Although PAU and IMH can present acutely with a clinical syndrome indistinguishable from dissection, increasingly asymptomatic cases are identified during work-up for other reasons [151]. The natural history of these asymptomatic lesions is not clear. There is increasing experience that suggests that the deeper the PAU, the greater the likelihood of developing complications (rupture or dissection).

Given that IMH is differentiated from acute dissection by thrombosis of the false lumen with no communication, it can be difficult to distinguish the two entities. Transesophageal echocardiogram and computed tomographic angiography (CTA) may not be able to distinguish between IMH, atherosclerotic plaque, and dissection [151,161]. MRI may be better able to distinguish between plaque and IMH [162]. In some instances, on further evaluation with intravascular ultrasound (IVUS) or other modalities, a communication is found. There are also clinical studies demonstrating that IMH can arise without any intimal process, however, probably most commonly because of rupture of vasa vasorum [163,164]. Regardless of the precise pathology, IMH has been estimated to be present in 5% to 20% of patients who have acute aortic syndromes [151,163,164].

In the acute setting, compared with patients who have dissection, patients who have IMH tend to be older and may have more severe pain, but rarely have malperfusion [159,163]. As is the case with dissection, with some exceptions, IMH involving the ascending aorta has a graver prognosis compared with IMH involving the arch or descending aorta [151,165]. The IRAD data suggested a fourfold increased mortality with type A IMH versus type B (42% versus 8%), supporting aggressive surgical repair of type A lesions [163,166,167]. Similar to dissection, type B lesions tend to be benign, with better prognosis than type A IMH and type B dissection [163,168–170]. Medical management is thus the primary management, with between 30% and 80% completely resolving [168,170,171]. As many as 54% develop aneurysms in follow-up, however, and 12% proceed to dissection [170]. Risk factors that seem to predict increased risk for these complications include atherosclerotic ulcers, increased aortic diameter greater than 40 mm, and lack of echogenicity in the false lumen [33,164,168,170]. Ulcers, particularly greater than 20 mm in maximum dimension, are a particular risk factor for the development of complications [164]. Intravascular ultrasound may be the most sensitive method of detecting ulcers in IMH that can be missed by CT or standard angiography [31]. Long-term follow-up is warranted, and the use of β-blockade is associated with improved outcomes [167,172]. Indications for intervention in the acute setting are similar to those for dissection, and whereas operative repair has been well described, there may be an increased role for endovascular approaches [151].

PAU may be the cause of nearly 8% of acute aortic syndromes [159]. As is the case with IMH, however, an increasing number are being detected during workup for other conditions [154]. They may be multiple, of varying depth, and are more common in the descending thoracic aorta [173]. CTA and IVUS are excellent tools for defining the specific anatomy [174]. As with IMH and dissection, there is greater conformity in recommending surgical resection for asymptomatic PAU of the ascending aorta because of the risk for rupture [2]. Because of the concern regarding the possibility of rupture, or less commonly dissection, operative resection or endovascular repair has been advocated, even in patients who have descending PAU [160,173]. Others have noted that with PAU in the arch or descending aorta β-blockade is sufficient and argue that in asymptomatic patients, or those in whom pain resolves with pressure control, medical management should be the first line of therapy [154,174,175]. There is increasing experience with endovascular stent grafting that seems to allow intervention in symptomatic patients with reduction in morbidity, and possibly in asymptomatic patients who may be at increased risk for complications because of depth of ulceration or presence of focal aortic dilation [176–180].

In summary, asymptomatic type B IMH or PAU can be managed medically. Symptomatic lesions require intervention. Asymptomatic IMH with PAU or PAU alone that are 20 mm or more in maximum dimension are reasonable candidates for elective repair. Endovascular approaches have been associated with results equaling surgical repair with reduced morbidity.

Combined procedures

There has been increasing interest in performing hybrid operations for the management of atherosclerotic aneurysms, including arch or visceral debranching accompanied by sequential or simultaneous endovascular stent grafting of the diseased aorta, which can be done in some cases without cardiopulmonary bypass [44,181]. These approaches are being extended to dissection also. In acute type A dissection, which extends into the descending aorta, because of the concern of persistent false lumen filling, especially in the setting of a compressed true lumen, some centers recommend placing an endograft into the true lumen and then use the proximal portion of the endograft to anchor the distal anastomosis of the ascending/arch replacement graft (an endovascular elephant trunk procedure) [182]. Uchida and colleagues [183] described 35 consecutive patients who underwent arch replacement with distal open endografting for acute type A dissection. There were two (5.5%) operative deaths, but the remainder survived. At mean follow-up of 55 months the false lumen was obliterated along the treated length (average 8.9 cm) in all, to the diaphragm in 20 (59%), and to the level of the superior mesenteric artery in 15 (44%), with reduced or stable aortic diameters in all. Preconstructed grafts in which the distal end of the elephant trunk (the "frozen elephant trunk") has a stent incorporated is another

form of this approach [184]. Acutely extending the elephant trunk by an endograft placed retrograde has also been described. This approach can also
be used in the chronic setting and is facilitated by having a relatively short
elephant trunk to avoid foreshortening or graft deformation. Marking the
end of the endograft with clips or pacer wires also helps, although occasionally a wire passed from the right brachial is needed to assist delivering the
endograft into the distal, open portion of the elephant trunk [136]. Aortic
debranching, which can take the form of a bifurcated graft arising from
the ascending aorta, or carotid–carotid–subclavian bypass, has been used
in chronic dissections involving the arch, and occasionally in the acute setting [131,185,186]. Visceral debranching followed by stenting of the thoracoabdominal aorta in patients who have chronic extensive dissections
deemed to be too high risk for open repair has also been described [46].

Future development

As is the case with atherosclerotic aneurysmal disease and traumatic rupture, there is ongoing development of medical, surgical, and endovascular
therapies for type B dissection. Aggressive β-blockade has been shown to re-
tard aortic root dilation in the case of Marfan disease, and may well have
the same benefit in the thoracoabdominal aorta [187]. Understanding the genetic basis for connective tissue disorders, including how variations may
predispose to specific complications, may permit better management, counseling, and possibly translation therapies [11,188].

Branch graft technology to permit endografting into the arch or visceral
segments continues to be actively researched for aneurysmal disease and
presumably could have an equally important role in chronic type B dissection cases [2,189–192]. With increasing interest in clinical trials of uncomplicated, but potentially at-risk patients, there may be an expanded role for
intervening in uncomplicated dissections. More disease-specific endografts
are currently being developed, which will allow various sizes, precurved skel-
etons to accept the arch better, and possibly bare stent configurations that
will reliably enhance false lumen thrombosis without an increased risk for
paralysis. Tapered distal endografts may prove useful in managing chronic
dissections when the septum is believed to be excessively stiff to avoid distal
graft collapse [124]. Biologic markers may be able to further identify patients who are at particular risk for developing later complications [54].

Summary

Type B dissection represents an acute aortic syndrome, along with PAU
and IMH. The cause predominantly involves atherosclerosis and hypertension, but in a significant proportion also involves connective tissue

disorders. In the acute setting and in uncomplicated patients, medical management with blood pressure control is the standard of care. Complicated dissection, manifested predominantly by malperfusion syndromes followed by rupture, requires a complication-specific approach. Acute surgical repair is associated with significant mortality and morbidity, increasing the attractiveness of endovascular approaches. Malperfusion syndromes are now predominantly managed by endovascular stent grafts, with fenestration, branch vessel stenting, operative bypass, and repair being reserved for failures, in anatomically suitable patients. Experience is still being gained into the exact role stent grafts play in the acute setting, but the results to date are encouraging compared with the surgical experience. It must be stressed, however, that surgical outcomes are to a large extent a reflection of experience, and some centers have superb operative results that approach the outcomes documented with endovascular repair and perhaps with more defined late outcome. Patients who are successfully managed during the acute phase medically still need close follow-up because a significant number develop complications. The issue of stenting certain high-risk subgroups of patients who are asymptomatic remains a question for further study. In the chronic setting, surgical repair has excellent results. There are encouraging preliminary data regarding the role of stent grafts but, at least in North America, there is concern that chronic dissections may not be as amenable to this approach. This also is an area of active investigation and it is hoped that the relative merits of both procedures will be clarified. Patients who have known connective tissue disorders, such as Marfan syndrome, should be carefully assessed because particularly in the acute setting there is concern that stent grafts will have a high failure rate, including acute rupture. At this time endovascular stent grafts are an exciting tool in the management of type B dissections, but are best considered as one of several tools, and the decision to use them ideally should be a team approach involving a team that has imaging, endovascular, and open operative skills required for all possibilities.

References

[1] Kouchoukos NT, Dougenis D. Surgery of the thoracic aorta. N Engl J Med 1997;336: 1876–88.

[2] Atkins MD Jr, Black JH 3rd, Cambria RP. Aortic dissection: perspectives in the era of stent-graft repair. J Vasc Surg 2006;43(Suppl A):30A–43A.

[3] Lauterbach SR, Cambria RP, Brewster DC, et al. Contemporary management of aortic branch compromise resulting from acute aortic dissection. J Vasc Surg 2001;33:1185–92.

[4] Meszaros I, Morocz J, Szlavi J, et al. Epidemiology and clinicopathology of aortic dissection. Chest 2000;117:1271–8.

[5] Cambria RP, Brewster DC, Gertler J, et al. Vascular complications associated with spontaneous aortic dissection. J Vasc Surg 1988;7:199–209.

[6] Hagan PG, Nienaber CA, Isselbacher EM, et al. The International Registry of Acute Aortic Dissection (IRAD): new insights into an old disease. JAMA 2000;283:897–903.

[7] Deeb GM, Williams DM, Bolling SF, et al. Surgical delay for acute type A dissection with malperfusion. Ann Thorac Surg 1997;64:1669–75 [discussion: 1675–77].

[8] Criado FJ, Abul-Khoudoud OR, Domer GS, et al. Endovascular repair of the thoracic aorta: lessons learned. Ann Thorac Surg 2005;80:857–63 [discussion: 863].

[9] Larson EW, Edwards WD. Risk factors for aortic dissection: a necropsy study of 161 cases. Am J Cardiol 1984;53:849–55.

[10] Coselli JS, Koksoy C. Aortic dissections. In: Franco KL, Verrier ED, editors. Advanced therapy in cardiac surgery. Hamilton (Ontario): B.C. Decker; 1999. p. 296–311.

[11] Ramirez F, Dietz HC. Therapy insight: aortic aneurysm and dissection in Marfan's syndrome. Nat Clin Pract Cardiovasc Med 2004;1:31–6.

[12] McDermott CD, Sermer M, Siu SC, et al. Aortic dissection complicating pregnancy following prophylactic aortic root replacement in a woman with Marfan syndrome. Int J Cardiol 2006;120:427–30.

[13] Neri E, Toscano T, Massetti M, et al. Cocaine-induced intramural hematoma of the ascending aorta. Tex Heart Inst J 2001;28:218–9.

[14] Hatzaras I, Tranquilli M, Coady M, et al. Weight lifting and aortic dissection: more evidence for a connection. Cardiology 2006;107:103–6.

[15] Williams JA, Loeys BL, Nwakanma LU, et al. Early surgical experience with Loeys-Dietz: a new syndrome of aggressive thoracic aortic aneurysm disease. Ann Thorac Surg 2007;83: S757–63 [discussion: S785–90].

[16] Loeys BL, Chen J, Neptune ER, et al. A syndrome of altered cardiovascular, craniofacial, neurocognitive and skeletal development caused by mutations in TGFBR1 or TGFBR2. Nat Genet 2005;37:275–81.

[17] Rasmus M, Huegli R, Jacob AL, et al. Extensive iatrogenic aortic dissection during renal angioplasty: successful treatment with a covered stent-graft. Cardiovasc Intervent Radiol 2007;30:497–500.

[18] Tsai TT, Evangelista A, Nienaber CA, et al. Partial thrombosis of the false lumen in patients with acute type B aortic dissection. N Engl J Med 2007;357:349–59.

[19] Khan IA, Nair CK. Clinical, diagnostic, and management perspectives of aortic dissection. Chest 2002;122:311–28.

[20] Williams DM, Lee DY, Hamilton BH, et al. The dissected aorta: percutaneous treatment of ischemic complications—principles and results. J Vasc Interv Radiol 1997;8: 605–25.

[21] Williams DM, Lee DY, Hamilton BH, et al. The dissected aorta: part III. Anatomy and radiologic diagnosis of branch-vessel compromise. Radiology 1997;203:37–44.

[22] Debakey ME, Henly WS, Cooley DA, et al. Surgical management of dissecting aneurysms of the aorta. J Thorac Cardiovasc Surg 1965;49:130–49.

[23] Daily PO, Trueblood HW, Stinson EB, et al. Management of acute aortic dissections. Ann Thorac Surg 1970;10:237–47.

[24] Fann JI, Smith JA, Miller DC, et al. Surgical management of aortic dissection during a 30-year period. Circulation 1995;92:II113–21.

[25] Januzzi JL, Movsowitz HD, Choi J, et al. Significance of recurrent pain in acute type B aortic dissection. Am J Cardiol 2001;87:930–3.

[26] Rosman HS, Patel S, Borzak S, et al. Quality of history taking in patients with aortic dissection. Chest 1998;114:793–5.

[27] Estrera AL, Miller CC, Goodrick J, et al. Update on outcomes of acute type B aortic dissection. Ann Thorac Surg 2007;83:S842–5 [discussion: S846–50].

[28] Januzzi JL, Sabatine MS, Choi JC, et al. Refractory systemic hypertension following type B aortic dissection. Am J Cardiol 2001;88:686–8.

[29] DeBakey ME, McCollum CH, Crawford ES, et al. Dissection and dissecting aneurysms of the aorta: twenty-year follow-up of five hundred twenty-seven patients treated surgically. Surgery 1982;92:1118–34.

[30] Suzuki T, Mehta RH, Ince H, et al. Clinical profiles and outcomes of acute type B aortic dissection in the current era: lessons from the International Registry of Aortic Dissection (IRAD). Circulation 2003;108(Suppl 1):II312–7.

[31] Wei H, Schiele F, Meneveau N, et al. Potential interest of intra-aorta ultrasound imaging for the diagnosis of aortic penetrating atherosclerotic ulcer. Int J Cardiovasc Imaging 2006; 22:653–6.

[32] Orihashi K, Sueda T, Okada K, et al. Perioperative diagnosis of mesenteric ischemia in acute aortic dissection by transesophageal echocardiography. Eur J Cardiothorac Surg 2005;28:871–6.

[33] Winnerkvist A, Lockowandt U, Rasmussen E, et al. A prospective study of medically treated acute type B aortic dissection. Eur J Vasc Endovasc Surg 2006;32:349–55.

[34] Winnerkvist A, Brorsson B, Radegran K. Quality of life in patients with chronic type B aortic dissection. Eur J Vasc Endovasc Surg 2006;32:34–7.

[35] Nienaber CA, Rehders TC, Ince H. Interventional strategies for treatment of aortic dissection. J Cardiovasc Surg (Torino) 2006;47:487–96.

[36] Schoder M, Czerny M, Cejna M, et al. Endovascular repair of acute type B aortic dissection: long-term follow-up of true and false lumen diameter changes. Ann Thorac Surg 2007;83:1059–66.

[37] Myrmel T, Lai DT, Miller DC. Can the principles of evidence-based medicine be applied to the treatment of aortic dissections? Eur J Cardiothorac Surg 2004;25:236–42 [discussion: 242–5].

[38] Umana JP, Miller DC, Mitchell RS. What is the best treatment for patients with acute type B aortic dissections—medical, surgical, or endovascular stent-grafting? Ann Thorac Surg 2002;74:S1840–3 [discussion: S1857–63].

[39] Tsai TT, Fattori R, Trimarchi S, et al. Long-term survival in patients presenting with type B acute aortic dissection: insights from the International Registry of Acute Aortic Dissection. Circulation 2006;114:2226–31.

[40] Elefteriades JA, Lovoulos CJ, Coady MA, et al. Management of descending aortic dissection. Ann Thorac Surg 1999;67:2002–5 [discussion: 2014–19].

[41] Song TK, Donayre CE, Walot I, et al. Endograft exclusion of acute and chronic descending thoracic aortic dissections. J Vasc Surg 2006;43:247–58.

[42] Panneton JM, Hollier LH. Dissecting descending thoracic and thoracoabdominal aortic aneurysms: Part II. Ann Vasc Surg 1995;9:596–605.

[43] Bernard Y, Zimmermann H, Chocron S, et al. False lumen patency as a predictor of late outcome in aortic dissection. Am J Cardiol 2001;87:1378–82.

[44] Czerny M, Zimpfer D, Fleck T, et al. Initial results after combined repair of aortic arch aneurysms by sequential transposition of the supra-aortic branches and consecutive endovascular stent-graft placement. Ann Thorac Surg 2004;78:1256–60.

[45] Dialetto G, Covino FE, Scognamiglio G, et al. Treatment of type B aortic dissection: endoluminal repair or conventional medical therapy? Eur J Cardiothorac Surg 2005;27:826–30.

[46] Greenberg R, Khwaja J, Haulon S, et al. Aortic dissections: new perspectives and treatment paradigms. Eur J Vasc Endovasc Surg 2003;26:579–86.

[47] Onitsuka S, Akashi H, Tayama K, et al. Long-term outcome and prognostic predictors of medically treated acute type B aortic dissections. Ann Thorac Surg 2004;78:1268–73.

[48] Kunishige H, Myojin K, Ishibashi Y, et al. Predictors of surgical indications for acute type B aortic dissection based on enlargement of aortic diameter during the chronic phase. Jpn J Thorac Cardiovasc Surg 2006;54:477–82.

[49] Eggebrecht H, Nienaber CA, Neuhauser M, et al. Endovascular stent-graft placement in aortic dissection: a meta-analysis. Eur Heart J 2006;27:489–98.

[50] Roseborough G, Burke J, Sperry J, et al. Twenty-year experience with acute distal thoracic aortic dissections. J Vasc Surg 2004;40:235–46.

[51] Resch TA, Delle M, Falkenberg M, et al. Remodeling of the thoracic aorta after stent grafting of type B dissection: a Swedish multicenter study. J Cardiovasc Surg (Torino) 2006;47:503–8.

[52] Greenberg R. Treatment of aortic dissections with endovascular stent grafts. Semin Vasc Surg 2002;15:122–7.

[53] Nathanson DR, Rodriguez-Lopez JA, Ramaiah VG, et al. Endoluminal stent-graft stabilization for thoracic aortic dissection. J Endovasc Ther 2005;12:354–9.

[54] Coselli JS. Panel discussion: session III-natural history and dissection. Ann Thorac Surg 2007;83:S846–50.

[55] Zipfel B, Hammerschmidt R, Krabatsch T, et al. Stent-grafting of the thoracic aorta by the cardiothoracic surgeon. Ann Thorac Surg 2007;83:441–8 [discussion: 448–9].

[56] Henke PK, Williams DM, Upchurch GR Jr, et al. Acute limb ischemia associated with type B aortic dissection: clinical relevance and therapy. Surgery 2006;140:532–9 [discussion: 539–40].

[57] Husmann MJ, Kickuth R, Ludwig K, et al. Intravascular ultrasound-guided creation of re-entry sites to improve intermittent claudication in patients with aortic dissection. J Endovasc Ther 2006;13:424–8.

[58] Leurs LJ, Bell R, Degrieck Y, et al. Endovascular treatment of thoracic aortic diseases: combined experience from the EUROSTAR and United Kingdom Thoracic Endograft registries. J Vasc Surg 2004;40:670–9 [discussion: 679–80].

[59] Gaxotte V, Thony F, Rousseau H, et al. Midterm results of aortic diameter outcomes after thoracic stent-graft implantation for aortic dissection: a multicenter study. J Endovasc Ther 2006;13:127–38.

[60] Fleck TM, Hutschala D, Tschernich H, et al. Stent graft placement of the thoracoabdominal aorta in a patient with Marfan syndrome. J Thorac Cardiovasc Surg 2003;125:1541–3.

[61] Coselli JS, LeMaire SA. Current status of thoracoabdominal aortic aneurysm repair in Marfan syndrome. J Card Surg 1997;12:167–72.

[62] Erbel R, Alfonso F, Boileau C, et al. Diagnosis and management of aortic dissection. Eur Heart J 2001;22:1642–81.

[63] Wheat MW Jr, Palmer RF, Bartley TD, et al. Treatment of dissecting aneurysms of the aorta without surgery. J Thorac Cardiovasc Surg 1965;50:364–73.

[64] Wheat MW Jr. Current status of medical therapy of acute dissecting aneurysms of the aorta. World J Surg 1980;4:563–9.

[65] Miller DC, Stinson EB, Oyer PE, et al. Operative treatment of aortic dissections. Experience with 125 patients over a sixteen-year period. J Thorac Cardiovasc Surg 1979;78: 365–82.

[66] Schor JS, Yerlioglu ME, Galla JD, et al. Selective management of acute type B aortic dissection: long-term follow-up. Ann Thorac Surg 1996;61:1339–41.

[67] Shimono T, Kato N, Tokui T, et al. Endovascular stent-graft repair for acute type A aortic dissection with an intimal tear in the descending aorta. J Thorac Cardiovasc Surg 1998;116: 171–3.

[68] Elefteriades JA, Hartleroad J, Gusberg RJ, et al. Long-term experience with descending aortic dissection: the complication-specific approach. Ann Thorac Surg 1992;53:11–20 [discussion: 20–1].

[69] Gurin D, Bulmer JW, Derby R. Dissecting aneurysm of the aorta: diagnosis and operative relief of acute arterial obstruction due to this cause. N Y State J Med 1935;35:1200–2.

[70] Umana JP, Lai DT, Mitchell RS, et al. Is medical therapy still the optimal treatment strategy for patients with acute type B aortic dissections? J Thorac Cardiovasc Surg 2002;124: 896–910.

[71] Glower DD, Fann JI, Speier RH, et al. Comparison of medical and surgical therapy for uncomplicated descending aortic dissection. Circulation 1990;82:IV39–46.

[72] Marui A, Mochizuki T, Mitsui N, et al. Toward the best treatment for uncomplicated patients with type B acute aortic dissection: a consideration for sound surgical indication. Circulation 1999;100:II275–80.

[73] Lansman SL, McCullough JN, Nguyen KH, et al. Subtypes of acute aortic dissection. Ann Thorac Surg 1999;67:1975–8 [discussion: 1979–80].

[74] Hata H, Takano H, Matsumiya G, et al. Late complications of gelatin-resorcin-formalin glue in the repair of acute type A aortic dissection. Ann Thorac Surg 2007;83:1621–6.

[75] Nakajima T, Kawazoe K, Kataoka T, et al. Midterm results of aortic repair using a fabric neomedia and fibrin glue for type A acute aortic dissection. Ann Thorac Surg 2007;83: 1615–20.

[76] Fann JI, Sarris GE, Mitchell RS, et al. Treatment of patients with aortic dissection presenting with peripheral vascular complications. Ann Surg 1990;212:705–13.

[77] Svensson LG, Crawford ES, Hess KR, et al. Dissection of the aorta and dissecting aortic aneurysms. Improving early and long-term surgical results. Circulation 1990;82:IV24–38.

[78] Kato M, Bai H, Sato K, et al. Determining surgical indications for acute type B dissection based on enlargement of aortic diameter during the chronic phase. Circulation 1995;92: II107–12.

[79] Sueyoshi E, Sakamoto I, Hayashi K, et al. Growth rate of aortic diameter in patients with type B aortic dissection during the chronic phase. Circulation 2004;110:II256–61.

[80] Sueyoshi E, Sakamoto I, Uetani M, et al. CT analysis of the growth rate of aortic diameter affected by acute type B intramural hematoma. AJR Am J Roentgenol 2006;186:S414–20.

[81] Laschinger JC, Cunningham JN Jr, Cooper MM, et al. Prevention of ischemic spinal cord injury following aortic cross-clamping: use of corticosteroids. Ann Thorac Surg 1984;38: 500–7.

[82] Kitamura M, Hashimoto A, Tagusari O, et al. Operation for type B aortic dissection: introduction of left heart bypass. Ann Thorac Surg 1995;59:1200–3.

[83] Coselli JS, LeMaire SA. Left heart bypass reduces paraplegia rates after thoracoabdominal aortic aneurysm repair. Ann Thorac Surg 1999;67:1931–4 [discussion: 1953–8].

[84] Coselli JS, LeMaire SA, Conklin LD, et al. Left heart bypass during descending thoracic aortic aneurysm repair does not reduce the incidence of paraplegia. Ann Thorac Surg 2004;77:1298–303 [discussion: 1303].

[85] Estrera AL, Miller CC 3rd, Chen EP, et al. Descending thoracic aortic aneurysm repair: 12-year experience using distal aortic perfusion and cerebrospinal fluid drainage. Ann Thorac Surg 2005;80:1290–6 [discussion: 1296].

[86] Safi HJ, Campbell MP, Miller CC 3rd, et al. Cerebral spinal fluid drainage and distal aortic perfusion decrease the incidence of neurological deficit: the results of 343 descending and thoracoabdominal aortic aneurysm repairs. Eur J Vasc Endovasc Surg 1997;14:118–24.

[87] Strauch JT, Lauten A, Spielvogel D, et al. Mild hypothermia protects the spinal cord from ischemic injury in a chronic porcine model. Eur J Cardiothorac Surg 2004;25:708–15.

[88] Kouchoukos NT, Masetti P, Murphy SF. Hypothermic cardiopulmonary bypass and circulatory arrest in the management of extensive thoracic and thoracoabdominal aortic aneurysms. Semin Thorac Cardiovasc Surg 2003;15:333–9.

[89] Kouchoukos NT, Masetti P, Rokkas CK, et al. Hypothermic cardiopulmonary bypass and circulatory arrest for operations on the descending thoracic and thoracoabdominal aorta. Ann Thorac Surg 2002;74:S1885–7 [discussion: S1892–8].

[90] Patel HJ, Shillingford MS, Mihalik S, et al. Resection of the descending thoracic aorta: outcomes after use of hypothermic circulatory arrest. Ann Thorac Surg 2006;82:90–5 [discussion: 95–6].

[91] Safi HJ, Miller CC 3rd, Subramaniam MH, et al. Thoracic and thoracoabdominal aortic aneurysm repair using cardiopulmonary bypass, profound hypothermia, and circulatory arrest via left side of the chest incision. J Vasc Surg 1998;28:591–8.

[92] Carrel TP, Berdat PA, Robe J, et al. Outcome of thoracoabdominal aortic operations using deep hypothermia and distal exsanguination. Ann Thorac Surg 2000;69:692–5.

[93] Svensson LG, Khitin L, Nadolny EM, et al. Systemic temperature and paralysis after thoracoabdominal and descending aortic operations. Arch Surg 2003;138:175–9 [discussion: 180].

[94] Rokkas CK, Sundaresan S, Shuman TA, et al. Profound systemic hypothermia protects the spinal cord in a primate model of spinal cord ischemia. J Thorac Cardiovasc Surg 1993;106: 1024–35.

[95]   Rokkas CK, Cronin CS, Nitta T, et al. Profound systemic hypothermia inhibits the release of neurotransmitter amino acids in spinal cord ischemia. J Thorac Cardiovasc Surg 1995; 110:27–35.

[96]   Coselli JS, Lemaire SA, Koksoy C, et al. Cerebrospinal fluid drainage reduces paraplegia after thoracoabdominal aortic aneurysm repair: results of a randomized clinical trial. J Vasc Surg 2002;35:631–9.

[97]   Crawford ES, Svensson LG, Hess KR, et al. A prospective randomized study of cerebrospinal fluid drainage to prevent paraplegia after high-risk surgery on the thoracoabdominal aorta. J Vasc Surg 1991;13:36–45 [discussion: 45–6].

[98]   Cina CS, Abouzahr L, Arena GO, et al. Cerebrospinal fluid drainage to prevent paraplegia during thoracic and thoracoabdominal aortic aneurysm surgery: a systematic review and meta-analysis. J Vasc Surg 2004;40:36–44.

[99]   Cheung AT, Pochettino A, McGarvey ML, et al. Strategies to manage paraplegia risk after endovascular stent repair of descending thoracic aortic aneurysms. Ann Thorac Surg 2005; 80:1280–8 [discussion: 1288–9].

[100] Cheung AT, Weiss SJ, McGarvey ML, et al. Interventions for reversing delayed-onset post-operative paraplegia after thoracic aortic reconstruction. Ann Thorac Surg 2002;74:413–9 [discussion: 420–1].

[101] Minatoya K, Karck M, Hagl C, et al. The impact of spinal angiography on the neurological outcome after surgery on the descending thoracic and thoracoabdominal aorta. Ann Thorac Surg 2002;74:S1870–2 [discussion: S1892–8].

[102] Griepp RB, Ergin MA, Galla JD, et al. Looking for the artery of Adamkiewicz: a quest to minimize paraplegia after operations for aneurysms of the descending thoracic and thoracoabdominal aorta. J Thorac Cardiovasc Surg 1996;112:1202–13 [discussion: 1213–5].

[103] Griepp RB, Griepp EB. Spinal cord perfusion and protection during descending thoracic and thoracoabdominal aortic surgery: the collateral network concept. Ann Thorac Surg 2007;83:S865–9 [discussion: S890–2].

[104] Etz CD, Homann TM, Plestis KA, et al. Spinal cord perfusion after extensive segmental artery sacrifice: can paraplegia be prevented? Eur J Cardiothorac Surg 2007;31:643–8.

[105] Biglioli P, Roberto M, Cannata A, et al. Upper and lower spinal cord blood supply: the continuity of the anterior spinal artery and the relevance of the lumbar arteries. J Thorac Cardiovasc Surg 2004;127:1188–92.

[106] Meylaerts SA, Jacobs MJ, van Iterson V, et al. Comparison of transcranial motor evoked potentials and somatosensory evoked potentials during thoracoabdominal aortic aneurysm repair. Ann Surg 1999;230:742–9.

[107] Dong CC, MacDonald DB, Janusz MT. Intraoperative spinal cord monitoring during descending thoracic and thoracoabdominal aneurysm surgery. Ann Thorac Surg 2002;74: S1873–6 [discussion: S1892–8].

[108] van Dongen EP, ter Beek HT, Schepens MA, et al. The relationship between evoked potentials and measurements of S-100 protein in cerebrospinal fluid during and after thoracoabdominal aortic aneurysm surgery. J Vasc Surg 1999;30:293–300.

[109] van Dongen EP, Schepens MA, Morshuis WJ, et al. Thoracic and thoracoabdominal aortic aneurysm repair: use of evoked potential monitoring in 118 patients. J Vasc Surg 2001;34: 1035–40.

[110] Elefteriades JA, Hammond GL, Gusberg RJ, et al. Fenestration revisited. A safe and effective procedure for descending aortic dissection. Arch Surg 1990;125:786–90.

[111] Morales DL, Quin JA, Braxton JH, et al. Experimental confirmation of effectiveness of fenestration in acute aortic dissection. Ann Thorac Surg 1998;66:1679–83.

[112] Panneton JM, Teh SH, Cherry KJ Jr, et al. Aortic fenestration for acute or chronic aortic dissection: an uncommon but effective procedure. J Vasc Surg 2000;32:711–21.

[113] Laas J, Heinemann M, Schaefers HJ, et al. Management of thoracoabdominal malperfusion in aortic dissection. Circulation 1991;84:III20–4.

[114] Hsu RB, Ho YL, Chen RJ, et al. Outcome of medical and surgical treatment in patients with acute type B aortic dissection. Ann Thorac Surg 2005;79:790–4 [author reply 794–5].

[115] Dake MD, Kato N, Mitchell RS, et al. Endovascular stent-graft placement for the treatment of acute aortic dissection. N Engl J Med 1999;340:1546–52.

[116] Bavaria JE, Appoo JJ, Makaroun MS, et al. Endovascular stent grafting versus open surgical repair of descending thoracic aortic aneurysms in low-risk patients: a multicenter comparative trial. J Thorac Cardiovasc Surg 2007;133:369–77.

[117] Matsumura JS. Worldwide survey of thoracic endografts: practical clinical application. J Vasc Surg 2006;43(Suppl A):20A–1A.

[118] Won JY, Suh SH, Ko HK, et al. Problems encountered during and after stent-graft treatment of aortic dissection. J Vasc Interv Radiol 2006;17:271–81.

[119] Schurink GW, Nijenhuis RJ, Backes WH, et al. Assessment of spinal cord circulation and function in endovascular treatment of thoracic aortic aneurysms. Ann Thorac Surg 2007; 83:S877–81 [discussion: S890–2].

[120] Dias NV, Sonesson B, Koul B, et al. Complicated acute type B dissections—an 8-years experience of endovascular stent-graft repair in a single centre. Eur J Vasc Endovasc Surg 2006;31:481–6.

[121] Fattori R, Napoli G, Lovato L, et al. Descending thoracic aortic diseases: stent-graft repair. Radiology 2003;229:176–83.

[122] Czermak BV, Waldenberger P, Fraedrich G, et al. Treatment of Stanford type B aortic dissection with stent-grafts: preliminary results. Radiology 2000;217:544–50.

[123] Yamaguchi M, Sugimoto K, Tsuji Y, et al. Percutaneous balloon fenestration and stent placement for lower limb ischemia complicated with type B aortic dissection. Radiat Med 2006;24:233–7.

[124] Mitchell RS. Invited commentary. Ann Thorac Surg 2007;83:1640.

[125] Shimono T, Shimpo H. [Transluminal stent-graft placement for the treatment of acute aortic dissection]. Kyobu Geka 2006;59:674–80 [in Japanese]

[126] Guo W, Gai LY, Liu XP, et al. [The endovascular repair of aortic dissection: early clinical results of 178 cases]. Zhonghua Wai Ke Za Zhi 2005;43:921–5 [in Chinese].

[127] Xu SD, Huang FJ, Yang JF, et al. Endovascular repair of acute type B aortic dissection: early and mid-term results. J Vasc Surg 2006;43:1090–5.

[128] Fattori R, Nienaber CA, Rousseau H, et al. Results of endovascular repair of the thoracic aorta with the Talent Thoracic stent graft: the Talent Thoracic Retrospective Registry. J Thorac Cardiovasc Surg 2006;132:332–9.

[129] Eggebrecht H, Herold U, Kuhnt O, et al. Endovascular stent-graft treatment of aortic dissection: determinants of post-interventional outcome. Eur Heart J 2005;26:489–97.

[130] Bockler D, Schumacher H, Ganten M, et al. Complications after endovascular repair of acute symptomatic and chronic expanding Stanford type B aortic dissections. J Thorac Cardiovasc Surg 2006;132:361–8.

[131] Czerny M, Zimpfer D, Rodler S, et al. Endovascular stent-graft placement of aneurysms involving the descending aorta originating from chronic type B dissections. Ann Thorac Surg 2007;83:1635–9.

[132] Nienaber CA, Zannetti S, Barbieri B, et al. INvestigation of STEnt grafts in patients with type B Aortic Dissection: design of the INSTEAD trial–a prospective, multicenter, European randomized trial. Am Heart J 2005;149:592–9.

[133] Nienaber CA, Kische S, Zeller T, et al. Provisional extension to induce complete attachment after stent-graft placement in type B aortic dissection: the PETTICOAT concept. J Endovasc Ther 2006;13:738–46.

[134] Wheatley GH 3rd, Gurbuz AT, Rodriguez-Lopez JA, et al. Midterm outcome in 158 consecutive Gore TAG thoracic endoprostheses: single center experience. Ann Thorac Surg 2006;81:1570–7, [discussion: 1577].

[135] Lee DY, Williams DM, Abrams GD. The dissected aorta: part II. Differentiation of the true from the false lumen with intravascular US. Radiology 1997;203:32–6.

[136] Spielvogel D, Cambria RP, Coselli JS, et al. Panel discussion: session IV-descending and thoracoabdominal aorta. Ann Thorac Surg 2007;83:S890–2.

[137] Fanelli F, Salvatori FM, Marcelli G, et al. Type A aortic dissection developing during endovascular repair of an acute type B dissection. J Endovasc Ther 2003;10:254–9.

[138] Bortone AS, De Cillis E, D'Agostino D, et al. Endovascular treatment of thoracic aortic disease: four years of experience. Circulation 2004;110:II262–7.

[139] Pamler RS, Kotsis T, Gorich J, et al. Complications after endovascular repair of type B aortic dissection. J Endovasc Ther 2002;9:822–8.

[140] Hansen CJ, Bui H, Donayre CE, et al. Complications of endovascular repair of high-risk and emergent descending thoracic aortic aneurysms and dissections. J Vasc Surg 2004; 40:228–34.

[141] Dong Xu S, Zhong Li Z, Huang FJ, et al. Treating aortic dissection and penetrating aortic ulcer with stent graft: thirty cases. Ann Thorac Surg 2005;80:864–8.

[142] Zhang R, Kofidis T, Baus S, et al. Iatrogenic type A dissection after attempted stenting of a descending aortic aneurysm. Ann Thorac Surg 2006;82:1523–5.

[143] Mossop PJ, McLachlan CS, Amukotuwa SA, et al. Staged endovascular treatment for complicated type B aortic dissection. Nat Clin Pract Cardiovasc Med 2005;2:316–21 quiz 322.

[144] Khoynezhad A, Donayre CE, Bui H, et al. Risk factors of neurologic deficit after thoracic aortic endografting. Ann Thorac Surg 2007;83:S882–9 [discussion: S890–2].

[145] Weigang E, Luehr M, Harloff A, et al. Incidence of neurological complications following overstenting of the left subclavian artery. Eur J Cardiothorac Surg 2007;31:628–36.

[146] Nojiri J, Matsumoto K, Kato A, et al. The Adamkiewicz artery: demonstration by intra-arterial computed tomographic angiography. Eur J Cardiothorac Surg 2007;31:249–55.

[147] Hutschala D, Fleck T, Czerny M, et al. Endoluminal stent-graft placement in patients with acute aortic dissection type B. Eur J Cardiothorac Surg 2002;21:964–9.

[148] Chaikof EL, Blankensteijn JD, Harris PL, et al. Reporting standards for endovascular aortic aneurysm repair. J Vasc Surg 2002;35:1048–60.

[149] Muhs BE, Balm R, White GH, et al. Anatomic factors associated with acute endograft collapse after Gore TAG treatment of thoracic aortic dissection or traumatic rupture. J Vasc Surg 2007;45:655–61.

[150] Flores J, Shiiya N, Kunihara T, et al. Reoperations after failure of stent grafting for type B aortic dissection: report of two cases. Surg Today 2005;35:581–5.

[151] Sundt TM. Intramural hematoma and penetrating atherosclerotic ulcer of the aorta. Ann Thorac Surg 2007;83:S835–41 [discussion: S846–50].

[152] Vilacosta I. Acute aortic syndrome. Rev Esp Cardiol 2003;56:29–39.

[153] Vilacosta I, Roman JA. Acute aortic syndrome. Heart 2001;85:365–8.

[154] Cho KR, Stanson AW, Potter DD, et al. Penetrating atherosclerotic ulcer of the descending thoracic aorta and arch. J Thorac Cardiovasc Surg 2004;127:1393–9 [discussion: 1399–401].

[155] Schneiderman J, Bordin GM, Adar R, et al. Patterns of expression of fibrinolytic genes and matrix metalloproteinase-9 in dissecting aortic aneurysms. Am J Pathol 1998;152:703–10.

[156] Lesauskaite V, Tanganelli P, Sassi C, et al. Smooth muscle cells of the media in the dilatative pathology of ascending thoracic aorta: morphology, immunoreactivity for osteopontin, matrix metalloproteinases, and their inhibitors. Hum Pathol 2001;32:1003–11.

[157] He R, Guo DC, Estrera AL, et al. Characterization of the inflammatory and apoptotic cells in the aortas of patients with ascending thoracic aortic aneurysms and dissections. J Thorac Cardiovasc Surg 2006;131:671–8.

[158] Coady MA, Rizzo JA, Hammond GL, et al. Penetrating ulcer of the thoracic aorta: what is it? How do we recognize it? How do we manage it? J Vasc Surg 1998;27:1006–15 [discussion: 1015–6].

[159] Coady MA, Rizzo JA, Elefteriades JA. Pathologic variants of thoracic aortic dissections. Penetrating atherosclerotic ulcers and intramural hematomas. Cardiol Clin 1999;17: 637–57.

[160] Stanson AW, Kazmier FJ, Hollier LH, et al. Penetrating atherosclerotic ulcers of the thoracic aorta: natural history and clinicopathologic correlations. Ann Vasc Surg 1986;1: 15–23.

[161] Ledbetter S, Stuk JL, Kaufman JA. Helical (spiral) CT in the evaluation of emergent thoracic aortic syndromes. Traumatic aortic rupture, aortic aneurysm, aortic dissection, intramural hematoma, and penetrating atherosclerotic ulcer. Radiol Clin North Am 1999;37: 575–89.

[162] Hayashi H, Matsuoka Y, Sakamoto I, et al. Penetrating atherosclerotic ulcer of the aorta: imaging features and disease concept. Radiographics 2000;20:995–1005.

[163] Evangelista A, Mukherjee D, Mehta RH, et al. Acute intramural hematoma of the aorta: a mystery in evolution. Circulation 2005;111:1063–70.

[164] Ganaha F, Miller DC, Sugimoto K, et al. Prognosis of aortic intramural hematoma with and without penetrating atherosclerotic ulcer: a clinical and radiological analysis. Circulation 2002;106:342–8.

[165] Kaji S, Nishigami K, Akasaka T, et al. Prediction of progression or regression of type A aortic intramural hematoma by computed tomography. Circulation 1999;100: II281–6.

[166] Robbins RC, McManus RP, Mitchell RS, et al. Management of patients with intramural hematoma of the thoracic aorta. Circulation 1993;88:II1–10.

[167] von Kodolitsch Y, Csosz SK, Koschyk DH, et al. Intramural hematoma of the aorta: predictors of progression to dissection and rupture. Circulation 2003;107:1158–63.

[168] Kaji S, Akasaka T, Katayama M, et al. Long-term prognosis of patients with type B aortic intramural hematoma. Circulation 2003;108(Suppl 1):II307–11.

[169] Tittle SL, Lynch RJ, Cole PE, et al. Midterm follow-up of penetrating ulcer and intramural hematoma of the aorta. J Thorac Cardiovasc Surg 2002;123:1051–9.

[170] Evangelista A, Dominguez R, Sebastia C, et al. Long-term follow-up of aortic intramural hematoma: predictors of outcome. Circulation 2003;108:583–9.

[171] Song JK, Kim HS, Song JM, et al. Outcomes of medically treated patients with aortic intramural hematoma. Am J Med 2002;113:181–7.

[172] Sueyoshi E, Imada T, Sakamoto I, et al. Analysis of predictive factors for progression of type B aortic intramural hematoma with computed tomography. J Vasc Surg 2002;35: 1179–83.

[173] Troxler M, Mavor AI, Homer-Vanniasinkam S. Penetrating atherosclerotic ulcers of the aorta. Br J Surg 2001;88:1169–77.

[174] Kazerooni EA, Bree RL, Williams DM. Penetrating atherosclerotic ulcers of the descending thoracic aorta: evaluation with CT and distinction from aortic dissection. Radiology 1992;183:759–65.

[175] Hussain S, Glover JL, Bree R, et al. Penetrating atherosclerotic ulcers of the thoracic aorta. J Vasc Surg 1989;9:710–7.

[176] Eggebrecht H, Herold U, Schmermund A, et al. Endovascular stent-graft treatment of penetrating aortic ulcer: results over a median follow-up of 27 months. Am Heart J 2006;151: 530–6.

[177] Sailer J, Peloschek P, Rand T, et al. Endovascular treatment of aortic type B dissection and penetrating ulcer using commercially available stent-grafts. AJR Am J Roentgenol 2001; 177:1365–9.

[178] Schoder M, Grabenwoger M, Holzenbein T, et al. Endovascular stent-graft repair of complicated penetrating atherosclerotic ulcers of the descending thoracic aorta. J Vasc Surg 2002;36:720–6.

[179] Pitton MB, Duber C, Neufang A, et al. Endovascular repair of a non-contained aortic rupture caused by a penetrating aortic ulcer. Cardiovasc Intervent Radiol 2002;25: 64–7.

[180] Brinster DR, Wheatley GH 3rd, Williams J, et al. Are penetrating aortic ulcers best treated using an endovascular approach? Ann Thorac Surg 2006;82:1688–91.

[181] Dambrin C, Marcheix B, Hollington L, et al. Surgical treatment of an aortic arch aneurysm without cardio-pulmonary bypass: endovascular stent-grafting after extra-anatomic bypass of supra-aortic vessels. Eur J Cardiothorac Surg 2005;27:159–61.

[182] Kato M. [Total arch graft implantation with open stent-graft placement for aortic arch aneurysm or dissection]. Kyobu Geka 2006;59:694–9.

[183] Uchida N, Ishihara H, Shibamura H, et al. Midterm results of extensive primary repair of the thoracic aorta by means of total arch replacement with open stent graft placement for an acute type A aortic dissection. J Thorac Cardiovasc Surg 2006;131:862–7.

[184] Baraki H, Hagl C, Khaladj N, et al. The frozen elephant trunk technique for treatment of thoracic aortic aneurysms. Ann Thorac Surg 2007;83:S819–23 [discussion: S824–31].

[185] Sorokin VA, Chong CF, Lee CN, et al. Combined open and endovascular repair of acute type A aortic dissection. Ann Thorac Surg 2007;83:666–8.

[186] Czerny M, Gottardi R, Zimpfer D, et al. Mid-term results of supraaortic transpositions for extended endovascular repair of aortic arch pathologies. Eur J Cardiothorac Surg 2007;31: 623–7.

[187] Shores J, Berger KR, Murphy EA, et al. Progression of aortic dilatation and the benefit of long-term beta-adrenergic blockade in Marfan's syndrome. N Engl J Med 1994;330: 1335–41.

[188] Chen L, Wang X, Carter SA, et al. A single nucleotide polymorphism in the matrix metalloproteinase 9 gene (-8202A/G) is associated with thoracic aortic aneurysms and thoracic aortic dissection. J Thorac Cardiovasc Surg 2006,131.1045 52.

[189] Hiramoto JS, Schneider DB, Reilly LM, et al. A double-barrel stent-graft for endovascular repair of the aortic arch. J Endovasc Ther 2006;13:72–6.

[190] Chuter TA, Reilly LM. Endovascular treatment of thoracoabdominal aortic aneurysms. J Cardiovasc Surg (Torino) 2006;47:619–28.

[191] Chuter TA. Branched and fenestrated stent grafts for endovascular repair of thoracic aortic aneurysms. J Vasc Surg 2006;43(Suppl A):111A–5A.

[192] Tse LW, Steinmetz OK, Abraham CZ, et al. Branched endovascular stent-graft for suprarenal aortic aneurysm: the future of aortic stent-grafting? Can J Surg 2004;47:257–62.

SURGICAL
CLINICS OF
NORTH AMERICA

Surg Clin N Am 87 (2007) 1087–1098

Hybrid Approaches to Repair of Complex Aortic Aneurysmal Disease

Benjamin W. Starnes, MD, FACS[a],*,
Nam T. Tran, MD[a],
Jerome M. McDonald, MD, FACS[b]

[a]Division of Vascular Surgery, University of Washington, Box 359796, 325 Ninth Avenue,
Seattle, WA 98104, USA
[b]Stockton Cardiothoracic Surgical Medical Group, Stockton, CA, USA

With the endovascular revolution upon us, the management of aortic aneurysmal disease has changed dramatically. This revolution was initiated when Juan Carlos Parodi implanted the first aortic stent graft in a human in Argentina in 1991[1]. Since then, more than 100,000 aneurysms worldwide have been repaired using early-generation and current-generation standardized grafts and this has dramatically reduced the 30-day mortality rates associated with open aortic surgery [2,3]. A new phenomenon has also arisen from this wonderful technology. The term hybrid means "of different origins" and hybrid approaches to vascular disease involve open and endovascular techniques to achieve a common goal, namely, to prevent death caused by aneurysmal rupture. In reality, the first aortic stent graft procedures were true hybrid procedures involving open bilateral femoral arterial exposure or, alternatively, a retroperitoneal conduit for access to the aorta for a subsequent endovascular approach. This article reviews novel approaches to the repair of complex aortic aneurysms and provides several illustrative examples.

Illustrative case one

A 62-year-old man who had severe chronic obstructive pulmonary disease (FEV-1 < 30% predicted), adult polycystic kidney disease, and baseline serum creatinine of 1.7 mg/dL presented with an asymptomatic 7.2-cm Crawford extent III thoracoabdominal aneurysm (Fig. 1). Hybrid approach

---

* Corresponding author.
E-mail address: starnes@u.washington.edu (B.W. Starnes).

0039-6109/07/$ - see front matter © 2007 Elsevier Inc. All rights reserved.
doi:10.1016/j.suc.2007.08.012
surgical.theclinics.com

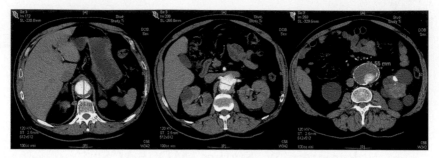

Fig. 1. Axial images depicting a Crawford extent III thoracoabdominal aneurysm in a patient who had severe chronic obstructive pulmonary disease and adult polycystic kidney disease. Note the representative axial slices at the diaphragm, renal artery origins, and infrarenal locations.

at repairing his aneurysm involved a two-stage procedure (Fig. 2). Stage one consisted of a midline laparotomy and left medial visceral rotation followed by multivisceral revascularization with a 12 × 7 mm bifurcated Dacron graft based from his left external iliac artery and bypassed to both renal arteries, the superior mesenteric artery, and celiac artery (Fig. 3). Ischemic time to each vascular bed was less than 12 minutes.

Stage two was conducted after a period of recovery and involved a totally percutaneous approach. This approach necessitated left arm access with

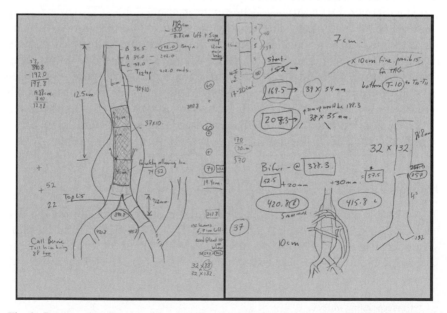

Fig. 2. Preoperative planning sheet depicting the detail required for eventual success. Note the drawing in the lower half of the right panel and its correlation with the intraoperative photo in Fig. 3.

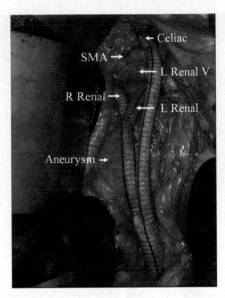

Fig. 3. Intraoperative photo with patient's head positioned at top. Note grafts to each of four visceral vessels and left renal vein crossing the aortic aneurysm.

placement of a pigtail catheter for contrast injections and main body graft deployment at the aortic bifurcation with the graft delivered through the right groin (20 French) (Cook Inc., Bloomington, Indiana). Cannulation of the contralateral gate and subsequent contralateral limb deployment was required to perfuse the visceral bypass graft during the remainder of the procedure. A 24-French sheath was then exchanged for the existing right 20-French sheath and delivered into the right ipsilateral limb. A 37 mm × 10 cm TAG (W.L. Gore, Flagstaff, Arizona) endoprosthesis was delivered into the descending thoracic aorta and deployed with adequate overlap in the previously placed bifurcated graft. A 40 mm × 10 cm TAG endoprosthesis was then deployed from the previously placed graft into the healthy descending thoracic aortic seal zone. Ballooning was then conducted to seat the graft and overlapping zones. Finally, the ipsilateral limb of the bifurcated graft was deployed into the right common iliac artery. The access sites were closed with a suture-mediated closure device. The patient recovered uneventfully and underwent postoperative CT angiography one month later confirming absence of endoleak (Fig. 4).

Illustrative case two

An 83-year-old man previously underwent three-vessel aortocoronary bypass grafting in the remote past. He had a history of moderate congestive heart failure with a calculated ejection fraction of 35%. He presented with

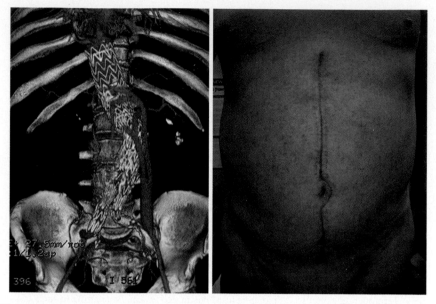

Fig. 4. Follow-up CTA depicting the final result of hybrid repair of this thoracoabdominal aneurysm and a corresponding photo demonstrating the patient's single cavitary healed incision with bilateral groin puncture wounds.

a rapidly enlarging, symptomatic 7.0-cm distal arch and proximal descending thoracic aortic aneurysm (Fig. 5) with intermittent, unrelenting interscapular back pain.

A hybrid approach was planned (Fig. 6). The patient underwent a two-stage procedure consisting of a redo sternotomy with left neck extension, application of a side biting clamp to the ascending aorta, and off-pump anastomosis of a 10-mm Dacron straight tube graft with a sharp bevel followed by bypass to the innominate artery, separate grafting to the left common carotid artery, and then left common carotid to subclavian artery

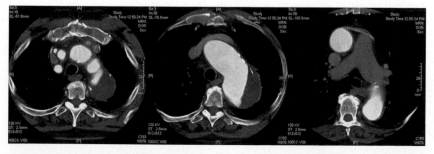

Fig. 5. Axial images depicting a large aortic arch and descending thoracic aortic aneurysm. Note the origin of a saphenous vein graft in the far right panel from a prior aortocoronary bypass.

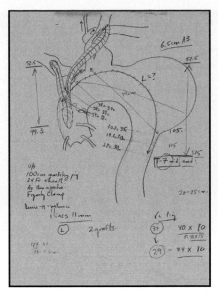

Fig. 6. Preoperative planning sheet showing measurements with origins of each of the previous coronary bypass grafts and planned debranching of the aortic arch.

bypass. Each great vessel origin was oversewn and a sponge marker band was placed around the origin of the original 10-mm bypass graft to make positioning of the stent graft easier during stage two.

Stage two consisted of left groin access with a 6-French sheath and a pigtail catheter placed in the arch. Right groin access with a 24-French sheath was achieved followed by insertion of a 34 mm × 15 cm TAG distally and then a 40 mm × 15 cm TAG proximally across the arch to the ascending aortic bypass graft. All seal sites were ballooned with a trilobed balloon and the patient was then closed. Follow-up CT angiography performed 3 months later demonstrated a successful result (Fig. 7).

Illustrative case three

A 66-year-old woman who had severe atherosclerotic peripheral vascular disease and tobacco abuse presented with complaints of dyspnea on exertion. CT scan of the chest revealed a 4.7-cm ascending aortic aneurysm and a 5.1-cm descending thoracic aortic aneurysm (Fig. 8). Echocardiography revealed mild to moderate aortic insufficiency. Interestingly, she weighed 51 kg with a body surface area of 1.54 m^2 and an aortic size index of 3.33, which would predict a high annual rupture risk [4]. Compounding this unique presentation were iliac access vessels of only 5 mm maximal diameter.

This patient underwent a single-stage procedure consisting of standard operative repair of her ascending aortic aneurysm through a median

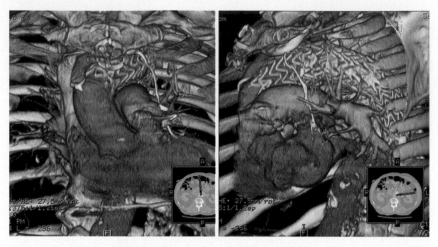

Fig. 7. Two follow-up CT reconstructed images showing the radiopaque marker at the base of the bypass graft (*left panel*) and exclusion of the aneurysm with two overlapping aortic stent grafts (*right panel*).

sternotomy and full cardiopulmonary bypass. The superior neck of the ascending aneurysm allowed arterial cannulation and clamp placement just proximal to the origin of the innominate artery (Fig. 9A). A 26-mm Dacron tube graft (Boston Scientific, Natick, Massachusetts) with a 10-mm pre-sewn side arm was used to repair the ascending aneurysm (Fig. 9B). The 10-mm side arm was positioned in a right anterolateral

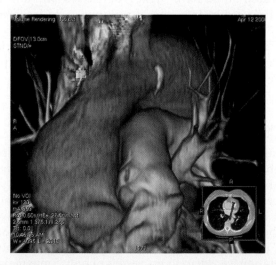

Fig. 8. Preoperative CT reconstructed image depicting an ascending and descending thoracic aortic aneurysm with relative sparing of the intervening segment of aorta encompassing the origins of the great vessels.

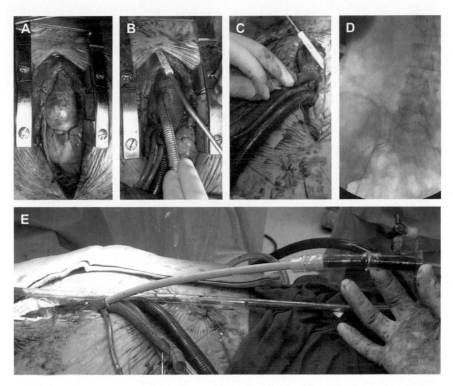

Fig. 9. Intraoperative photos. (*A*) Median sternotomy depicting ascending aneurysm, (*B*) after ascending replacement with a 26-mm Dacron tube graft with 10-mm side branch factory presewn, (*C*) access of side branch with 11-French sheath and wire directed antegrade across aortic arch, (*D*) wire snared through right groin for complete wire control, and (*E*) delivery of aortic stent graft antegrade through chest and across aortic arch (off pump).

dimension and clamped to facilitate subsequent antegrade delivery of a stent graft endoprosthesis. The arterial cannula was removed and the venous cannula left in place for transfusion of any blood loss occurring with endograft delivery.

The right common femoral artery was then accessed using Seldinger technique and a 6-French sheath placed for delivery of a snare device. Similarly, the left common femoral artery was accessed with a 5-French sheath for placement in the arch of a marking pigtail catheter for contrast injections. The sternal retractor was removed to facilitate imaging and the 10-mm side-arm graft was accessed with an 18-gauge needle and an 11-French sheath (Fig. 9C). A hydrophilic wire was then passed across the arch and directly into the right common iliac artery under fluoroscopic guidance whereupon it was easily snared and delivered through the 6-French sheath (Fig. 9D). The 11-French sheath was then exchanged for a 22-French sheath, which was then delivered into the 10-mm side arm but not beyond its origin from the 26-mm tube graft (Fig. 9E). Standard arch aortography confirmed a dominant right vertebral artery and short proximal landing zone.

A 26 mm × 15 cm TAG endoprosthesis was then prepared and delivered antegrade through the sheath and into appropriate position using oblique imaging. The graft was deployed with excellent result and partial coverage of the left subclavian artery (Fig. 10). The graft was then ballooned to profile distally and then proximally. Completion imaging demonstrated a successful result. The 10-mm side-arm graft was clamped with a vascular clamp and amputated followed by pledgeted repair using 5-0 Prolene. Total time for the endovascular portion of the case was 15 minutes and total estimated blood loss was less than 50 mL.

The patient had an uncomplicated postoperative course. Postoperative CT angiography was performed, which confirmed the absence of aortic dissection and complete exclusion of the descending aortic aneurysm (See Fig. 10). She was discharged to home on postoperative day seven and follow-up two-dimensional echocardiogram revealed absence of the aforementioned aortic insufficiency.

Discussion

Hybrid open and endovascular approaches for the repair of aortic pathology offer a patient-specific approach with the ultimate goal of preventing eventual rupture-related morbidity and mortality. With new endovascular technology and device design, the human aorta has become almost completely approachable with a variety of exclusively minimally invasive alternatives [5]. Specific regions of the aorta that remain challenging for a successful endovascular-only approach include the aortic arch and

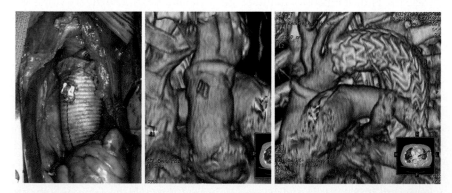

Fig. 10. From left to right: Completion intraoperative photo after ligation and oversewing of graft side branch, corresponding CT reconstructed image showing remarkable detail as compared with first image, and completion sagittal reconstruction of this successful hybrid procedure.

para-visceral aorta. Operative "debranching" or translocation of the origin of certain named vessels to alternative or remote locations allows for subsequent repair of the aorta with endovascular means in these difficult locations. On review of current literature, there are a limited number of small case series and individual case reports that make firm conclusions suspect regarding the durability and efficacy of these hybrid procedures. A few notable exceptions deserve mention, however, and include reports of more than 10 patients each [6–15].

Surgery to correct aneurysms involving the aortic arch have typically required a combination of cardiopulmonary bypass, deep hypothermia, and circulatory arrest, which can carry a substantial morbidity and mortality risk [16]. Novel approaches to treating aortic arch pathology without use of these adjunctive techniques have been described with small numbers of patients [11,13–15,17–21]. A few studies have evaluated the effectiveness of completing a traditional elephant trunk procedure, originally described by Borst and colleagues in 1983 [22], with subsequent endovascular placement of a stent graft [13,18]. Mortality with a traditional elephant trunk procedure has been quoted as high as 20% with up to 30% of patients never receiving the second and final stage of the procedure involving separate thoracotomy [18]. Greenberg and colleagues [13] recently described the Cleveland Clinic experience with 22 patients who required elephant trunk and endovascular completion. There were no strokes or cases of paraplegia in this series and 30-day mortality was 4.5%. They concluded that endovascular completion was feasible and could be accomplished with minimal morbidity and mortality in this small subset of patients. Avoidance of a required thoracotomy in this patient population highlights the power of a hybrid approach in this clinical scenario.

Surgical results for the correction of thoracoabdominal aortic aneurysms (Crawford extent I–IV) carry a mean 30-day mortality of 14% [23–26] and in contemporary series at centers of excellence, a permanent paraplegia risk of between 2.4% and 6.8% [27]. Similar data from the same series define a cumulative rate of permanent neurologic deficits for the repair of thoracoabdominal aneurysms at 3.3% [28]. This year, Donas and colleagues [12] published an article entitled "Hybrid open-endovascular repair for thoracoabdominal aortic aneurysms: current status and level of evidence" and evaluated 13 separate published series involving detailed data on 58 patients. The overall incidence of permanent paraplegia and stroke was 0% and overall 30-day mortality was 15.5%. The authors cautioned that their data did not allow for robust conclusions regarding long-term outcome. A review of recently published case series and respective morbidity and mortality rates is depicted in Table 1.

Some authors have expressed caution at adopting these hybrid techniques for broad application to all patients who have thoracoabdominal aneurysms [8,10]. Resch and colleagues [10] described their experience with 13 patients undergoing visceral debranching before total endovascular exclusion of

Table 1
Contemporary hybrid series of greater than 10 patients each with respective morbidity and mortality data

Author	Year	N	Permanent paraplegia	Stroke	30-Day mortality (n/%)
Chiesa et al	2007	13	0	0	4/23
Bockler et al	2007	19	0	0	3/17
Zhou et al	2006	15	0	0	0/0
Black et al	2006	26	0	1	3/13
Resch et al	2006	13	2	0	3/23
Fulton et al	2005	10	0	0	0/0
Total		99	2/2%	1/1%	13/13%

thoracoabdominal aneurysms. Two patients developed paraplegia (15%) and the 30-day mortality rate was 23%. The authors cautioned that this approach still carried a significant perioperative risk and that newer, less-invasive alternatives should be explored [10]. One must consider, however, that a large percentage of these patients (38%) had extensive Crawford extent II thoracoabdominal aneurysms, which carry the highest perioperative risk.

The ultimate goal in any endeavor at repairing an aortic aneurysm is to prevent death caused by rupture. If one can achieve this goal with less perioperative morbidity, the application of this technology can be applied to patients who would in the past have never been offered any option for repair. The attractiveness of these hybrid approaches relates to the level and duration of the open surgery required, blood loss, ischemic time to respective vascular beds, and avoidance of additional cavitary incisions.

The question of whether to stage a procedure has been debated in the literature with proponents for and against. Each procedure must be tailored to the individual patient's anatomy and comorbidities. In our third illustrative case, single-stage repair allowed for delivery of the endovascular device through the open chest in an antegrade fashion at the time of ascending aortic replacement. This approach avoided what would have required a retroperitoneal conduit because of small access vessels. The endovascular portion of the case added a mere 15 minutes to the open portion of the procedure.

Evident in the illustrative cases presented was the level of preoperative planning required for a successful outcome in each case. Preoperative detailed imaging is essential and has been touted as such by all authors describing hybrid approaches. Detailed and precise preoperative planning with the use of three-dimensional workstations and appropriate software for sizing is mandatory. Other factors, such as room set-up, access options, device delivery to minimize ischemic time, intraoperative imaging, combining stent graft products from various manufacturers, and a host of other factors, must be considered before embarking on such hybrid adventures.

All of the illustrative cases described were conducted by a multidisciplinary team led by vascular and cardiothoracic surgeons. The importance of collaboration in these endeavors cannot be overemphasized because the future fully trained vascular and endovascular specialist has yet to be defined in the modern era. Requisite skills will involve the ability to perform a full array of open vascular and cardiac surgery, a robust complement of advanced endovascular skills, including microcatheter manipulation, and the ability to interpret and manipulate advanced imaging modalities for accuracy in endograft sizing.

Newer stent graft designs on the near horizon involve multibranched and fenestrated stent grafts. Hybrid approaches, however, will not go away any time soon because these multibranch and fenestrated procedures involve custom-made grafts that take time (weeks) to manufacture. New and clever approaches to hybrid repairs will come to light with standardization and separate classification schemes.

Summary

Hybrid approaches to aortic pathology offer the advantages of versatility, avoidance of bicavitary surgical incisions and exposures, and a combination of open and endovascular techniques, and potentially offer a broader range of therapies to a patient population that would not otherwise be considered for aortic surgical repair. The durability of these procedures currently remains in question. The common goal of any of these procedures, when conducted for repair of aneurysmal disease, remains to prevent death caused by rupture of the aortic aneurysm. The procedure need only be as durable as to exceed the patient's life span if he or she were to die of other causes. Hybrid approaches to aortic pathology require an experienced and dedicated team with adequate resources in modern facilities.

References

[1] Parodi JC, Palmaz JC, Barone HD. Transfemoral intraluminal graft implantation for abdominal aortic aneurysms. Ann Vasc Surg 1991;5(6):491–9.
[2] Prinssen M, Verhoeven EL, Buth J, et al. A randomized trial comparing conventional and endovascular repair of abdominal aortic aneurysms. N Engl J Med 2004;351(16):1607–18.
[3] Greenhalgh RM, Brown LC, Kwong GP, et al. Comparison of endovascular aneurysm repair with open repair in patients with abdominal aortic aneurysm (EVAR trial 1), 30-day operative mortality results: randomised controlled trial. Lancet 2004;364(9437):843–8.
[4] Davies RR, Gallo A, Coady MA, et al. Novel measurement of relative aortic size predicts rupture of thoracic aortic aneurysms. Ann Thorac Surg 2006;81(1):169–77.
[5] Moon MC, Morales JP, Greenberg RK. The aortic arch and ascending aorta: are they within the endovascular realm? Semin Vasc Surg 2007;20(2):97–107.
[6] Black SA, Wolfe JH, Clark M, et al. Complex thoracoabdominal aortic aneurysms: endovascular exclusion with visceral revascularization. J Vasc Surg 2006;43(6):1081–9.
[7] Bockler D, Schumacher H, Klemm K, et al. Hybrid procedures as a combined endovascular and open approach for pararenal and thoracoabdominal aortic pathologies. Langenbecks Arch Surg 2007; [epub ahead of print].

[8] Chiesa R, Tshomba Y, Melissano G, et al. Hybrid approach to thoracoabdominal aortic aneurysms in patients with prior aortic surgery. J Vasc Surg 2007;45(6):1128–35.

[9] Fulton JJ, Farber MA, Marston WA, et al. Endovascular stent-graft repair of pararenal and type IV thoracoabdominal aortic aneurysms with adjunctive visceral reconstruction. J Vasc Surg 2005;41(2):191–8.

[10] Resch TA, Greenberg RK, Lyden SP, et al. Combined staged procedures for the treatment of thoracoabdominal aneurysms. J Endovasc Ther 2006;13(4):481–9.

[11] Zhou W, Reardon M, Peden EK, et al. Hybrid approach to complex thoracic aortic aneurysms in high-risk patients: surgical challenges and clinical outcomes. J Vasc Surg 2006; 44(4):688–93.

[12] Donas KP, Czerny M, Guber I, et al. Hybrid open-endovascular repair for thoracoabdominal aortic aneurysms: current status and level of evidence. Eur J Vasc Endovasc Surg 2007; [epub ahead of print].

[13] Greenberg RK, Haddad F, Svensson L, et al. Hybrid approaches to thoracic aortic aneurysms: the role of endovascular elephant trunk completion. Circulation 2005;112(17): 2619–26.

[14] Saleh HM. Hybrid repair of aortic arch aneurysm. Acta Chir Belg 2007;107(2):173–80.

[15] Schumacher H, Von Tengg-Kobligk H, Ostovic M, et al. Hybrid aortic procedures for endoluminal arch replacement in thoracic aneurysms and type B dissections. J Cardiovasc Surg (Torino) 2006;47(5):509–17.

[16] Brueck M, Heidt MC, Szente-Varga M, et al. Hybrid treatment for complex aortic problems combining surgery and stenting in the integrated operating theater. J Interv Cardiol 2006; 19(6):539–43.

[17] Antona C, Vanelli P, Petulla M, et al. Hybrid technique for total arch repair: aortic neck reshaping for endovascular-graft fixation. Ann Thorac Surg 2007;83(3):1158–61.

[18] Herold U, Tsagakis K, Kamler M, et al. [Change of paradigms in the surgical treatment of complex thoracic aortic disease]. Herz 2006;31(5):434–42 [in German].

[19] Matalanis G, Durairaj M, Brooks M. A hybrid technique of aortic arch branch transposition and antegrade stent graft deployment for complete arch repair without cardiopulmonary bypass. Eur J Cardiothorac Surg 2006;29(4):611–2.

[20] Melissano G, Civilini E, Marrocco-Trischitta MM, et al. Hybrid endovascular and off-pump open surgical treatment for synchronous aneurysms of the aortic arch, brachiocephalic trunk, and abdominal aorta. Tex Heart Inst J 2004;31(3):283–7.

[21] Shah A, Coulon P, de CT, et al. Novel technique: staged hybrid surgical and endovascular treatment of acute Type A aortic dissections with aortic arch involvement. J Cardiovasc Surg (Torino) 2006;47(5):497–502.

[22] Borst HG, Walterbusch G, Schaps D. Extensive aortic replacement using "elephant trunk" prosthesis. Thorac Cardiovasc Surg 1983;31(1):37–40.

[23] Elefteriades JA, Hartleroad J, Gusberg RJ, et al. Long-term experience with descending aortic dissection: the complication-specific approach. Ann Thorac Surg 1992;53(1):11–20.

[24] Svensson LG, Crawford ES, Hess KR, et al. Experience with 1509 patients undergoing thoracoabdominal aortic operations. J Vasc Surg 1993;17(2):357–68.

[25] Kouchoukos NT, Daily BB, Rokkas CK, et al. Hypothermic bypass and circulatory arrest for operations on the descending thoracic and thoracoabdominal aorta. Ann Thorac Surg 1995;60(1):67–76.

[26] Cambria RP, Davison JK, Carter C, et al. Epidural cooling for spinal cord protection during thoracoabdominal aneurysm repair: A five-year experience. J Vasc Surg 2000;31(6): 1093–102.

[27] Safi HJ, Miller CC III, Huynh TT, et al. Distal aortic perfusion and cerebrospinal fluid drainage for thoracoabdominal and descending thoracic aortic repair: ten years of organ protection. Ann Surg 2003;238(3):372–80.

[28] Estrera AL, Miller CC III, Huynh TT, et al. Neurologic outcome after thoracic and thoracoabdominal aortic aneurysm repair. Ann Thorac Surg 2001;72(4):1225–30.

SURGICAL
CLINICS OF
NORTH AMERICA

Surg Clin N Am 87 (2007) 1099–1114

Ischemic Colitis Complicating
Major Vascular Surgery

Scott R. Steele, MD, FACS

Department of Surgery, Madigan Army Medical Center, Fort Lewis, WA 98431, USA

Ischemic colitis is a well-described complication of major vascular surgery, mostly following open abdominal aortic aneurysm (AAA) repair and endovascular aneurysm repair (EVAR), but also with aortoiliac surgery, aortic dissection, and thoracic aneurysm repair [1,2]. Although Boley and colleagues [3] described ischemia of the colon in 1963 as a reversible process secondary to vascular occlusion, the term was not coined until 1966, when Marston and colleagues [4] described its three stages of evolution (transient ischemia, late ischemic stricture, and gangrene), along with the natural history of the disease. Furthermore, the development of colonic ischemia as a result of major vascular and aortic surgery has only been well described since the 1970s [5–9]. The original reports were scattered and mostly consisted of autopsy studies, depicting not only the high mortality associated with this condition but also, in retrospect, the relative lack of insight as to explanations for its onset and progression. Unfortunately, recent outcomes have not shown much improvement. Luckily, the overall incidence remains low, estimated at between 0.6% and 3.1%, with higher rates attributed to ruptured aneurysms, open repair, and emergent surgery [10]. Following the development of ischemic colitis, mortality has been reported to be as high as 67%, highlighting the need for rapidly identifying the commencement of symptoms and, perhaps more importantly, those patients at risk, in attempt to prevent its onset [10,11]. Further emphasizing the seriousness of the development of this condition, in a study of 222 aortic aneurysm repairs, colonic ischemia was the most common cause of death, even more than multisystem organ failure and myocardial infarction [12]. Thus, the physician tasked with treating patients who have vascular disease needs to be well versed in this condition, not only to recognize its occurrence and course but to be aware of how to manage this highly lethal condition.

E-mail address: docsteele@hotmail.com

doi:10.1016/j.suc.2007.07.007

This article reviews the causes, presentation, and diagnostic strategies of colonic ischemia. It also covers the operative management and outcomes for bowel resection and vascular repair. Finally, some of the research regarding alternative options for diagnosing this condition is discussed.

Pathogenesis

Simply stated, ischemic colitis occurs when blood flow is interrupted and supply does not equal colonic demand. Most commonly, this interruption is not associated with occlusion of any of the major abdominal vessels, because the collateral circulation of the colonic blood supply from the superior mesenteric, inferior mesenteric, hypogastric, and meandering mesenteric arteries is extensive. Regardless of the cause, the earliest dysfunction is seen at the mucosal level, furthest away from the vasa recta, creating a secondary disruption of the mucosal barrier that can lead to bacterial translocation and sepsis [13]. Ischemic colitis may occur with many different conditions, including embolism from cardiac disease, low-flow states such as congestive heart failure, sepsis, and vasopressor use. However, major vascular surgery, especially involving the abdominal aorta, is a well-known risk factor [14]. As such, ischemic colitis is recognized as a potential complication of both open AAA repair and EVAR, with its development associated with high mortality not only from the colonic insult but from the subsequent physiologic derangements that follow [15]. When occurring in the context of major vascular repair, the pathogenesis may be unique in that, in many cases, an isolated interruption of inferior mesenteric artery (IMA) blood flow may be the sole underlying cause [8]. Following open repair, many different variables can play major roles in its onset, including larger perioperative fluid shifts, cross-clamping of the aorta, compressive retroperitoneal hematomas, and prolonged hypotension [16]. On the other hand, the exact pathogenesis following endovascular repair has yet to be elicited completely. Although multiple theories exist, the most common one involves embolization of cholesterol plaque following implantation of the stent graft or manipulation of catheters and guidewires within the aneurysm sac [17].

Regardless of the method of repair, presentation of the underlying vascular disease also significantly affects the rate and prevalence of ischemic colitis, with 60% of ruptured AAAs developing colonic ischemia [18]. Other factors that have been shown to have a higher association with the development of colonic ischemia are increased intraoperative blood loss, hypotension, and prior pelvic radiation [12,19]. Because radiation damage is progressive and cumulative over time, it may be a precipitating factor not only in early disease but also with chronic changes such as stricture. Damage occurs directly to the bowel wall, in addition to causing secondary hyaline deposition and fibrosis of the microvasculature at the arteriole level [20]. Thus, prior radiation therapy may decrease the major and collateral circulation of the colonic blood supply that is at most risk during aortic repair, in addition to creating a primary impairment to the colon [19].

On the contrary, established collateral circulation appears to portend a protective effect, with one study showing that a patent meandering mesenteric artery (arc of Riolan) was not associated with any cases of ischemia [6]. Clearly, however, the most important factor in curtailing its morbid effects is to prevent, or at least minimize, all potential variables that can lead to secondary injury.

Diagnosis

Regrettably, the clinical manifestations of ischemic colitis are inconsistent. Most commonly, patients present with abdominal pain, fever, distension, and diarrhea anywhere from hours to days following surgery [16]. The diarrhea may be bloody or nonbloody, depending on the location, degree, and extent of the colon affected. Abdominal examination may show widely variable findings, ranging from mild localized tenderness to diffuse peritonitis. Rectal examination may be completely normal or may demonstrate blood, ranging from bright red to melena. Laboratory examination is often noteworthy for a leukocytosis and metabolic acidosis, and may also present with significant electrolyte abnormalities.

Although any area of the colon may be affected, the watershed areas of the rectosigmoid (Sudeck's point) and splenic flexure (Griffith's point) are commonly involved because of the often incomplete anastomoses of the marginal artery in these locations. The next most common area afflicted is the cecum, secondary to low blood flow in the terminal branches of the ileocolic artery combined with varying competency of the right colic artery [21]. Longo and colleagues [22] found a much higher rate of right colonic involvement than most other studies did, with 46% of their 47 patients having this portion affected. Unfortunately, as reported in his large study of almost 5000 Veterans Administration patients, regardless of the presentation, the mean time to diagnosis was 5.5 days following aortic surgery (range 1–21 days) [14]. This time was secondary to not only the slow evolution of the disease but also, in other cases, to the lack of acumen of the caretaker. Therefore, identifying patients at the onset of their clinical course entails a high index of suspicion. Complete history and physical examination, focusing on the abdominal examination and evaluation for peritoneal signs, is of utmost importance. Any peritonitis mandates emergent exploratory laparotomy for evaluation for bowel viability. Again, because of the high morbidity and mortality once ischemic colitis following major vascular surgery precipitates, the ultimate goal remains to avoid this condition altogether.

In the absence of that, early diagnosis remains the key, and has been the work of several investigators. The early setting may show few clinical symptoms, leading to a delay in diagnosis and increasing the likelihood of complications, or even death. Efforts have therefore been made to identify changes on both a clinical and biochemical front. Although some of these methods are still often only investigational or not yet widely used, they represent a potentially important adjunct to the currently available diagnostic tools. One of these markers is plasma D-lactate. In a study of 12 patients who had histologically confirmed ischemic colitis after undergoing either elective or emergent open aortic aneurysm surgery, plasma D-lactate was found to be elevated in patients as early as 2 hours postoperatively, with a peak on days 1 and 2 [13]. Lange and colleagues [23] had similar findings, with plasma lactate exceeding the normal level in all 20 patients who had mesenteric ischemia; however, sensitivity for the entire cohort with acute abdominal disease was much lower, at less than 50%.

Although early serum markers are promising and may prove effective, intraoperative assessment may lead to even earlier manifestations and may provide the surgeon with the opportunity to address the issue before leaving the operating room. In a study of 22 patients sustaining a ruptured aneurysm, laser Doppler flowmetry was used to evaluate the erythrocyte flux to the potentially ischemic area of the colon following repair of the rupture [18]. With an overall ischemic incidence of 41%, the investigators were able to identify 100% of these patients when finding erythrocyte flux to be significantly decreased (defined as < 50 perfusion units). Thus, using this value as the lowest threshold tolerable, the investigators proposed an algorithm for revascularization of the colon at the time of aortic repair when this level was reached. Laser Doppler flowmetry has also been used to monitor serosal blood flow in the sigmoid colon during open repair, to evaluate whether revascularization should be performed [24]. Similarly, colonic mucosal oxygen saturation measured by way of a spectrophotometer probe inserted into the rectum has been evaluated during aortic surgery to detect changes in the colonic blood flow [25]. It has been shown to be a sensitive indicator of decreases in colonic flow in both the endovascular and open settings, and correlates with aortic balloon occlusion during EVAR and aortic cross clamping with open repair. Techniques such as this may provide easily detectable and continuous intraoperative monitoring of the changes in the colon blood flow and may serve as indicators of the potential need for revascularization or resection, or may help identify those patients at risk who require further work-up, should the levels not return to normal. The plethora of information alone regarding investigational and research endeavors into techniques to diagnose ischemic colitis speak to the degree of its importance and the high potential for morbidity and mortality.

Aside from the more investigational methods, endoscopy remains a commonly used method for diagnosis when patients present with clinical symptoms or, for some centers, as a part of routine postoperative screening. Ischemia has a wide extent of changes and characteristics when viewed endoscopically (Table 1). Biopsy is rarely useful and is more likely to demonstrate either nonspecific ischemic or inflammatory changes rather than the ghost cells that are classic for ischemia [16]. Supporters of the routine use of

Table 1
Endoscopic findings of ischemic colitis

Stage	Endoscopic findings
Acute	Hyperemia, edema, friable mucosa, superficial ulcerations, petechial hemorrhage, gangrene[a]
Subacute	Edema, exudate, ulceration
Chronic	Stricture, mass, segmental involvement

[a] Irreversible damage characterized by gray, green, or black appearance.

endoscopy suggest that the classic pattern of rectal and distal sigmoid sparing, along with varying degrees of more proximal mucosally based changes, is quite helpful in this select patient population [26]. Others point to the potential risks of the procedure, including perforation, along with its inability to predict accurately the degree of necrosis to the bowel wall, as reasons not to perform it routinely. In a review of seven prospective, nonrandomized series evaluating the role of routine colonoscopy following abdominal aortic surgery, endoscopy was able to diagnose ischemic colitis accurately on appearance, but failed to differentiate mucosal-only injury from full-thickness ischemia reliably [27]. Furthermore, some question the importance of the information gathered by endoscopy, suggesting it rarely adds anything beyond that which could be easily identified on routine clinical examination alone, and does not change the eventual management. In a study of 105 patients over 3 years undergoing routine scheduled endoscopy within 72 hours of aortic surgery, only 12 patients were found to have ischemic colitis (11.4%), of which 7 were symptomatic and carried a diagnosis of ischemic colitis before undergoing the procedure [28]. Findings in this cohort included the typical wide spectrum, ranging from superficial ulcerations and mucosal erythema to mucosal sloughing, muscle death, and even full-thickness necrosis. The investigators suggested that routine endoscopy should only be a part of the care of the postaortic surgery patient for whom postoperative clinical symptoms dictate, or for whom intraoperative assessment of the colonic viability is in question. Other investigators have used more of a selective approach to determine which patients are in need of postoperative endoscopy, and find it useful as a confirmatory test only. Brandt and associates [29] found the most common indications for endoscopy to include bloody stools, hemodynamic instability, sepsis, and acidosis. In this light, the scope is used more to corroborate the clinical examination. Overall, despite these differing views, endoscopy has a definite role in the evaluation of these patients, may provide useful information (especially when findings may suggest a worse insult than initially suspected), and should be a part of the surgeon's armamentarium.

Other radiology tests may provide additional insight into the diagnosis or the degree of insult to the bowel. In general, angiography does not help in patients who have acute ischemic changes, although it may be useful occasionally in the patient who has previously undergone reimplantation of the

IMA, to evaluate for patency or collateral circulation. Much more commonly, angiography is used in conjunction with duplex ultrasonography in the chronic setting, to identify the patency status of the major visceral vessels before a proposed revascularization procedure. Multiplanar CT imaging has been used to diagnose ischemic colitis, with associated changes in the bowel wall more often offering clues to the diagnosis (Fig. 1) [30]. Being able to evaluate the bowel and surrounding tissue aids in diagnosis by indicating findings such as wall thickening, mesenteric fat stranding, mucosal enhancement, intramural air, and dilatation, or even more ominous signs such as portal venous gas.

Open aortic aneurysm repair

The incidence of ischemic colitis following elective open AAA repair is approximately 1% to 7% and is thought to be due to patient factors (ie, advanced age, medical comorbidities) and the physiologic insult from prolonged operative times and blood loss associated with an open operation [12,14,31,32]. Although potentially the most devastating complication, colonic ischemia is often the least common gastrointestinal complication following open aortic surgery. In a study of 120 consecutive patients undergoing open aortic aneurysm repair, 25 patients also developed ileus (n = 12), upper gastrointestinal bleeding (n = 5), Clostridium difficile enterocolitis (n = 5), acute cholecystitis (n = 2), mechanical obstruction (n = 2), and ascites (n = 2), with only 1 case of ischemic colitis [33]. These conditions can occur in conjunction with, or independent of, one another; therefore, a thorough evaluation is required because treatment can be very different for each.

Risk factors for the development of ischemic colitis include prolonged aortic cross clamp time and loss of patency of the IMA and hypogastric arteries [28]. In a study of 2824 patients undergoing aortoiliac surgery,

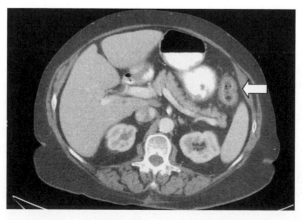

Fig. 1. Ischemic colitis of the splenic flexure.

including 62 patients who developed ischemic colitis, rupture and shock on admission were the primary factors associated with the development of ischemic colitis [32]. Large retrospective series have found these risk factors to be more commonly associated with an open repair, which may be related in part to a paucity of surgeons being comfortable approaching these extremely high-risk patients with an endovascular approach. Other risk factors found to be independently associated with an open approach and the development of ischemic colitis include renal disease, emergency surgery, advanced age, aortobifemoral graft placement, prolonged operative time, and ligation of the hypogastric arteries.

During open repair, surgeons directly evaluate the IMA blood flow when opening the aneurysm sac. Whether or not to reconstruct or reimplant the IMA as a routine component of aortic repair is controversial. Indications for reimplantation include slow oozing from the IMA, borderline perfusion of the sigmoid colon as demonstrated intraoperatively, or decreased stump pressure of the transected pedicle [34]. Yet many investigators have found that routine reimplantation provides no benefit over maintaining stable cardiac output and blood pressure support alone [35,36]. Others have found that IMA reimplantation is helpful under certain conditions. In a study of 151 patients comparing selective ligation with reimplantation of patent IMAs (based on clinical bowel inspection, Doppler signals, and IMA stump pressures), Seeger and colleagues [37] found the rate of colonic ischemia to be 2.7% and 0% ($P < .05$) for selective ligation and reimplantation, respectively, and recommended routine reimplantation for all patent IMAs to limit colonic infarction. Despite the multiple studies evaluating this question, the data remain contradictory, with strong opinions on both sides. Most importantly, surgeons must make every attempt to preserve colonic blood supply and evaluate the viability of the colon at the time of the operation, rather than adhere to the dictum of a "wait and see" approach.

Endovascular aneurysm repair

In 1991, Parodi and colleagues [38] were the first to demonstrate EVAR as a feasible option for the repair of AAA. Since that time, multiple studies have documented the benefit of EVAR in reducing mortality, postoperative complications, and hospital length of stay [39,40]. Relatively small reports of ischemic colitis following EVAR have also demonstrated an incidence of approximately 0% to 6%, depending on the sample size, the aneurysm presentation (ie, elective versus ruptured), and the definition of ischemic colitis (Table 2) [41–46]. Patients presenting with ruptured aneurysms are at a significant risk for ischemic changes, although EVAR appears to be somewhat protective compared with the open approach. In a study of ruptured aneurysms treated with EVAR, the incidence was higher, at 24%, albeit much lower than a similar cohort undergoing open repair (44%) [47]. Although the exact pathophysiology of ischemic colitis following EVAR is still

Table 2
Ischemic colitis following endovascular aortic aneurysm repair

Author	No. patients	No. with ischemic colitis	Early diagnosis (≤3 days)	Colectomy	Revascularization	Mortality
Champagne et al 2007[a] [47]	36	8 (23%)	8 (100)	3 (38%)	0	0%
Nevelsteen et al 2006 [41]	1	1	0	1	0	1 (100%)
Mehta et al 2006[a] [42]	40	2 (5%)	—	—	—	—
Lee et al 2006[b] [43]	24	1 (4.2%)	1	0	0	0%
Mehta et al 2005 [44]	175	—	—	1	—	—
Maldonado et al 2004 [50]	311	4 (1.2%)	3 (75%)	3 (75%)	0	2 (50%)
Axelrod et al 2004 [45]	102	0	0	—	—	—
Geraghty et al 2004 [49]	233	4 (1.7%)	3	3	1[c]	2 (50%)
Verhoeven et al 2002 [46]	17	1 (5.8%)	N/A	0	0	0%
Dadian et al 2001 [48]	278	8 (2.9%)	N/A	2 (25%)	0	3 (38%)

Abbreviation: N/A, not available.
[a] All cases of ruptured aneurysms.
[b] EVAR with concomitant unilateral iliac artery embolization.
[c] Unsuccessful attempt at preserving hypogastric patency at initial surgery (patient lived).

controversial, it is thought to result primarily from embolism of particulate thrombus within the aneurysm sac rather than from a global physiologic insult [48–51]. Occlusion of the hypogastric arteries has led to the development of severe buttock claudication and pelvic ischemia, and this has also been hypothesized to be an additional potential factor in the development of colonic ischemia, by way of occlusion of one of the collateral pathways [49]. In addition, perioperative contributing factors similar to those for open repair, such as hypotension, blood loss, and occlusion of the IMA following graft deployment, are suggested causative sources.

The benefits of EVAR in reducing perioperative complications and hospital length of stay have been clearly demonstrated. The relatively small number of case series reporting the incidence of ischemia in EVAR suggests that EVAR is associated with, on average, a lower risk of developing ischemic colitis than open AAA repair, but the nationwide incidence of ischemia following EVAR compared with open AAA repair is unknown. If continued experience with EVAR demonstrates a lower risk than open AAA repair, this will yield yet another benefit of EVAR in the treatment of AAA. Endovascular repair should not preclude the ability to preserve the potential collateral blood supply by maintaining vascular flow to at least one internal iliac artery [52]. Unfortunately, the advent of catheter-based technology has also led to the development of known complications though new means that have not yet been described. For example, ischemic colitis has recently been reported following translumbar injection with 8000 units of thrombin for the treatment of an endoleak into the native aneurysm sac from the originating lumbar vessel [53]. This case of ischemic colitis was felt to originate from an embolization of the rectosigmoid arcade through the IMA, leaving the investigators to speculate about the need for IMA outflow occlusion before thrombin injection. Again, as further experience with minimally invasive and catheter-based procedures takes place, one can anticipate increased knowledge into not only the mechanisms of injury but also ways to avoid this complication.

Treatment

Supportive

The mainstay of therapy for ischemic colitis remains supportive therapy, with adequate fluid hydration and blood pressure support. Vasopressor support is controversial because it is also a contributing factor. Low-flow states and sepsis may require improvement in blood pressure; however, in general, because of the vasoconstriction of the splanchnic vessels, vasopressors may add to the ischemic process, worsening the situation. Should pressor support be necessary, beta-adrenergic agonists that also improve cardiac output are preferred, and one should make every attempt to avoid alpha-agonists if possible. Additionally, broad spectrum antibiotics such as fluoroquinolones and flagyl, or monotherapy with Unasyn or Imipenem have been shown to decrease bacterial translocation and morbidity, and should be added empirically [54]. Most of the studies emphasizing the value of nonoperative therapy do have a degree of self-selection, because those patients "healthy" enough to undergo a trial of nonoperative management by definition are likely to be in a more stable condition and have not manifested signs of overt bowel infarction. Yet they are still at high risk for complications and death, with Longo reporting a single death in a study of 16 patients who had ischemic colitis following nonoperative therapy [22]. With rare exceptions, all patients who have evidence of bowel infarction require surgical therapy.

Surgery

Surgical options generally fall into two categories: bowel resection and vascular reconstruction. Typically, when patients require operative intervention, the surgeon must first determine bowel viability. Caution, however, must ensue because often, in cases with less than full-thickness injury and frank necrosis, the serosal appearance of the bowel does not accurately reflect the degree of ischemic changes to the entire bowel wall. Therefore, surgeons must either rely on the endoscopic appearance and extent of the ischemic changes (which, as stated, is not always accurate) or use adjunctive measures to evaluate the viability of the bowel.

Intraoperatively, several different methods have been described for providing surgeons with additional useful information regarding blood flow. The surgeon must balance the need to avoid leaving behind necrotic bowel with the potential morbidity of overzealous resection leading to short-bowel syndrome. Clinically, unlike mesenteric ischemia of the small bowel, motility does not provide as much help when dealing with the colon. The intraoperative judgment of the well-trained surgeon remains one of the most important factors. Palpation of mesenteric pulses or detecting Doppler signals on the antimesenteric portion of the bowel wall also provides valuable information. Woods lamp evaluation of the bowel wall following administration of fluorescein dye intravenously can also aid in separating perfused from nonperfused bowel. Surgeons have classically mandated a second-look operation in 12 to 48 hours, regardless of the patient's clinical condition, to evaluate the need for further resection and to aid in being less aggressive at resecting potentially viable bowel at the initial surgery [55]. The already elevated mortality of 50% to 67% is even higher, should surgical resection of infarcted bowel be present at the second operation. Longo and colleagues [14] found an 89% mortality for patients meeting this condition. Further highlighting the need for early diagnosis, in 1991 van Vroonhoven and colleagues [56] published a series of 20 patients who had ischemic colitis following ruptured aortic aneurysm. Eighteen patients required a laparotomy for transmural involvement, with all 20 patients dying during the hospitalization. Although the investigators questioned the usefulness of bowel resection in these patients, it may simply suggest that diagnosis delayed past a certain point in the pathologic process portends almost certain mortality.

Vascular repair involves two separate components and is performed in the acute and chronic ischemia settings. First, patency of the IMA supplying the most at-risk portion of the left colon must be assured. Should the ischemic changes be present in other areas of the colon, attention is focused on that particular region's vascular supply. In addition, determining the antegrade flow to the iliac vessels that provide potential pelvic collaterals needs to be a routine part of both the open and endovascular techniques. Although the technical aspects of vascular reconstruction are beyond the scope of this article, options for dealing with the IMA or other major visceral vessel include resection of the base of the IMA along with a small cuff of aortic wall (Carrell patch) and reimplanting it in the aortic graft, patch angioplasty of the stenotic opening, bypass grafting, or endarterectomy of the atherosclerotic plaque [57,58]. Finally, with the development of improved technology, endovascular approaches have also been described in the treatment of segmental ischemic colitis [59]. However, in the absence of further data, the role that this technology plays in this setting remains undefined.

Review of the literature

Outcome

When reviewing the literature on this topic, two points become apparent. First, most published series are retrospective in nature and, in general, contain a small cohort of patients. Second, the degree and extent of colitis have a large impact on overall outcome. In a study of 43 patients over 6 years, segmental colitis was present in most patients (72%) [15]. Those patients in whom the entire colon was affected with ischemic changes had a much worse prognosis, with all requiring surgery and an overall mortality of 75%. Fortunately, ischemic colitis most often affects only the mucosa and most patients are able to be treated successfully using nonoperative means. Surgery is then relegated only to those in the direst of clinical conditions or those presenting with frank peritonitis from infarcted bowel. Those patients who are well enough to be treated with nonoperative means have better outcomes. In a series of 278 patients undergoing EVAR, only 8 developed ischemic colitis [48]. Two patients died immediately, with an additional death in one of the two undergoing surgery, for a mortality of 38% in those with ischemic changes. Yet all four patients who were treated nonoperatively survived. Although results like these are difficult to compare across different series secondary to a large selection bias, they do underscore the wide range of disease severity that occurs in these patients.

Reimplantation of the IMA has also had varied results. In a study of 10 colonic ischemia patients over a 10-year period, reimplantation was deemed necessary in 5 patients because of inadequate colonic perfusion at the time of open aortic repair. Ultimately, transmural (versus limited mucosal) necrosis occurred in 60%, including four of the five patients who were felt to have a technically successful reimplantation [60]. In all six of these cases, intraoperative hypotension was also felt to be a contributing factor. A drawback to this study is the investigators' lack of reporting of the total rate of IMA reimplantation that did not develop ischemic changes over the course of the study; thus, the overall success rate is unknown. However, these results emphasize the need for preventing the factors that may lead to ischemic changes, because in some cases the initial ischemic insult may be nonreversible, even with a technically successful attempt that improves blood flow to the ischemic segment.

A small percentage of patients develop ischemic colitis following surgery, require an initial operative bowel resection, survive, and then go on to require a second operative procedure apart from a "planned take-back." These patients have an even higher mortality, with one study reporting death in seven of eight patients [61]. Indications for the second exploration include sepsis of unknown origin, attempt at further revascularization, and evidence of additional infarcted bowel. Yet the end result remains similar, with a very high mortality rate. Thus, despite an initial stabilization, the at-risk patient requires continued high-intensity monitoring, with efforts directed at controlling blood pressure, sepsis, and secondary injury.

Chronic changes

Patients sustaining a bout of ischemic colitis who are able to recover fully may have varying degrees of symptoms, ranging from completely asymptomatic, mild constipation, or near-obstructing colonic strictures (Fig. 2). Because of the overall high mortality with fulminate disease and the lack of presentation with milder forms, the true rate of colonic stricture following nonoperative management is unknown. Similarly, the rate of recurrent ischemic colitis has not been well delineated. Longo and colleagues [22] found no rate of relapse at a mean follow-up of 5.3 years in his 47 patients. Yet high-quality, longitudinal studies with adequate follow-up are lacking. Therefore, patients should be counseled on discharge about the potential future ramifications of this disease.

Other patients may develop chronic visceral ischemia, which is manifested by abdominal pain, especially with eating, when supply does not equal demand; this condition may lead to relative bowel ischemia, which may result ultimately in food fear and weight loss. Complete visceral artery revascularization of celiac, superior mesenteric, and inferior mesenteric arteries is often required to alleviate symptoms. Occasionally, however, patients will only be able to have a single IMA revascularization because of technical failures or other considerations. Although data on this procedure are limited, a study of 11 patients over a 6-year period in which isolated IMA repair was performed showed 10 patients with improved or cured symptoms perioperatively and 70% still with patent repairs and symptomatic improvement at longer follow-up [57]. For this procedure to be a success, a well-developed pattern of collateral circulation for the IMA system is required and this should be evaluated before considering this option.

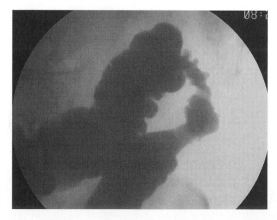

Fig. 2. Barium enema, demonstrating splenic flexure stricture from chronic ischemic colitis.

Finally, concerns regarding infection of the aortic prosthetic graft leading to higher mortality and subsequent complications are present not only in the acute but also in the chronic setting. Infection of the graft has been shown to lead to complications such as need for graft explantation, revascularization including extra-anatomic bypass, aortoduodenal fistula, sepsis, and death following both the open and EVAR settings [62–64]. Yet endovascular graft placement along with prolonged antibiotics has also been described in case reports as a potential treatment for patients who have known infected aneurysms, although recommendation awaits further data collection [65]. Although the comparative rates of graft infection for the endovascular and open settings following ischemic colitis are unknown, theoretic advantages to the endovascular approach include preservation of natural tissue planes secondary to lack of opening up the retroperitoneum during repair. Thus, the graft is never exposed to topical contamination. Should this be borne out in the future, it will provide a further advantage to the endovascular method in this unique setting.

Summary

Ischemic colitis following vascular surgery continues to carry a high morbidity and mortality. Extensive effort has gone into the development of new techniques to diagnose and treat this condition at earlier stages. Physicians need to carry a high degree of suspicion as to the diagnosis because, unfortunately, many patients may have a paucity of symptoms early, leading to a delay in work-up and worse outcomes. Supportive treatment remains the mainstay, including blood pressure, fluid support, and broad-spectrum antibiotics. Although surgical therapy, including bowel resection or vascular reconstruction, remains an option, the development of this condition unfortunately still portends a poor prognosis.

References

[1] Michael H, Brandt LJ, Hochsztein JG. Ischemic colitis complicating aortic dissection. Gastrointest Endosc 2002;55(3):442–4.
[2] Najibi S, Terramani TT, Weiss VJ, et al. Endoluminal versus open treatment of descending thoracic aortic aneurysms. J Vasc Surg 2002;36(4):732–7.
[3] Boley SJ, Schwartz S, Lash J, et al. Reversible vascular occlusion of the colon. Surg Gynecol Obstet 1963;116:53–60.
[4] Marston A, Pheils MT, Thomas ML, et al. Ischemic colitis. Gut 1966;7(1):1–15.
[5] Rausis C, Mirkovitch V, Robinson JW, et al. Colonic ischaemia after prosthetic replacement of the abdominal aorta and other forms of ischaemic colitis. Schweiz Rundsch Med Prax 1974;63(18):545–9.
[6] Ernst CB, Hagihara PF, Daugherty ME, et al. Ischemic colitis incidence following abdominal aortic reconstruction: a prospective study. Surgery 1976;80(4):417–21.
[7] Ernst CB, Hagihara PF, Daugherty ME, et al. Inferior mesenteric artery stump pressure: a reliable index for safe IMA ligation during abdominal aortic aneurysmectomy. Ann Surg 1978; 187:641–6.

[8] Hagihara PF, Ernst CB, Griffen WO Jr. Incidence of ischemic colitis following abdominal aortic reconstruction. Surg Gynecol Obstet 1979;149:571–3.

[9] Connolly JE, Stammer EA. Intestinal gangrene as the result of mesenteric arterial steal. Am J Surg 1973;126:197–204.

[10] Jarvinen O, Laurikka J, Salenius JP, et al. Mesenteric infarction after aortoiliac surgery on the basis of 1752 operations from the National Vascular Registry. World J Surg 1999;23(3): 243–7.

[11] Porcellini M, Renda A, Selvetella L, et al. Intestinal ischemia after aortic surgery. Int Surg 1996;81(2):195–9.

[12] Sandison AJ, Panayiotopoulos Y, Edmondson RC, et al. A 4-year prospective audit of the cause of death after infrarenal aortic aneurysm surgery. Br J Surg 1996;83(10):1386–9.

[13] Assadian A, Assadian O, Senekowitsch C, et al. Plasma D-lactate as a potential early marker for colon ischaemia after open aortic reconstruction. Eur J Vasc Endovasc Surg 2006;31(5): 470–4.

[14] Longo WE, Lee TC, Barnett MG, et al. Ischemic colitis complicating abdominal aortic aneurysm surgery in the U.S. veteran. J Surg Res 1996;60(2):351–4.

[15] Longo WE, Ward D, Vernava AM III, et al. Outcome of patients with total colonic ischemia. Dis Colon Rectum 1997;40(12):1448–54.

[16] Gandhi SK, Hanson MM, Vernava AM, et al. Ischemic colitis. Dis Colon Rectum 1996; 39(1):88–100.

[17] Jaeger HJ, Mathias KD, Gissler HM, et al. Rectum and sigmoid colon necrosis due to cholesterol embolization after implantation of an aortic stent-graft. J Vasc Interv Radiol 1999;10(6):751–5.

[18] Redaelli CA, Schilling MK, Carrel TP. Intraoperative assessment of intestinal viability by laser Doppler flowmetry for surgery of ruptured abdominal aortic aneurysms. World J Surg 1998;22(3):283–9.

[19] Israeli D, Dardik H, Wolodiger F, et al. Pelvic radiation therapy as a risk factor for ischemic colitis complicating abdominal aortic reconstruction. J Vasc Surg 1996;23(4):706–9.

[20] Wellwood JM, Jackson BT. The intestinal complications of radiotherapy. Br J Surg 1973; 60(10):814–8.

[21] Yamazaki T, Shirai Y, Tada T, et al. Ischemic colitis arising in watershed areas of the colonic blood supply: a report of two cases. Surg Today 1997;27(5):460–2.

[22] Longo WE, Ballantyne GH, Gusberg RJ. Ischemic colitis: patterns and prognosis. Dis Colon Rectum 1992;35(8):726–30.

[23] Lange H, Jackel R. Usefulness of plasma lactate concentration in the diagnosis of acute abdominal disease. Eur J Surg 1994;160(6–7):381–4.

[24] Sakakibara Y, Jikuya T, Saito EM, et al. Does laser Doppler flowmetry aid the prevention of ischemic colitis in abdominal aortic aneurysm surgery? Thorac Cardiovasc Surg 1997;45(1): 32–4.

[25] Lee ES, Bass A, Arko FR, et al. Intraoperative colon mucosal oxygen saturation during aortic surgery. J Surg Res 2006;136(1):19–24.

[26] Forde KA, Lebwohl O, Wolff M, et al. Reversible ischemic colitis: correlation of colonoscopic and pathologic changes. Am J Gastroenterol 1979;72:182–5.

[27] Houe T, Thorboll JE, Sigild U, et al. Can colonoscopy diagnose transmural ischaemic colitis after abdominal aortic surgery? An evidence-based approach. Eur J Vasc Endovasc Surg 2000;19(3):304–7.

[28] Fanti L, Masci E, Mariani A, et al. Is endoscopy useful for early diagnosis of ischemic colitis after aortic surgery? Results of a prospective trial. Ital J Gastroenterol Hepatol 1997;29(4): 357–60.

[29] Brandt CP, Piotrowski JJ, Alexander JJ. Flexible sigmoidoscopy. A reliable determinant of ischemia following ruptured abdominal aortic aneurysm. Surg Endosc 1997;11(2):113–5.

[30] Wiesner W, Mortele KJ, Glickman JN, et al. CT findings in isolated ischemic proctosigmoiditis. Eur Radiol 2002;12(7):1762–7.

[31] Bjorck M, Bergqvist D, Troeng T. Incidence and clinical presentation of bowel ischaemia after aortoiliac surgery–2930 operations from a population-based registry in Sweden. Eur J Vasc Endovasc Surg 1996;12:139–44.

[32] Bjorck M, Troeng T, Bergqvist D. Risk factors for intestinal ischaemia after aortoiliac surgery: a combined cohort and case-control study of 2824 operations. Eur J Vasc Endovasc Surg 1997;13:531–9.

[33] Valentine RJ, Hagino RT, Jackson MR, et al. Gastrointestinal complications after aortic surgery. J Vasc Surg 1998;28(3):404–11.

[34] Killen DA, Reed WA, Gorton ME, et al. Is routine postaneurysmectomy hemodynamic assessment of the inferior mesenteric artery helpful? Ann Vasc Surg 1999;13(5):533–8.

[35] Kaiser MM, Wenk H, Sassen R, et al. Ischemic colitis after vascular surgery reconstruction of an abdominal aortic aneurysm. Chirurg 1996;67(4):380–6.

[36] Piotrowski JJ, Ripepi AJ, Yuhas JP, et al. Colonic ischemia: the Achilles heel of ruptured aortic aneurysm repair. Am Surg 1996;62(7):557–60.

[37] Seeger JM, Coe DA, Kaelin LD, et al. Routine reimplantation of patent inferior mesenteric arteries limits colon infarction after aortic reconstruction. J Vasc Surg 1992;15(4):635–41.

[38] Parodi JC, Palmaz JC, Barone HD. Transfemoral intraluminal graft implantation for abdominal aortic aneurysms. Ann Vasc Surg 1991;5:491–9.

[39] Dillavou ED, Muluk SC, Makaroun MS. Improving aneurysm-related outcomes: nationwide benefits of endovascular repair. J Vasc Surg 2006;43:446–51.

[40] Lee WA, Carter JW, Upchurch G, et al. Perioperative outcomes after open and endovascular repair of intact abdominal aortic aneurysms in the United States during 2001. J Vasc Surg 2004;39:491–6.

[41] Nevelsteen I, Duchatcau J, De Vleeschauwer P, et al. Ischaemic colitis after endovascular repair of an infrarenal abdominal aortic aneurysm: a case report. Acta Chir Belg 2006;106(5): 588–91.

[42] Mehta M, Taggert J, Darling RC 3rd, et al. Establishing a protocol for endovascular treatment of ruptured aortic aneurysms: outcomes of a prospective analysis. J Vasc Surg 2006; 44(1):1–8.

[43] Lee C, Dougherty M, Calligaro K. Concomitant unilateral internal iliac artery embolization and endovascular infrarenal aortic aneurysm repair. J Vasc Surg 2006;43(5):903–7.

[44] Mehta M, Roddy SP, Darling RC 3rd, et al. Infrarenal abdominal aortic aneurysm repair via endovascular versus open retroperitoneal approach. Ann Vasc Surg 2005;19(3):374–8.

[45] Axelrod DJ, Lookstein RA, Guller J, et al. Inferior mesenteric artery embolization before endovascular aneurysm repair: technique and initial results. J Vasc Interv Radiol 2004; 15(11):1263–7.

[46] Verhoeven EL, Prins TR, van den Dungen JJ, et al. Endovascular repair of acute AAAs under local anesthesia with bifurcated endografts: a feasibility study. J Endovasc Ther 2002;9(6):729–35.

[47] Champagne BJ, Lee EC, Valerian B, et al. Incidence of colonic ischemia after repair of ruptured abdominal aortic aneurysm with endograft. J Am Coll Surg 2007;204:597–602.

[48] Dadian N, Ohki T, Veith FJ, et al. Overt colon ischemia after endovascular aneurysm repair: the importance of microembolization as an etiology. J Vasc Surg 2001;34(6):986–96.

[49] Geraghty PJ, Sanchez LA, Rubin BG, et al. Overt ischemic colitis after endovascular repair of aortoiliac aneurysms. J Vasc Surg 2004;40(3):413–8.

[50] Maldonado TS, Rockman CB, Riles E, et al. Ischemic complications after endovascular abdominal aortic aneurysm repair. J Vasc Surg 2004;40(4):703–9.

[51] Zhang WW, Kuyaylat MN, Anain PM, et al. Embolization as cause of bowel ischemia after endovascular abdominal aortic aneurysm repair. J Vasc Surg 2004;40(5):867–72.

[52] Welborn MB 3rd, Seeger JM. Prevention and management of sigmoid and pelvic ischemia associated with aortic surgery. Semin Vasc Surg 2001;14(4):255–65.

[53] Gambaro E, Abou-Zamzam AM Jr, Teruya TH, et al. Ischemic colitis following translumbar thrombin injection for treatment of endoleak. Ann Vasc Surg 2004;18(1):74–8.

[54] van Saene HK, Percival A. Bowel microorganisms—a target for selective antimicrobial control. J Hosp Infect 1991;19(Suppl C):19–41.

[55] Kaminsky O, Yampolski I, Aranovich D, et al. Does a second-look operation improve survival in patients with peritonitis due to acute mesenteric ischemia? A five-year retrospective experience. World J Surg 2005;29(5):645–8.

[56] van Vroonhoven TJ, Verhagen HJ, Broker WF, et al. Transmural ischaemic colitis following operation for ruptured abdominal aortic aneurysm. Neth J Surg 1991;43(3):56–9.

[57] Schneider DB, Nelken NA, Messina LM, et al. Isolated inferior mesenteric artery revascularization for chronic visceral ischemia. J Vasc Surg 1999;30(1):51–8.

[58] Rapp JH, Reilly LM, Qvarfordt PG, et al. Durability of endarterectomy and antegrade grafts in the treatment of chronic visceral ischemia. J Vasc Surg 1986;3(5):799–806.

[59] Bailey JA, Jacobs DL, Bahadursingh A, et al. Endovascular treatment of segmental ischemic colitis. Dig Dis Sci 2005;50(4):774–9.

[60] Mitchell KM, Valentine RJ. Inferior mesenteric artery reimplantation does not guarantee colon viability in aortic surgery. J Am Coll Surg 2002;194(2):151–5.

[61] Parish KL, Chapman WC, Williams LF Jr. Ischemic colitis. An ever-changing spectrum? Am Surg 1991;57(2):118–21.

[62] Ruby BJ, Cogbill TH. Aortoduodenal fistula 5 years after endovascular abdominal aortic aneurysm repair with the Ancure stent graft. J Vasc Surg 2007;45(4):834–6.

[63] DeBast Y, Creemers E. Infection of an abdominal aortic stent graft with suprarenal attachment. Ann Vasc Surg 2006;20(6):736–8.

[64] Ghosh J, Murray D, Khwaja N, et al. Late infection of an endovascular stent graft with septic embolization, colonic perforation, and aortoduodenal fistula. Ann Vasc Surg 2006; 20(2):263–6.

[65] Lee KH, Won JY, Lee do Y, et al. Stent-graft treatment of infection aortic and arterial aneurysms. J Endovasc Ther 2006;13(3):338–45.

SURGICAL
CLINICS OF
NORTH AMERICA

ELSEVIER
SAUNDERS

Surg Clin N Am 87 (2007) 1115–1134

Acute and Chronic Mesenteric Ischemia

Garth S. Herbert, MD, Scott R. Steele, MD, FACS*

Madigan Army Medical Center, Department of Surgery, Fort Lewis, Tacoma, WA 98431, USA

Although advances in diagnostic imaging, surgical technique, asepsis, and antibiotics have improved outcomes in most surgical diseases over the last several decades, mesenteric ischemia remains a highly morbid condition. Fortunately it remains a rare occurrence, accounting for less than 1 in every 1000 hospital admissions [1]. Likewise, mortality rates remain elevated at 30% to 90%, depending on the etiology [2–6], and may in fact be even higher if deaths in patients who have undiagnosed mesenteric ischemia are considered. In one review, only one third of patients who had acute mesenteric ischemia were correctly diagnosed before surgical exploration or death [5]. Another review of autopsy cases in Sweden suggested true mortality rates may exceed 90% for mesenteric ischemia, and in only 33% was the diagnosis even considered before death [7]. Despite its relative infrequency, the high morbidity and mortality rates thus underscore the need for surgeons to be acutely aware of the presentation and management of this disease process.

Mesenteric ischemia occurs when visceral tissues receive inadequate blood flow. This may be a consequence of an arterial embolus or thrombosis, venous thrombosis limiting arterial inflow, or even extrinsic compression of mesenteric vessels. Smooth muscle tone within the mesenteric vessels is heavily autoregulated, increasing splanchnic blood flow after a large meal from 10% of cardiac output at rest to up to 35% [8]. When demand exceeds the capacity of the mesenteric circulation because of intrinsic or extrinsic lesions, the bowel becomes ischemic, with the mucosa being most vulnerable to inadequate blood flow.

The diagnosis of mesenteric ischemia is often one of exclusion, made after eliminating more common possibilities. Patients most often present with abdominal pain, unfortunately a vague complaint common to scores of other diagnoses. Other associated symptoms, such as nausea, vomiting,

* Corresponding author.
E-mail address: docsteele@hotmail.com (S.R. Steele).

0039-6109/07/$ - see front matter. Published by Elsevier Inc.
doi:10.1016/j.suc.2007.07.016

diarrhea, and bloating may also be present in various combinations [5,9,10], although their presence is likewise nonspecific. The differential diagnosis in patients presenting with these symptoms thus remains broad and includes ulcer disease, bowel obstruction, complications of cholelithiasis, pancreatitis, inflammatory bowel disease, appendicitis, diverticulitis, or simply gastroenteritis. Elevated anion gap, elevated lactate levels, and leukocytosis may be found on laboratory analysis. Elevated lactate levels, a reflection of ongoing anaerobic metabolism, is suggestive of an ischemic process. Like most other laboratory studies that may be measured in the evaluation of a patient who has abdominal pain, however, it is not specific for mesenteric ischemia [11]. Additional information can then be garnered from primary diagnostic imaging modalities, including computed tomographic angiography (CTA), duplex ultrasonography, and magnetic resonance angiography (MRA). Although suspicion of bowel infarction mandates urgent surgical therapy directed at potential resection of nonviable bowel, the underlying etiology of mesenteric ischemia may be managed by open and endovascular techniques.

This article briefly reviews the various etiologies, presentation, and diagnosis of different types of mesenteric ischemia. Operative management techniques and the applicability of percutaneous endovascular intervention are discussed. Finally, the authors explore emerging technologies that have the potential to further improve diagnosis and treatment of this frequently lethal disease process.

Types of mesenteric ischemia

Embolic

Embolism to the visceral vessels is the most common cause of mesenteric ischemia, responsible for approximately 30% to 50% of cases [3,12]. Risk factors for visceral emboli include atrial fibrillation, myocardial infarction with subsequent impaired wall motion, and structural heart defects (ie, right-to-left shunts). The acute nature of embolic disease results in rapid progression of symptoms, because collateral blood supply is limited with acute occlusion. The acuity of the presentation in combination with frequent delays in diagnosis contributes to a high mortality rate, which averages 70% for visceral emboli in a review of several published reports [2]. The superior mesenteric artery (SMA) is more commonly involved than the celiac axis (CA) or inferior mesenteric artery (IMA) because of its less acute angle of takeoff from the aorta. Emboli typically lodge distal to the takeoff of the middle colic artery, sparing the duodenum and the transverse colon—a characteristic that can often help differentiate it from thrombosis that typically occurs more proximally [11,13]. The typical patient who has visceral ischemia from an embolic source reports the sudden onset of severe pain. Physical examination is often notable for the lack of guarding or peritoneal signs, so-called "pain out of proportion" to examination. Peritoneal findings may occur late, following embolic occurrences, after the development of infarcted bowel, and typically portend worse outcomes. Despite the classic description, only one third of patients who have embolic disease present with the triad of abdominal pain, bloody stools, and fever associated with acute mesenteric ischemia [12]. Clearly mesenteric ischemia must be considered early, especially in patients who have risk factors for atherosclerotic disease, and should be worked up aggressively in those presenting with abdominal pain and other associated symptoms that do not rapidly conform to another diagnosis.

Thrombotic

Thrombosis of arterial mesenteric inflow accounts for only 15% to 30% of cases of mesenteric ischemia. It is the most morbid of the various types, however, with an accompanying 90% mortality in a review of several studies [2]. This high mortality rate has been postulated to be a consequence of proximal thromboses affecting a greater percentage of the overall bowel. One study attempting to correlate the length of bowel with the site of thrombosis or embolus in the SMA (proximal versus distal), however, found no association between the site of occlusion and length of nonviable bowel [13]. With regard to presenting symptoms, most patients suffering from acute mesenteric arterial thrombosis have a history of chronic mesenteric ischemia (CMI) [3,14], with symptoms of weight loss, abdominal pain, and food fear predating the acute episode of mesenteric ischemia.

Venous thrombosis accounts for a minority of cases but is associated with a mortality rate between 20% and 50% [15,16]. Although many cases are associated with cirrhosis or portal hypertension, other etiologies include malignancy, pancreatitis, oral contraceptive use, inheritable hypercoagulable states to include factor V Leiden, protein C deficiency, or prothrombin 20,210 mutation, and a history of recent surgery [4,12,16,17]. In fact, approximately half of patients presenting with venous thrombosis have had a deep venous thrombosis or pulmonary embolus in the past [16]. Presentations vary from acute to chronic, depending on the rapidity with which the clot develops. Pain is more prominent in acute thrombosis, and bowel infarction is more likely in this group. Those patients who have chronic thrombosis rarely have pain, and development of esophageal or gastric varices is far more likely than bowel infarction [4]. Most important, mesenteric venous thrombosis should be considered and ruled out early in patients who have a history of a venous thrombosis or other hypercoagulable states who present with abdominal pain.

Nonocclusive ischemia

In the absence of arterial or venous occlusion, mesenteric ischemia may still occur in low-flow states. As atherosclerosis remains a systemic disease, those patients manifesting disease elsewhere often have plaque involving the SMA, IMA, and CA. In fact, autopsy studies suggest the prevalence of atherosclerotic involvement of these vessels is between 30% and 50% [18]. Clearly most of these patients are asymptomatic, because retrospective autopsy studies evaluating the cause of death suggest the incidence of mesenteric ischemia is less than 0.01% in the general population [19,20]. Other contributing factors to nonocclusive mesenteric ischemia include the use of vasopressors, digitalis, and cocaine, which have been documented to exacerbate ischemia in the setting of pre-existing lesions [3].

Patients who have CMI typically present with postprandial abdominal pain and associated weight loss, consistent with a supply-demand mismatch process. Women are more commonly affected than men, with the stereotypical patient suffering from mesenteric ischemia being a cachectic woman in her sixth to seventh decade of life. Physical examination may reveal an epigastric bruit in 48% to 63% of patients [18,21], indicative of turbulent flow through an area of vascular narrowing. A history of smoking, peripheral vascular disease, and hypertension is also frequently present [14,22]. In addition, patients may demonstrate evidence of gallbladder dysmotility, gastroparesis, or gastric ulcers as a reflection of disease in the CA [14].

Finally, although CMI is most commonly caused by atherosclerotic disease, extrinsic compression of the CA can lead to mesenteric ischemia. Most commonly this results from impingement of the diaphragm on the CA, although the surrounding nerve plexus may also contribute to compression [23]. This syndrome, more commonly occurring in females, is known as the median arcuate ligament syndrome, also referred to as celiac compression syndrome [18,24]. This diagnosis should be considered in young patients who have unexplained abdominal pain and normal upper endoscopy, normal liver, pancreatic, and gastric laboratory studies, and particularly in those patients who have an abdominal bruit (from partially obstructed flow in the CA) [23].

Diagnosis

Angiography

Angiography was traditionally the gold standard for the diagnosis of mesenteric ischemia. The development of multidetector row computed tomography (CT), however, has permitted detailed analysis of vascular flow that was never before possible, thereby relegating angiography to more of a confirmatory role [25]. Furthermore, angiography remains an invasive technique that requires the availability of an endovascular specialist, a luxury not consistently available emergently at most medical centers. These weaknesses aside, angiography is the lone diagnostic modality that offers the potential therapeutic options for mesenteric ischemia (see section on treatment).

Typically aortography is performed with anterior and lateral views. Lateral films provide optimal visualization for detecting proximal disease, permitting analysis of the takeoff of the CA, the SMA, and the IMA [18]. Anterior views, however, are essential to diagnose ischemia caused by poor perfusion in the distal mesenteric vessels [11]. When nonocclusive ischemia is suggested by angiography, intra-arterial infusion of vasodilators such as papaverine or prostaglandin E1 may also be used to augment blood flow if a test dose suggests the limitations in flow are reversible by augmenting arterial flow [26]. Mesenteric venous thrombosis may be suggested by a slowing in arterial inflow and filling defects in mesenteric veins or absent flow in veins with reliance on collateral routes of drainage [26]. Digital subtraction angiography can be helpful in improving resolution of the images and in reducing the contrast load necessary to permit adequate evaluation [18]. Finally, angiography may be the best diagnostic modality to confirm the diagnosis of median arcuate ligament syndrome, in which dynamic compression of the CA is demonstrated with a combination of inspiratory and expiratory images (Fig. 1) [27].

Ultrasound

Advances in resolution of commercially available ultrasound devices have permitted the identification of mesenteric vessels transabdominally. Doppler waveform analysis has further permitted the detailed

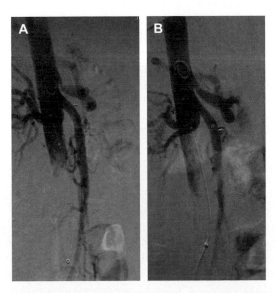

Fig. 1. These lateral aortogram images demonstrate arcuate median ligament syndrome (also referred to as celiac compression syndrome). (*A*) Relatively unobstructed flow through the celiac axis at end inspiration. (*B*) At end expiration, pronounced reduction in the diameter of the proximal celiac axis.

characterization of blood flow necessary for identification of stenotic or occluded mesenteric vessels. Duplex ultrasonography, combining B-mode ultrasonography with Doppler waveform analysis, has thus led to the emergence of ultrasound as a diagnostic option in mesenteric ischemia. The examiner not only receives an anatomic view of the vessel, but also flow detail corroborating the findings.

Established criteria for the diagnosis of mesenteric stenosis focus on the peak systolic velocity (PSV) and end diastolic velocity (EDV) as measured by duplex ultrasonography. Zwolak and colleagues [28] found an EDV greater than 45 cm/s to be 100% sensitive for detecting greater than 50% stenosis of the SMA, with retrograde common hepatic flow being the most sensitive indicator of stenosis of the CA. Other studies argue that the PSV offers greater sensitivity than EDV in diagnosing stenosis of the SMA or CA, with respective velocities greater than 275 cm/s and 200 cm/s indicating greater than 70% stenosis in these vessels [29,30]. Duplex evaluation following a meal (similar to exercise when evaluating cardiac flow) provided no increase in sensitivity in one study evaluating SMA stenoses; therefore, it is not commonly performed [31].

Although ultrasound diagnosis of mesenteric ischemia remains promising, the technique has several shortcomings. First, the IMA is often difficult to visualize with duplex ultrasonography; nonetheless, mesenteric ischemia is rare in the presence of normal flow in the CA and SMA [14]. Ultrasonography requires the availability of a skilled registered vascular technologist or physician capable of producing reliable images. Next, ultrasound evaluation may be limited by patient body habitus (obesity in particular makes evaluation more challenging), previous intra-abdominal surgeries, patient compliance, and the presence of bowel gas [30]. Evaluation following abstinence from oral intake for 8 hours is often recommended for an optimal study [30]. Yet this is rarely the situation encountered in practice, especially in the emergent setting. Ultrasound may therefore remain more suitable for evaluation of CMI until there are further enhancements in technology and technique for this diagnostic modality.

Computed tomography

CT evaluation for mesenteric ischemia remains an attractive choice, because the examination is rapid, noninvasive, and widely available in most hospitals. Early evaluations of mesenteric ischemia by CT, however, showed a disappointing sensitivity of only 64% [32]. Subsequently the development of multidetector row CT has greatly improved the images obtained with this technique. In one recent prospective study involving 62 patients undergoing biphasic multidetector row CT (involving arterial and portal phase evaluations), mesenteric ischemia was identified as a possible diagnosis in all 26 who were ultimately determined to have mesenteric ischemia [33]. Of note, only eight of these patients had arterial abnormalities noted on the CT angiogram, demonstrating the importance of associated bowel findings in making the diagnosis [33]. Although the diagnosis made by CT altered treatment in only 5 patients (19% of those with mesenteric ischemia), this prospective study confirmed the ability of CT to accurately diagnose acute mesenteric ischemia, contradicting earlier reports that questioned its usefulness [33].

Although findings of vessel occlusion or significant narrowing may be seen on CT angiogram, associated changes in the bowel wall more often offer clues to the diagnosis. By providing the ability to evaluate the bowel also, a diagnosis of mesenteric ischemia can be aided by findings such as wall thickening, mucosal enhancement, intramural air, or dilatation, in addition to ominous signs such as portal venous gas (Fig. 2) [25,33–35]. In isolation, the sensitivity of these findings varies widely. Kirkpatrick and colleagues [33], however, suggest that the presence of portal venous gas, pneumatosis, or a combination of bowel wall thickening with venous thrombosis, solid organ infarction, or focal lack of enhancement of bowel wall seen on CTA as criteria for the diagnosis of mesenteric ischemia results in sensitivity of 96% and specificity of 94%.

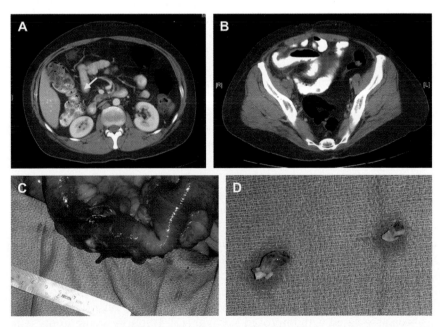

Fig. 2. These selected images are from a CT scan of a patient who had acute mesenteric ischemia secondary to a nearly occluded SMA from an embolic source (*arrow, A*) and resultant small bowel thickening in the ischemic ileum (*B*). At laparotomy, the distal ileum was found to be ischemic (*C*) and was resected; an SMA thrombectomy (*D*) and patch angioplasty was performed.

Magnetic resonance imaging

Several reports have established the usefulness of MRI in making the diagnosis of CMI. One study demonstrated significant postprandial reduction in the amount of blood flow in the SMA in healthy volunteers as compared with patients who had documented SMA stenosis [36]. Burkart and colleagues [37] documented a similar reduction in superior mesenteric and portal venous flow in patients who had CMI when compared with healthy volunteers. Finally, Lauenstein and associates [38] demonstrated decreased bowel wall enhancement following contrast administration in patients who had symptoms of mesenteric ischemia and stenosis documented angiographically. The time required to perform MRI examinations and the possible need for bowel stimulation with a meal limit the usefulness of MRI in the diagnosis of acute mesenteric ischemia, making it more appropriate for evaluating the chronic state. Even so, CTA is likely a better examination than MRI for the diagnosis of CMI because of its capacity for higher resolution in combination with faster scans [39].

Management of mesenteric ischemia

Patients who have suspected mesenteric ischemia must receive adequate fluid resuscitation, because capillary leak in the setting of visceral ischemia may lead to significant fluid shifts. To avoid exacerbating visceral ischemia, a preference should be given to β-adrenergic agonists such as dopamine when vasopressors are required [3]. In addition, empiric, broad-spectrum antibiotics such as imipenem [3] are recommended, because ischemia leads to more frequent translocation of bacteria through the intestinal wall [11]. Anticoagulation, most commonly in the form of an unfractionated heparin drip to permit rapid titration should surgery be required, is recommended to prevent further propagation of thrombus [3,10,40]. Surgical therapy is indicated for all patients who have evidence of bowel ischemia, regardless of the underlying etiology. Arterial disease has been addressed with various techniques, with a standard open approach and the emergence of endovascular repair.

Mesenteric venous thrombosis (MVT) in the absence of peritoneal findings suggestive of bowel necrosis may be managed nonoperatively. Unfortunately a significant percentage of patients require surgery, with most of these patients needing bowel resection. In a review of 72 patients who had MVT by Rhee and colleagues [16], 64% of patients required surgical exploration, of whom 85% required resection of infarcted bowel. Systemic anticoagulation remains the mainstay of nonoperative therapy, and early use of heparin has been associated with improved survival [15]. Heparin is commonly reinstituted postoperatively when safe; long-term anticoagulation is strongly recommended for those who have ischemia caused by embolic events or MVT to prevent reoccurrence [3,6]. Some investigators report the use of vasodilators such as papaverine as an adjunct [4,12]. Surgical thrombectomy

[41], thrombolysis [42,43], and percutaneous transhepatic thrombectomy [44] have also been described in isolated reports as treatments for mesenteric thrombosis. All patients should undergo a work-up for hypercoagulable states, which, as mentioned, are common contributors to the development of mesenteric venous thrombosis.

Surgical therapy

In the setting of arterial insufficiency, whether in the acute or chronic form, mesenteric bypass is commonly performed. Bypass may be performed in an antegrade fashion, with inflow from the supraceliac aorta (more commonly free of atherosclerotic disease), or retrograde from the iliac vessels. Some investigators suggest that the former is more anatomically favorable, because retrograde grafts may be more prone to kinking [12,22,45]. At exploration, unless bowel is frankly necrotic, revascularization should be performed before bowel resection. Once revascularized, the bowel can be re-examined to determine if restoration of blood flow has reversed the ischemic process. Similarly, views differ on the choice of bypass grafts. Although reversed saphenous vein grafts are more appropriate in the setting of gross contamination from infarcted bowel [46], prosthetic grafts may in fact be more durable for mesenteric artery bypass. Although no randomized trials exist regarding the use of prosthetic versus endogenous grafts, most modern series indicate a preference for the use of prosthetic grafts in this setting [3,14,22,47–50]. Synthetic grafts also offer the benefit of facilitating simultaneous revascularization of the CA and SMA through a single aortotomy with the use of bifurcated grafts.

Technique

In performing antegrade bypass, a transabdominal approach can be used, gaining access to the aorta by dividing the triangular ligament over the left lobe of the liver and dividing the diaphragmatic crus (Fig. 3). Unless the SMA disease is proximal, a retropancreatic window is created for the aorto-SMA graft before anticoagulation. Proximal and distal control of the aorta are gained before administration of heparin, cross-clamping, and performance of an aortotomy. A bifurcated graft (most commonly made of polytetrafluoroethylene, or PTFE) is then sewn end-to-side to the aorta, after which aortic flow is restored. Alternatively a side-biting clamp may be used to avoid distal (in particular renal) ischemia. The graft is then sewn end-to-side to the common hepatic artery. The second limb may be passed behind the pancreas for distal SMA disease or anterior to the pancreas to the SMA for proximal disease, and anastomosed end-to-end or end-to-side to the SMA (Fig. 4) [14,46].

Alternatively retrograde bypass may be performed using the iliac arteries for inflow (Fig. 5). This technique may be appropriate in patients who have had a previous antegrade bypass or in patients whose distal thoracic aorta is

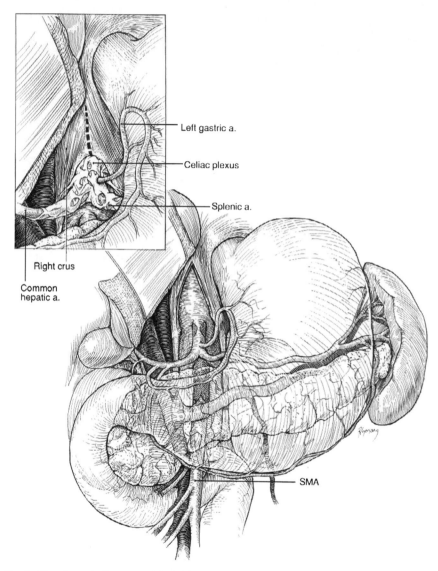

Fig. 3. The triangular ligament of the left lobe of the liver has been divided. Subsequently the right crus of the diaphragm is divided to provide access to the supraceliac aorta. (*From* Kazmers A. Operative management of chronic mesentric ischemia. Ann Vasc Surg 1998;12:302; with permission.)

not appropriate for inflow to an antegrade bypass [14]. For the surgeon unfamiliar with this anatomy and less experienced performing this procedure, the retrograde technique also offers the advantage of being less technically complicated [45].

Short of mesenteric arterial bypass, other options for mesenteric ischemia include thrombectomy and embolectomy. Cunningham and colleagues

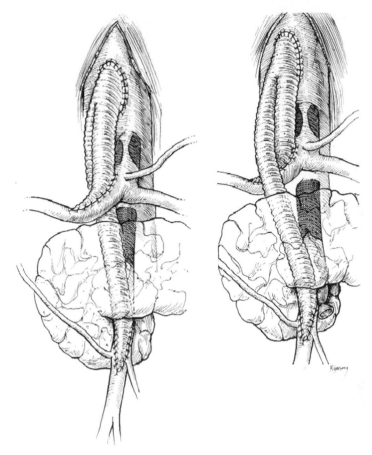

Fig. 4. When performing an antegrade bypass, a bifurcated graft is anastomosed end-to-side to the common hepatic artery, with the second limb passing either anterior or posterior to the common hepatic artery and then following a retropancreatic course. (*From* Kazmers A. Operative management of chronic mesentric ischemia. Ann Vasc Surg 1998;12:305; with permission.)

[51] obtained comparable results to mesenteric bypass using a trap-door, transaortic endarterectomy technique, facilitating revascularization of the CA and the SMA through a single aortotomy. In this technique, creation of the trap-door involves cutting three sides of a rectangle that surrounds the CA and the SMA (with one of the long sides being left intact). In a single study reviewing transaortic and local endarterectomy, local endarterectomy was associated with a higher rate of failure, and practice has shifted accordingly [52]. Fogarty catheter embolectomy remains an option if preoperative imaging definitively suggests embolic disease. Because thrombosis at the site of arteriotomy may occur in up to 17% of patients postoperatively [13], consideration should be given to closure with patch angioplasty.

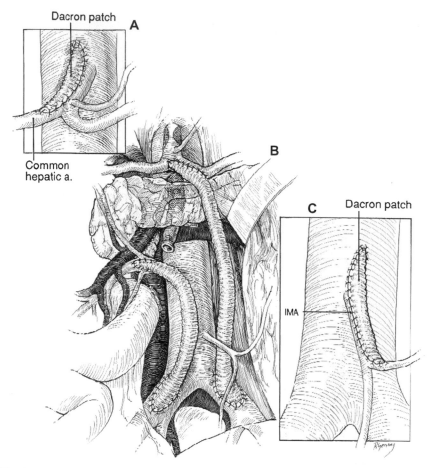

Fig. 5. (*A*) and (*C*) Technique for patch angioplasty repair of the celiac trunk and inferior mesenteric artery. (*B*) Typical orientation of a retrograde bypass, which may be technically easier to perform than antegrade bypass but more prone to kinking. (*From* Kazmers A. Operative management of chronic mesentric ischemia. Ann Vasc Surg 1998;12:307; with permission.)

Results

Results following mesenteric bypass graft are largely favorable. Jimenez and colleagues [49] had 94% 5-year primary-assisted patency rates among 47 patients undergoing aortomesenteric bypass. Similarly, McMillan and colleagues [53] documented 89% patency at 6 years in a total of 38 bypass grafts as followed by serial duplex scanning or arteriography. Notably, most patients in these two studies underwent revascularization of the CA and the SMA [49,53]. Although not proven by randomized studies, it seems likely that revascularization of both vessels provides for redundancy in the event that one repair subsequently fails. For this reason, revascularization of both vessels is encouraged if flow through both is impaired. Other studies, although not necessarily following objective measures of graft patency rates, document symptom-free survival rates (whether patients who are still alive remain free of symptoms) ranging from 57% to 86% at 5 years [21,22,51,52]. Owing to the overall rarity of mesenteric ischemia (or lack of difference between the two techniques), no studies were able to document differences in patency rates between antegrade and retrograde bypass. Although few studies report results of bypass for acute and chronic mesenteric ischemia, patency results following intervention for both disease forms are similar [52,53].

Assessment of bowel viability

Determination of bowel viability is a critical component of surgical therapy for mesenteric ischemia. Although the need for bowel resection is paradoxically associated with higher survival rates (likely because patients who have widely necrotic bowel and poor prognoses undergo no resection) [9], it remains critical to determine which bowel is salvageable to avoid the morbidity and mortality associated with extensive resections. Several different methods have been used to determine bowel viability intraoperatively. Clinical assessment by evaluating the color and motility of the bowel remains one of the most important tools of the surgeon in evaluating intestinal viability. Other techniques, including antimesenteric Doppler interrogation, and observation of perfusion following administration of intravenous fluorescein dye are also commonly used. None of these techniques, however, have proven to be thoroughly reliable in predicting future intestinal viability. One limited study evaluating these three techniques found the sensitivity for each to be less than 60% [54].

Because of the inability to accurately predict which segments of bowel remain viable, a second-look operation 24 to 48 hours after the initial procedure has been historically recommended [6,54]. In support of this opinion, one review of 43 patients undergoing open mesenteric revascularization noted that 11 of the 23 patients undergoing a second-look operation required bowel resection [9]. Realizing the morbidity associated with a negative laparotomy, exploratory laparoscopy has been suggested. One group evaluated 23 patients who had laparoscopy at 24 hours after the initial surgery, avoiding repeat laparotomy in 20 patients (87%) [55]. Increased technical skill, however, is required for thorough evaluation of what is commonly edematous, friable, dilated bowel, to avoid increasing morbidity and mortality through inadvertent perforation or overlooking of critical disease. In addition, as the rationale for a second exploration is not documented in most retrospective reviews, others suggest that only selective re-exploration should be performed. Kaminsky and colleagues [56] suggest that the yield of re-exploration is low (only 17% of patients in their review benefited from a second-look procedure), and that judgment of the surgeon based on findings at the initial surgery should guide decisions regarding a second-look. Whatever method of evaluation is eventually used, the surgeon needs to balance overzealous resection and potential for development of short bowel syndrome with the risk of leaving behind potentially ischemic bowel.

Endovascular therapy

The use of endovascular therapy for mesenteric ischemia is predominantly limited to treatment of the chronic form of the disease. The first report of endovascular therapy for mesenteric vascular disease documented relief of symptoms of CMI following angioplasty of the SMA [57]. Although one study documenting outcome following percutaneous transluminal angioplasty (PTA) of mesenteric vessels versus PTA with stenting found no difference in outcome [58], the overall trend has been toward increased use of PTA with stenting in endovascular therapy for CMI. Some investigators suggest this tendency results from extrapolation of data regarding endovascular treatment of renal artery stenosis, in which PTA and stenting remain more durable than PTA alone [27,59].

Several small series have been published documenting outcome following endovascular therapy following PTA with stenting of mesenteric vessels, primarily for CMI (Table 1). For each of the studies, technical success was defined as residual stenosis of less than 30%, and relief of symptoms was considered clinical success. Long-term patency of the mesenteric vessels varied in assessment; some studies relied on duplex ultrasound, others on angiography, and still others on presence of symptoms alone. Proponents of endovascular therapy over open surgical intervention cite the low morbidity and mortality rates and shorter hospital stay. Although initial technical success rates following percutaneous intervention are high, however (88%–100%), patency rates at 1 year decreased to 70% to 80% [27,58–60].

Few studies have attempted to directly compare percutaneous intervention with surgery for mesenteric ischemia. In one review of 28 patients undergoing percutaneous intervention compared with a total of 85 patients treated with various surgical procedures (mesenteric artery bypass, endarterectomy, or patch angioplasty), the morbidity and mortality between the two groups did not differ, although recurrence of symptoms was higher in the group treated percutaneously [61]. Of note, the morbidity and mortality rates for PTA and stenting in this study, 17.9% and 10.7%, respectively, were much higher than previously summarized [61]. In addition, there was a significant difference between the average number of vessels revascularized in the PTA/stenting group as compared with the surgery group (1.1 versus 1.5, respectively, $P < .01$) [61]. In this limited study comparing endovascular therapy with open surgical therapy, surgery therefore seemed to offer more durable results with comparable peri-procedure morbidity and mortality. Unfortunately the higher complication rates with PTA call into question their experience with the procedure and may have affected the results of the comparison.

Table 1
Outcomes following endovascular therapy for chronic mesenteric ischemia

Author	No. of patients	No. of interventions	Technical success	Clinical success	Morbidity (%)	Mortality (%)	Patency rates		F/U (mo)
							1°	1° asst.	
Shih [58]	33	47	87	88%	13	3.4	83	—	11
Sharafuddin [27]	25	28	96	88%	12	4	83	92	15
AbuRahama [62]	22	24	96	95%	0	0	30	—	26
Landis [60]	29	63	97	90%	13.7	6	70.1	87.9	12
Silva [59]	59	61	96	88%	3.4	1.7	71	100	14

In a second smaller study, nine patients who underwent mesenteric bypass grafting were compared with eight patients who underwent angioplasty alone. There was no difference in mortality, because one patient died in each group [47]. Technical success, however, defined as residual stenosis less than 30%, was achieved in only 30% of the angioplasty procedures compared with 100% in the surgical group [47]. Long-term pain relief occurred in 88% of the operative bypass group at 34.5 months, as compared with 67% in the angioplasty group at just 9 months [47]. In this small study, operative repair again seems to be more durable than endovascular therapy for mesenteric ischemia.

Although these two studies directly comparing surgery to percutaneous intervention for mesenteric ischemia failed to find a difference between morbidity and mortality rates, comparison of the individual series as reported in this review suggests that morbidity and mortality and length of hospital stay are greater for patients undergoing surgical intervention. The long-term patency rates following surgical bypass, however, remain higher than those after angioplasty, with and without stenting. One particular area of weakness of percutaneous intervention is among patients who have median arcuate ligament syndrome. Several investigators note a failure of PTA and stenting among patients in which compression of the CA by the diaphragm contributes to ischemic symptoms [6,47,62]. Surgical therapy with release of the median arcuate ligament should be the primary treatment of choice in these cases.

Thrombolytic therapy

Thrombolytic therapy as an adjunct to endovascular techniques has been explored to a limited degree for acute mesenteric ischemia. As with other endovascular techniques, peritoneal examination findings suggestive of bowel infarction remain a contraindication to thrombolytic therapy and mandate surgical exploration. Other contraindications are recent surgery, trauma, cerebrovascular or gastrointestinal bleed, and uncontrolled hypertension. Highlighting a need for more data, a recent systematic review of mesenteric arterial thrombolysis found the largest series describing this technique to consist of just 10 patients [1]. In this study, Simo and colleagues used urokinase by way of catheter-directed thrombolysis in a small cohort with SMA embolism [60]. Clinical success was achieved in seven patients, one of whom later required laparotomy after abdominal pain worsened, but there was no mortality secondary to bowel ischemia [60]. All patients in whom thrombolysis was successful had resolution of abdominal pain within 1 hour of starting therapy [60]. The authors agree with the conclusion by Schoots and colleagues [1] that preliminary results suggest this technique may hold promise, but further investigation regarding safety and durability of the technique is warranted before including thrombolysis as a valid therapeutic option in mesenteric ischemia.

Emerging diagnostic technology

As bowel mucosa is the intestinal layer most vulnerable to ischemia, measurement of mucosal oxygen tension has been proposed as one means of diagnosing mesenteric ischemia earlier and more accurately. Friedland and colleagues [63] describe an oximetric device using white-light reflectance spectrophotometry used during endoscopy to measure mucosal hemoglobin saturation in the colon. Preliminary data gathered in animals revealed an oxygen saturation of 72%, which decreased more than 40% following ligation of the arterial supply of the left colon and hypoxic ventilation [63]. Further human studies demonstrated the normal level of mucosal oxygen saturations range between 60% and 70% [64]. Analysis of three patients who had CMI revealed saturations between 16% and 30%, which increased to between 51% and 60% following revascularization by mesenteric arterial angioplasty and stenting [64]. The particular role endoscopy with mucosal oximetry measurement plays remains unknown. Likely, it may prove to be an effective means of evaluating for CMI, in cases in which arteriolar disease may not be readily evident on traditional angiography or CT angiography. This technique may also gain applicability to acute mesenteric ischemia, however, with planned development of a handheld probe that could permit intraoperative measurement of mucosal perfusion [64]. Although this would currently require an enterotomy, it could be used to assess the surrounding bowel when ischemia necessitates resection of one portion of bowel.

Similarly, other investigations have included oximetric measurements of SMV flow using MRI. This technique takes advantage of the paramagnetic properties of deoxygenated hemoglobin in contrast to oxygenated hemoglobin. Li and colleagues [65] describe measurement of oxygen saturation of blood flowing through the SMV before and after ingestion of a meal. SMV oxygen saturation in patients who do not have mesenteric ischemia (as determined by angiography and a lack of symptoms) increased an average of 4.6% following a meal, whereas saturation decreased 8.8% postprandially in those patients who had clinical and radiographic evidence of mesenteric ischemia [65]. Given the time required to perform magnetic resonance oximetry, to including the need for postprandial studies, applicability of this technique remains limited to evaluation of patients who have CMI.

Summary

Mesenteric ischemia in chronic and acute forms carries a high morbidity and mortality rate, each increased by frequent delays in diagnosis [66]. Although laboratory studies have low specificity for diagnosing mesenteric ischemia, CT angiography and traditional angiography remain sensitive diagnostic imaging techniques. Once diagnosed, prompt surgical therapy and anticoagulation remain cornerstones of therapy. Although prosthetic grafts in an antegrade or retrograde fashion provide the most durable means of repair, endovascular stenting and angioplasty have high early success rates and may be preferable for patients who have prohibitive risk factors for open surgery and who do not have evidence of infarcted bowel. In cases in which bowel viability is questionable, multiple options including second-look operations are available and should be used, despite the relative lack of data showing improved outcomes. Emerging diagnostic technologies may permit earlier diagnosis, allowing urgent treatment for mesenteric ischemia and potentially reducing the high mortality rates currently seen with this condition.

References

[1] Schoots IG, Levi MM, Reekers JA, et al. Thrombolytic therapy for acute superior mesenteric artery occlusion. J Vasc Interv Radiol 2005;16(3):317–29.
[2] Schoots IG, Koffeman GI, Legemate DA, et al. Systematic review of survival after acute mesenteric ischaemia according to disease aetiology. Br J Surg 2004;91(1):17–27.
[3] Falkensammer J, Oldenburg WA. Surgical and medical management of mesenteric ischemia. Curr Treat Options Cardiovasc Med 2006;8(2):137–43.
[4] Kumar S, Sarr MG, Kamath PS. Mesenteric venous thrombosis. N Engl J Med 2001; 345(23):1683–8.
[5] Mamode N, Pickford I, Leiberman P. Failure to improve outcome in acute mesenteric ischaemia: seven-year review. Eur J Surg 1999;165(3):203–8.
[6] Bradbury AW, Brittenden J, McBride K, et al. Mesenteric ischaemia: a multidisciplinary approach. Br J Surg 1995;82(11):1446–59.
[7] Acosta S, Ogren M, Sternby NH, et al. Incidence of acute thrombo-embolic occlusion of the superior mesenteric artery—a population-based study. Eur J Vasc Endovasc Surg 2004; 27(2):145–50.
[8] Rosenblum JD, Boyle CM, Schwartz LB. The mesenteric circulation. Anatomy and physiology. Surg Clin North Am 1997;77(2):289–306.
[9] Park WM, Gloviczki P, Cherry KJ Jr, et al. Contemporary management of acute mesenteric ischemia: factors associated with survival. J Vasc Surg 2002;35(3):445–52.
[10] Endean ED, Barnes SL, Kwolek CJ, et al. Surgical management of thrombotic acute intestinal ischemia. Ann Surg 2001;233(6):801–8.
[11] Oldenburg WA, Lau LL, Rodenberg TJ, et al. Acute mesenteric ischemia: a clinical review. Arch Intern Med 2004;164(10):1054–62.
[12] Chang RW, Chang JB, Longo WE. Update in management of mesenteric ischemia. World J Gastroenterol 2006;12(20):3243–7.
[13] Ottinger LW. The surgical management of acute occlusion of the superior mesenteric artery. Ann Surg 1978;188(6):721–31.
[14] Kazmers A. Operative management of chronic mesenteric ischemia. Ann Vasc Surg 1998; 12(3):299–308.
[15] Abdu RA, Zakhour BJ, Dallis DJ. Mesenteric venous thrombosis—1911 to 1984. Surgery 1987;101(4):383–8.
[16] Rhee RY, Gloviczki P, Mendonca CT, et al. Mesenteric venous thrombosis: still a lethal disease in the 1990s. J Vasc Surg 1994;20(5):688–97.
[17] Steele SR, Martin MJ, Garafalo T, et al. Superior mesenteric vein thrombosis following laparoscopic Nissen fundoplication. JSLS 2003;7(2):159–63.
[18] Moawad J, Gewertz BL. Chronic mesenteric ischemia. Clinical presentation and diagnosis. Surg Clin North Am 1997;77(2):357–69.
[19] Acosta S, Ogren M, Sternby NH, et al. Clinical implications for the management of acute thromboembolic occlusion of the superior mesenteric artery: autopsy findings in 213 patients. Ann Surg 2005;241(3):516–22.

[20] Acosta S, Ogren M, Sternby NH, et al. Fatal nonocclusive mesenteric ischaemia: population-based incidence and risk factors. J Intern Med 2006;259(3):305–13.

[21] Mateo RB, O'Hara PJ, Hertzer NR, et al. Elective surgical treatment of symptomatic chronic mesenteric occlusive disease: early results and late outcomes. J Vasc Surg 1999; 29(5):821–31 [discussion: 832].

[22] Moawad J, McKinsey JF, Wyble CW, et al. Current results of surgical therapy for chronic mesenteric ischemia. Arch Surg 1997;132(6):613–8 [discussion: 618–19].

[23] Bech FR. Celiac artery compression syndromes. Surg Clin North Am 1997;77(2):409–24.

[24] Rogers DM, Thompson JE, Garrett WV, et al. Mesenteric vascular problems. A 26-year experience. Ann Surg 1982;195(5):554–65.

[25] Horton KM, Fishman EK. Multi-detector row CT of mesenteric ischemia: can it be done? Radiographics 2001;21(6):1463–73.

[26] Clark RA, Gallant TE. Acute mesenteric ischemia: angiographic spectrum. AJR Am J Roentgenol 1984;142(3):555–62.

[27] Sharafuddin MJ, Olson CH, Sun S, et al. Endovascular treatment of celiac and mesenteric arteries stenoses: applications and results. J Vasc Surg 2003;38(4):692–8.

[28] Zwolak RM, Fillinger MF, Walsh DB, et al. Mesenteric and celiac duplex scanning: a validation study. J Vasc Surg 1998;27(6):1078–87 [discussion: 1088].

[29] Moneta GL, Yeager RA, Dalman R, et al. Duplex ultrasound criteria for diagnosis of splanchnic artery stenosis or occlusion. J Vasc Surg 1991;14(4):511–8 [discussion: 518–20].

[30] Nicoloff AD, Williamson WK, Moneta GL, et al. Duplex ultrasonography in evaluation of splanchnic artery stenosis. Surg Clin North Am 1997;77(2):339–55.

[31] Gentile AT, Moneta GL, Lee RW, et al. Usefulness of fasting and postprandial duplex ultrasound examinations for predicting high-grade superior mesenteric artery stenosis. Am J Surg 1995;169(5):476–9.

[32] Taourel PG, Deneuville M, Pradel JA, et al. Acute mesenteric ischemia: diagnosis with contrast-enhanced CT. Radiology 1996;199(3):632–6.

[33] Kirkpatrick ID, Kroeker MA, Greenberg HM. Biphasic CT with mesenteric CT angiography in the evaluation of acute mesenteric ischemia: initial experience. Radiology 2003;229(1):91–8.

[34] Chou CK, Mak CW, Tzeng WS, et al. CT of small bowel ischemia. Abdom Imaging 2004; 29(1):18–22.

[35] Zandrino F, Musante F, Gallesio I, et al. Assessment of patients with acute mesenteric ischemia: multi-slice computed tomography signs and clinical performance in a group of patients with surgical correlation. Minerva Gastroenterol Dietol 2006;52(3):317–25.

[36] Li KC, Whitney WS, McDonnell CH, et al. Chronic mesenteric ischemia: evaluation with phase-contrast cine MR imaging. Radiology 1994;190(1):175–9.

[37] Burkart DJ, Johnson CD, Reading CC, et al. MR measurements of mesenteric venous flow: prospective evaluation in healthy volunteers and patients with suspected chronic mesenteric ischemia. Radiology 1995;194(3):801–6.

[38] Lauenstein TC, Ajaj W, Narin B, et al. MR imaging of apparent small-bowel perfusion for diagnosing mesenteric ischemia: feasibility study. Radiology 2005;234(2):569–75.

[39] Shih MC, Hagspiel KD. CTA and MRA in mesenteric ischemia: part 1, role in diagnosis and differential diagnosis. AJR Am J Roentgenol 2007;188(2):452–61.

[40] McKinsey JF, Gewertz BL. Acute mesenteric ischemia. Surg Clin North Am 1997;77(2):307–18.

[41] Ghaly M, Frawley JE. Superior mesenteric vein thrombosis. Aust N Z J Surg 1986;56(3): 277–9.

[42] Robin P, Gruel Y, Lang M, et al. Complete thrombolysis of mesenteric vein occlusion with recombinant tissue-type plasminogen activator. Lancet 1988;1(8599):1391.

[43] Bilbao JI, Rodriguez-Cabello J, Longo J, et al. Portal thrombosis: percutaneous transhepatic treatment with urokinase—a case report. Gastrointest Radiol 1989;14(4):326–8.

[44] Naganuma M, Inoue N, Hosoda Y, et al. [A case of superior mesenteric vein thrombosis treated by percutaneous transhepatic thrombectomy]. Nippon Shokakibyo Gakkai Zasshi 1995;92(2):158–63 [in Japanese].

[45] Johnston KW, Lindsay TF, Walker PM, et al. Mesenteric arterial bypass grafts: early and late results and suggested surgical approach for chronic and acute mesenteric ischemia. Surgery 1995;118(1):1–7.

[46] Shanley CJ, Ozaki CK, Zelenock GB. Bypass grafting for chronic mesenteric ischemia. Surg Clin North Am 1997;77(2):381–95.

[47] Rose SC, Quigley TM, Raker EJ. Revascularization for chronic mesenteric ischemia: comparison of operative arterial bypass grafting and percutaneous transluminal angioplasty. J Vasc Interv Radiol 1995;6(3):339–49.

[48] Park WM, Cherry KJ Jr, Chua HK, et al. Current results of open revascularization for chronic mesenteric ischemia: a standard for comparison. J Vasc Surg 2002;35(5):853–9.

[49] Jimenez JG, Huber TS, Ozaki CK, et al. Durability of antegrade synthetic aortomesenteric bypass for chronic mesenteric ischemia. J Vasc Surg 2002;35(6):1078–84.

[50] Calderon M, Reul GJ, Gregoric ID, et al. Long-term results of the surgical management of symptomatic chronic intestinal ischemia. J Cardiovasc Surg (Torino) 1992;33(6):723–8.

[51] Cunningham CG, Reilly LM, Rapp JH, et al. Chronic visceral ischemia. Three decades of progress. Ann Surg 1991;214(3):276–87 [discussion: 287–8].

[52] Cho JS, Carr JA, Jacobsen G, et al. Long-term outcome after mesenteric artery reconstruction: a 37-year experience. J Vasc Surg 2002;35(3):453–60.

[53] McMillan WD, McCarthy WJ, Bresticker MR, et al. Mesenteric artery bypass: objective patency determination. J Vasc Surg 1995;21(5):729–40 [discussion: 740–1].

[54] Ballard JL, Stone WM, Hallett JW, et al. A critical analysis of adjuvant techniques used to assess bowel viability in acute mesenteric ischemia. Am Surg 1993;59(5):309–11.

[55] Anadol AZ, Ersoy E, Taneri F, et al. Laparoscopic "second-look" in the management of mesenteric ischemia. Surg Laparosc Endosc Percutan Tech 2004;14(4):191–3.

[56] Kaminsky O, Yampolski I, Aranovich D, et al. Does a second-look operation improve survival in patients with peritonitis due to acute mesenteric ischemia? A five-year retrospective experience. World J Surg 2005;29(5):645–8.

[57] Furrer J, Gruntzig A, Kugelmeier J, et al. Treatment of abdominal angina with percutaneous dilatation of an arterial mesenteric superior stenosis. Preliminary communication. Cardiovasc Intervent Radiol 1980;3(1):43–4.

[58] Shih MC, Angle JF, Leung DA, et al. CTA and MRA in mesenteric ischemia: part 2, normal findings and complications after surgical and endovascular treatment. AJR Am J Roentgenol 2007;188(2):462–71.

[59] Silva JA, White CJ, Collins TJ, et al. Endovascular therapy for chronic mesenteric ischemia. J Am Coll Cardiol 2006;47(5):944–50.

[60] Landis MS, Rajan DK, Simons ME, et al. Percutaneous management of chronic mesenteric ischemia: outcomes after intervention. J Vasc Interv Radiol 2005;16(10):1319–25.

[61] Kasirajan K, O'Hara PJ, Gray BH, et al. Chronic mesenteric ischemia: open surgery versus percutaneous angioplasty and stenting. J Vasc Surg 2001;33(1):63–71.

[62] AbuRahma AF, Stone PA, Bates MC, et al. Angioplasty/stenting of the superior mesenteric artery and celiac trunk: early and late outcomes. J Endovasc Ther 2003;10(6):1046–53.

[63] Friedland S, Benaron D, Parachikov I, et al. Measurement of mucosal capillary hemoglobin oxygen saturation in the colon by reflectance spectrophotometry. Gastrointest Endosc 2003; 57(4):492–7.

[64] Friedland S, Benaron D, Coogan S, et al. Diagnosis of chronic mesenteric ischemia by visible light spectroscopy during endoscopy. Gastrointest Endosc 2007;65(2):294–300.

[65] Li KC, Dalman RL, Ch'en IY, et al. Chronic mesenteric ischemia: use of in vivo MR imaging measurements of blood oxygen saturation in the superior mesenteric vein for diagnosis. Radiology 1997;204(1):71–7.

[66] Boley SJ, Brandt LJ, Sammartano RJ. History of mesenteric ischemia. The evolution of a diagnosis and management. Surg Clin North Am 1997;77(2):275–88.

SURGICAL
CLINICS OF
NORTH AMERICA

Surg Clin N Am 87 (2007) 1135–1147

Current Trends in Lower Extremity Revascularization

Ganesha B. Perera, MD, Sean P. Lyden, MD*

Department of Vascular Surgery, Desk S40, Cleveland Clinic Foundation, 9500 Euclid Avenue, Cleveland, OH 44195, USA

Current estimates show that peripheral arterial disease affects approximately 8 to 12 million people in the United States; this number will undoubtedly grow as the geriatric patient population increases [1]. Most patients who have peripheral arterial disease are asymptomatic, with intermittent claudication being the first symptom. Of those with intermittent claudication, 30% will progress to rest pain and critical limb ischemia (CLI), and approximately 18% will require lower extremity revascularization over a 10-year period [2,3].

In 2000, the Trans Atlantic Inter-Societal Consensus (TASC) statement classified arterial lesions in the femoropopliteal segment (FP), to allow for the study of outcomes and to suggest the best management strategies based on published outcomes (Fig. 1) [4]. The TASC classifications were expected to evolve over time as physician experience and technologies advanced. In the past decade, the liberal application of endovascular technologies to the FP segment has generated a large amount of published data on these techniques, leading to a revision of the document and subsequent publication of TASC II [4,5]. Now, longer stenoses and short occlusions are considered best treated with endovascular means. As understanding of endovascular technologies and outcomes advance, further revisions to this document may be expected.

Although useful, the TASC morphologic classification does not take into consideration many factors that affect the success of treating lesions for short-term and midterm outcomes. The authors believe that understanding the strengths and weaknesses of each modality is essential. As long as surgical reconstruction options are not lost when performing percutaneous

* Corresponding author.
E-mail address: lydens@ccf.org (S.P. Lyden).

0039-6109/07/$ - see front matter © 2007 Elsevier Inc. All rights reserved.
doi:10.1016/j.suc.2007.07.004   *surgical.theclinics.com*

Type A lesions

· Single stenosis ≤10 cm in length
· Single occlusion ≤5 cm in length

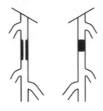

Type B lesions:

· Multiple lesions (stenoses or occlusions), each ≤5 cm
· Single stenosis or occlusion ≤15 cm not involving the
  infrageniculate popliteal artery
· Single or multiple lesions in the absence of continuous
  tibial vessels to improve inflow for a distal bypass
· Heavily calcified occlusion ≤5 cm in length
· Single popliteal stenosis

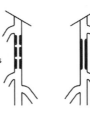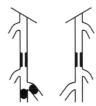

Type C lesions

· Multiple stenoses or occlusions totaling >15 cm with or
  without heavy calcification
· Recurrent stenoses or occlusions that need treatment
  after two endovascular interventions

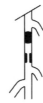

Type D lesions

· Chronic total occlusions of CFA or SFA (>20 cm,
  involving the popliteal artery)
· Chronic total occlusion of popliteal artery and proximal
  trifurcation vessels

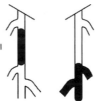

Fig. 1. TASC II classification of femoral popliteal lesions. CFA, common femoral artery; SFA, superficial femoral artery. (*From* Norgren L, Hiatt WR, Dormandy JA, et al. Inter-society consensus for the management of peripheral arterial disease (TASC II). J Vasc Surg 2007; 45(Suppl S):S5–67; with permission.)

interventions, endovascular treatment of FP lesions should be the first approach. The physician and patient must understand that the reduced morbidity and mortality may come at a cost of diminished durability and a potential need for reintervention. The authors have found that, when used appropriately, an open procedure can follow an endovascular procedure that has failed; similarly, an endovascular procedure can follow an open procedure after failure. Adjunctive dual antiplatelet therapy with aspirin and clopidogrel is commonly used without level I supportive evidence to justify its use.

Percutaneous transluminal angioplasty

The FP interventional technique with the longest follow-up and most data is percutaneous transluminal angioplasty (PTA), which involves a controlled injury to plaque in the arterial wall, creating a localized dissection while stretching the medial and adventitial layers. Important determinants of successful PTA are lesion location, length, plaque composition, and morphology [6,7]. Eccentric and ostial lesions do not respond well to PTA. A higher vessel rupture rate has also been noted with PTA of circumferentially calcified lesions [7]. Longer stenoses and occlusions in the FP segment are more likely to have flow-limiting dissection or suboptimal expansion caused by elastic recoil, compared with short, focal lesions. Dissections occur with all angioplasties but do not require further treatment if not flow limiting. Longer balloon inflation times (180 seconds versus 30 seconds) have been shown to decrease major dissections but not to improve late outcomes [8]. When a dissection is flow limiting, repeat low-pressure angioplasty can often resolve the situation or, if not, the flap should be covered with a nitinol self-expanding stent.

Pooled results of femoropopliteal PTA indicate 1-, 3-, and 5-year primary patency rates of 65% to 77%, 48% to 66%, and 42% to 55%, respectively, without delineation of TASC lesion status [9]. However, many of the individual studies with the best long-term outcomes for angioplasty were performed for short stenoses or short occlusions. Johnston and colleagues [10] prospectively reported femoropopliteal PTA results performed in the 1980s in 254 limbs. Predictors of success were claudication, proximal lesion location, and greater than two-vessel runoff. For stenoses with good runoff, the success rate (as measured by improvement in clinical grade and ankle brachial index [ABI]) was 53% at 5 years, whereas for occlusions with poor runoff, the success rate was only 16% at 5 years. Data from the STAR registry identified poor tibial runoff, diabetes, and renal failure as factors associated with long-term failure of femoropopliteal PTA [11]. Primary patency at 1, 3, and 5 years for 219 limbs was 87%, 69%, and 55%, respectively. Poor tibial runoff was most predictive of late occlusion.

When FP PTA is performed for CLI, patency rates are much lower. Lofberg and colleagues [12] reported 121 procedures performed on 92 patients having CLI, with a mean ABI of 0.3 before intervention. Initial technical success was 88%, and cumulative primary success rates at 1 and 5 years were 40% and 27%, respectively. For superficial femoral artery (SFA) occlusions longer than 5 cm, the primary success rate at 5 years was only 12%, compared with 32% if the occlusion was shorter than 5 cm [12].

Recently, VIVA Physicians, Inc. published performance goals and end-point assessment with respect to PTA alone versus nitinol stenting [13]. Data were derived from the PTA control arm of three unpublished, randomized industry trials and five published trials in the medical literature [13]. Using this aggregate data, the expected vessel patency rate for PTA of lesions 4 to 15 cm in length at 1 year is 33%. This rate is much lower than those of the aforementioned studies, and may be due to treatment of longer lesion lengths by these newer studies or to more rigorous assessment of primary patency using duplex ultrasonography.

Subintimal angioplasty

Subintimal angioplasty, described by Bolia in 1989, is a variant of PTA that allows the treatment of long occlusions when intraluminal wire crossing is not possible [14]. Briefly, an extraluminal dissection is created and advanced past the occlusion, with re-entry into the true lumen distally. This path is then balloon dilated and angiography is used to confirm the new path of blood flow. Technical failure is mainly due to an inability to re-enter the true lumen; however, adjuncts such as the new re-entry devices are decreasing the failure rate. Technical success, 12-month primary patency, and limb salvage rates have ranged from 74% to 92%, 22% to 92%, and 50% to 94%, respectively, in recent series [15]. Lazaris and colleagues [16] prospectively evaluated 46 patients who had CLI whose only other options were bypass or amputation. Ninety percent of the 51 subintimal angioplasties were performed in TASC D lesions, with skin ulceration or necrosis present in 73%. Twelve-month primary patency and limb salvage rates were 50% and 92%, respectively. Similar to conventional PTA, the number of runoff vessels significantly predicted late occlusion, one-vessel runoff having a 12-month patency of 25%, compared with an 81% patency with at least two-vessel runoff. Length of occlusion also predicted reocclusion, with a hazard ratio of 1.02 for every 1 cm of occlusion traversed.

Endovascular cryoplasty

Suboptimal expansion due to elastic recoil and flow-limiting dissection, and intimal hyperplasia causing late restenosis, are common in SFA after standard angioplasty. Endovascular cryoplasty is a new technique that attempts to decrease the inadequate dilatation and late restenosis. Cryoplasty couples cold thermal energy with balloon angioplasty. The ice field created in the arterial wall causes interstitial saline to freeze, resulting in plaque microfracture and decreased elasticity within the media, and leading to more uniform dilatation during PTA, with a markedly decreased rate of flow-limiting dissection. In experimental models, cryoplasty induces intracellular dehydration and rehydration and initiates smooth muscle cell apoptosis, leading to noninflammatory remodeling, which, theoretically, should lead to decreased intimal hyperplasia and thus, decreased rates of restenosis. The PolarCath (Boston Scientific, Natick, Massachusetts) is an FDA-approved device for endovascular cryoplasty. An initial use of this technique in femoropopliteal lesions was presented by Fava and colleagues [17].

Fifteen patients were treated who had a mean lesion length, diameter stenosis, and tibioperoneal runoff of 6.5 cm, 86%, and 1.7 vessels, respectively. Fourteen-month follow-up demonstrated a primary patency of 83% and a 17% restenosis rate, with two patients having late occlusions. A multicenter, nonrandomized registry by Laird and colleagues [18,19] included 102 patients who had SFA lesions with a mean length of 4.8 cm, with 15 (14.7%) occlusions. Most of the lesions (84%) were de novo in the SFA. Patients who had rest pain, gangrene, in-stent restenoses, and heavily calcified lesions were excluded. The technical success rate was 86% and freedom from target vessel revascularization was 83% at 9 months [19]. Adjunctive stenting was required in only nine target lesions (8.8%), remarkably less than seen in PTA alone.

Nitinol stents

Because of the limitations of angioplasty, adjunctive or primary nitinol (nickel titanium alloy) self-expanding stents have been used by many physicians. Nitinol stents have demonstrated greater radial force, increased resistance to crush deformity, and reduced foreshortening, which allows for greater precision of placement, when compared with the prior generation of stainless-steel stents [20]. Primary patency for nitinol self-expanding stents in the femoropopliteal arteries has been encouraging, with recent reviews having 1- and 3-year primary patencies in the range of 76% to 97% and 60% to 76%, respectively [21–25]. Mewissen and colleagues [25] evaluated the use of self-expanding nitinol stents in 137 limbs with FP TASC A, B, and C lesions (125 TASC B and C). The mean lesion length was 12.2 cm, with a mean follow-up of 302 days. Duplex-derived primary patency at 1 and 2 years was 76% and 60%, respectively. Similar results come from the control arm of the SIROCCO trial, which demonstrated restenosis of 21% at 24 months with preserved ABIs for self-expanding nitinol stents in the FP segment [26,27]. In a recent randomized trial, Schillinger and colleagues [20] compared PTA with primary implantation of nitinol stents in the SFA. Both cohorts had approximately 50 patients, with most patients (88%) being claudicants. Target lesion length was 9 to 10 cm, with approximately 35% in each group having total occlusions. Most patients in both cohorts (range 75%–86%) had at least two-vessel runoff. Seventeen patients in the original PTA-only group crossed over to the stenting group during the index procedure: nine because of a flow-limiting dissection and eight because of a residual stenosis of greater than 30% after PTA alone. Angiographic restenosis rates were higher for angioplasty by intent-to-treat (43% PTA versus 24% stenting) and as-treated (50% PTA versus 25% stenting) analysis at 6 months. One-year rates of restenosis by duplex also favored primary nitinol stenting, at 37% versus 63% (PTA).

In a retrospective series, Surowiec and colleagues [28] compared the results of PTA with selective stenting (37% in this series), as analyzed by

TASC lesion type. Unfortunately, stenting was not broken down by TASC category. They found that primary patency rates were highly dependent on TASC lesion type. At 1 year, TASC A lesions had a primary patency higher than 80%, whereas that of TACD D lesions was less than 40%. These results appear to be superior to those afforded by PTA and first-generation stents. However, it appears that the severity of TASC classification does diminish the overall patency of PTA-treated lesions.

The VIVA physicians' objective performance criteria, which was discussed previously regarding angioplasty, suggested that a 66% 12-month primary patency (for patients with Rutherford class 2–4 symptoms with 4- to 15-cm-long lesions) should be the new benchmark for SFA nitinol stent outcomes [13].

Late restenosis secondary to intimal hyperplasia also remains an issue. In an effort to address intimal hyperplasia further, drug-eluting nitinol stents are now being studied. The only published trial evaluating this potential therapy is a randomized, controlled trial comparing the sirolimus-eluting SMART stent (Cordis, Miami Lakes, Florida) with the bare SMART stent for TASC C SFA lesions [26]. At 24 months, the restenosis rates were no different between the two treatment arms (22.9% and 21.1% for drug-eluting and bare stents, respectively). This finding may be due to lack of selection of the most appropriate drug or drug-elution profile, or to problems with the materials used to bond the drugs to the stents. Stent fractures were noted in 36% of the drug-eluting group and in 20% of the bare stent group, without any demonstrable clinical significance. This study was one of the first to raise awareness of late nitinol stent fracture. Current data now suggest that, despite encouraging results for nitinol stents, stent fractures increase the risk of restenosis. Scheinert and colleagues [29] analyzed 261 self-expanding nitinol stents implanted in the FP segment of 93 patients at a mean follow-up of 10.7 months. Stent fractures were noted in 64 cases (24.5%), with complete strut separation noted in 16 (25%). A diameter reduction of more than 50% was seen at the site of stent fracture in 33%, and in 34%, stent occlusion was noted at the site of fracture. Additionally, a greater incidence of fractures was noted with increasing lengths of the stented segment (13.2% versus 52% for less than 8 cm and longer than 16 cm, respectively). The primary patency at 12 months was significantly lower for those with stent fractures (41.1% versus 84.3%, $P < .0001$).

Level I evidence comparing surgical bypass with angioplasty with or without stenting is sparse. The BASIL trial was a multicenter trial in the United Kingdom that randomized patients who had CLI (rest pain, rest pain with tissue loss, and ankle pressures above or below 50 mmHg) to surgical bypass or angioplasty [30]. Approximately 225 patients were in both arms, with the primary end points being amputation-free survival and all-cause mortality. More than 90% in both groups had rest pain and more than 75% had tissue loss. Two thirds of both groups were not on statin therapy and just over one-half were on antiplatelet therapy. Most

(58% in both groups) were not diabetic and approximately one third (32%–40%) were current smokers. In the surgical cohort, 75% of the bypasses used the long saphenous vein, with the distal anastomosis being evenly distributed between the above-knee popliteal artery, the below-knee popliteal artery, and the crural arteries. The length of the target lesion in the angioplasty group was not specified; however, PTA involved the SFA in 80% and more distal vessels in 62% of patients. The use of adjuvant stenting, either at the index intervention or later reintervention, was not discussed. Amputation-free survival at 1 year was 68% and 71% for the surgical and PTA cohorts, respectively. At 3 years, it was 57% and 52% in the surgical and PTA group, respectively. A post-hoc analysis at the 2-year mark showed a decreased hazard ratio for all-cause mortality favoring the surgical group. These investigators concluded that, in this population of patients, an angioplasty-first strategy had similar outcomes in amputation-free survival.

Polytetrafluoroethylene-covered nitinol stents

The risk of developing diffuse neointimal hyperplasia in uncovered nitinol stents also led to consideration of stents covered with material such as expanded polytetrafluoroethylene (ePTFE). The theoretic advantage of an ePTFE-covered nitinol stent is the elimination of neointimal hyperplasia. A potential problem with this idea is the occlusion of collateral vessels and the inability to prevent edge restenosis. The Viabahn endoprosthesis (W.L. Gore & Associates, Flagstaff, Arizona) is an ePTFE self-expanding nitinol stent graft that has been studied and is approved for use in the SFA.

In an initial safety and efficacy study, 80 femoral arteries in 74 patients were treated with a mean device length of 13 cm [31]. Primary patency at 1 year was 79%, with three early thromboses and 14 late restenoses or occlusions. A midterm study evaluated 63 grafts implanted in the FP segment of 52 patients, with a mean lesion length of 8.5 cm [32]. Primary patency at 1 and 2 years was 78.4% and 74.1%, with no difference in patency noted for increasing lesion length. A 7.7% rate of distal embolization was successfully treated with catheter aspiration or local lysis. A small, single-center evaluation of long-term results was published by Saxon and colleagues [33]. These investigators evaluated the ePTFE stent graft in 15 patients and found a primary patency of 87% at 2 years.

Kedora and colleagues [34] recently conducted a prospective, randomized study comparing covered ePTFE/nitinol self-expanding stent-grafts with prosthetic above-the-knee femoropopliteal bypass. Fifty limbs were randomized into each group. Primary patency at 1 year was approximately 74% for both cohorts, with a mean follow-up of 18 months. The covered nitinol ePTFE stent graft in the SFA had a 1-year patency comparable to surgical bypass, with a significantly shorter hospital stay (0.9 versus 3.1 days).

Table 1
Summary of femoropopliteal endovascular intervention results

Intervention	Author	Year	No. limbs	1° patency (%)						Limb salvage 1 y (%)
				6 mo	1 y	1.5 y	2 y	3 y	5 y	
PTA alone										
	Norgren [5]	2007	Pooled data	—	65–77	—	—	48–66	42–55	—
	Rocha-Singh [13]	2007	—	—	33	—	—	—	—	—
	Clark [11]	2001	219	—	87	—	—	69	55	—
	Lofberg [12]	2001	121	—	40[a]	—	—	—	27[a]	—
	Johnston [10]	1987	254	—	—	—	—	—	16–53	—
PTA with nitinol stents										
	Pooled data [18–22]	—	—	—	76–97	—	—	60–76	—	—
	Schillinger [20]	2006	51	76[b]	63[b]	—	—	—	—	—
	SIROCCO II [27]	2005	28	92	—	82	—	—	—	—
	Surowiec [28]	2005	—	—	40–80	—	—	—	—	—
	Mewissen [25]	2004	137	—	76	—	60	—	—	—
PTFE nitinol stents										
	Kedora [34]	2007	50	—	74	—	—	—	—	—
	Jahnke [32]	2003	63	—	78	—	74	—	—	—
	Saxon [33]	2003	15	—	—	—	87	—	—	—
	Lammer [31]	2000	80	—	79	—	—	—	—	—

SIA								
Lazaris [16]	2006	51	—	50	—	—	—	92
Lipsitz [15]	2005	—	—	22–92	—	—	—	50–94
Cryoplasty								
Laird [18,19]	2005	102	—	83[c]	—	75	—	—
Fava [17]	2004	15	—	83[d]	—	—	—	—
Mechanical atherectomy								
Ramaiah [36]	2006	1258	90[e]	80[e]	—	—	—	96
Zeller [35]	2004	71	63–80	—	—	—	—	—
Laser angioplasty								
Bosiers [40]	2005	51	—	—	—	—	—	90 (6 mo)
Laird [39]	2004	155	—	—	—	—	—	93 (6 mo)
Scheinert [38]	2001	411	—	34	—	—	—	—

Abbreviation: SIA, subintimal angioplasty.

[a] Success rate.

[b] Freedom from restenosis.

[c] At 300 days.

[d] 14-month data.

[e] Freedom from target vessel revascularization.

Debulking technologies

Directional mechanical atherectomy

Originally described and used in the coronary circulation, mechanical atherectomy has also found renewed interest in the peripheral vascular system. The technique of directional mechanical atherectomy currently available uses the SilverHawk device (FoxHollow, Redwood City, California). Studies have thus far been small, retrospective series or registry data, with the primary end point often being freedom from target vessel revascularization, as opposed to the more robust measure of duplex-derived vessel patency. Zeller and colleagues [35] reported on 71 femoropopliteal de novo, restenotic, or in-stent restenotic lesions with a mean length of 4.8 cm. After atherectomy alone, they had a less than 30% residual stenosis in 76% of lesions. However, additional balloon angioplasty was needed in 58%, and stents were implanted in 6%. At 6-month follow-up, primary lesions fared best. Primary patency at 6 months ranged from 63% to 80%. Most data regarding the SilverHawk device come from the self-reported multicenter TALON registry [36] and comprise 601 patients having 1258 lesions with a mean treated length of 7.6 cm. Nearly one third had CLI and one half were diabetics. Stand-alone success was present in 74% of treated lesions, whereas 26% required adjunctive therapy. Freedom from target vessel revascularization at 6 and 12 months was 90% and 80%, respectively. Multiple lesions and increasing Rutherford stage predicted less favorable outcomes. Overall 1-year amputation rate and mortality were 4%.

Newer reports have suggested inferior outcomes in long TASC C and D lesions in patients who have CLI, using the SilverHawk device [37]. However many patients in this series had infrageniculate lesions that were not concomitantly treated, which may explain the poor long-term patency results.

Laser atherectomy

The initial use of lasers to treat peripheral arterial lesions used wavelengths that created thermal injury and significant collateral damage. New excimer laser technology (CliRpath Excimer Laser, Spectranetics, Colorado Springs, Colorado) uses photochemical (rather than thermal) energy, which is absorbed over a very short distance and potentially eliminates any heat generation. Laser technology is ideally suited to long, concentric, chronic occlusions that cannot be traversed by other means. The drawbacks of the laser are that it is not directional (forward-facing only) and the largest probe size is 2.5 mm. Thus, any treatment of the SFA and likely popliteal artery needs adjunctive measures.

Laser atherectomy has demonstrated usefulness in specific situations. Scheinert and colleagues [38] demonstrated its use in 318 patients who had chronic occlusions of the SFA. Four hundred and eleven occlusive lesions with a mean length of 19 cm were treated, with an initial technical success rate of 83%. Adjunctive PTA was necessary in all cases and stenting was required in 7.3%. Primary patency at 1 year was only 33.6%, with most failures occurring between 6 and 9 months postintervention. Primary assisted patency and secondary patency were 65.1% and 75.9%, respectively. Aggressive surveillance and a low threshold to reintervene were thus mandatory to maintain patency in this cohort with long SFA occlusions.

Two large series have looked at laser-assisted angioplasty in those with CLI. Laird and colleagues [39], in the multicenter LACI trial, studied 145 patients (155 limbs) with CLI in a high-risk population (46% American Society of Anesthesiologists (ASA) class 4), with the primary end point being limb salvage at 6 months. Most patients (60%) had TASC D lesions. The median total lesion length treated per limb was 11 cm and their procedural success was 85%. Adjunctive PTA was used in 95%, with stents implanted in 70 limbs (45%). The 6-month limb salvage rate was 93%. Freedom from CLI was approximately 66% at 6 months. Bosiers and colleagues [40], in a similar but smaller study, in Belgium, found congruent results, with a 90.5% limb salvage rate at 6 months and freedom from CLI of 86%. Long-term data on laser atherectomy are lacking, but it appears that, at least in the short term, it has demonstrated benefit in crossing difficult femoropopliteal occlusions and in promoting limb salvage in those who have CLI with prohibitive surgical risk. Table 1 reflects a summary of the studies reviewed.

Summary

Endovascular technology has revolutionized the approach to, and treatment algorithm for, atherosclerotic lower extremity vascular disease. Despite its limitations, available data demonstrate success in improving vessel patency, with decreased morbidity and mortality, compared with surgical procedures. TASC lesion severity correlates with endovascular or open surgical success. Although not a panacea, endovascular strategies are being applied increasingly to more complex femoropopliteal TASC lesions, often driven by the overall cardiovascular morbidity of the patient population in question. As long as open surgical reconstruction is not summarily precluded, an endovascular-first strategy is reasonable, regardless of TASC classification, accepting potentially decreased durability as the trade-off. Proper patient selection and awareness of the indications and limitations of this new technology are paramount to maximizing the preservation of life and limb.

References

[1] Das TS, Beregi JP, Garcia LA, et al. Infrainguinal lesion-specific device choices: round-table discussion. J Endovasc Ther 2006;13(Suppl 2):II60–71.

[2] Muluk SC, Muluk VS, Kelley ME, et al. Outcome events in patients with claudication: a 15-year study in 2777 patients. J Vasc Surg 2001;33(2):251–7 [discussion: 257–8].

[3] Aquino R, Johnnides C, Makaroun M, et al. Natural history of claudication: long-term serial follow-up study of 1244 claudicants. J Vasc Surg 2001;34(6):962–70.

[4] Dormandy JA, Rutherford RB. Management of peripheral arterial disease (PAD). TASC Working Group. TransAtlantic Inter-Society Consensus (TASC). J Vasc Surg 2000; 31(1 Pt 2):S1–296.

[5] Norgren L, Hiatt WR, Dormandy JA, et al. Inter-Society Consensus for the Management of Peripheral Arterial Disease (TASC II). J Vasc Surg 2007;45(Suppl S):S5–67.

[6] Capek P, McLean GK, Berkowitz HD. Femoropopliteal angioplasty. Factors influencing long-term success. Circulation 1991;83(Suppl 2):I70–80.

[7] Johnston KW. Femoral and popliteal arteries: reanalysis of results of balloon angioplasty. Radiology 1992;183(3):767–71.

[8] Zorger N, Manke C, Lenhart M, et al. Peripheral arterial balloon angioplasty: effect of short versus long balloon inflation times on the morphologic results. J Vasc Interv Radiol 2002; 13(4):355–9.

[9] Norgren L, Hiatt WR, Dormandy JA, et al. Inter-society consensus for the management of peripheral arterial disease. Int Angiol 2007;26(2):81–157.

[10] Johnston KW, Rae M, Hogg-Johnston SA, et al. 5-year results of a prospective study of percutaneous transluminal angioplasty. Ann Surg 1987;206(4):403–13.

[11] Clark TW, Groffsky JL, Soulen MC. Predictors of long-term patency after femoropopliteal angioplasty: results from the STAR registry. J Vasc Interv Radiol 2001;12(8):923–33.

[12] Lofberg AM, Karacagil S, Ljungman C, et al. Percutaneous transluminal angioplasty of the femoropopliteal arteries in limbs with chronic critical lower limb ischemia. J Vasc Surg 2001; 34(1):114–21.

[13] Rocha-Singh KJ, Jaff MR, Crabtree TR, et al. Performance goals and endpoint assessments for clinical trials of femoropopliteal bare nitinol stents in patients with symptomatic peripheral arterial disease. Catheter Cardiovasc Interv 2007;69(6):910–9.

[14] Bolia A, Brennan J, Bell PR. Recanalisation of femoro-popliteal occlusions: improving success rate by subintimal recanalisation. Clin Radiol 1989;40(3):325.

[15] Lipsitz EC, Veith FJ, Ohki T. Subintimal angioplasty in the management of critical lower-extremity ischemia: value in limb salvage. Perspect Vasc Surg Endovasc Ther 2005;17(1): 11–20.

[16] Lazaris AM, Salas C, Tsiamis AC, et al. Factors affecting patency of subintimal infrainguinal angioplasty in patients with critical lower limb ischemia. Eur J Vasc Endovasc Surg 2006;32(6):668–74.

[17] Fava M, Loyola S, Polydorou A, et al. Cryoplasty for femoropopliteal arterial disease: late angiographic results of initial human experience. J Vasc Interv Radiol 2004;15(11):1239–43.

[18] Laird J, Jaff MR, Biamino G, et al. Cryoplasty for the treatment of femoropopliteal arterial disease: results of a prospective, multicenter registry. J Vasc Interv Radiol 2005;16(8): 1067–73.

[19] Laird JR, Biamino G, McNamara T, et al. Cryoplasty for the treatment of femoropopliteal arterial disease: extended follow-up results. J Endovasc Ther 2006;13(Suppl 2):II52–9.

[20] Schillinger M, Sabeti S, Loewe C, et al. Balloon angioplasty versus implantation of nitinol stents in the superficial femoral artery. N Engl J Med 2006;354(18):1879–88.

[21] Lugmayr HF, Holzer H, Kastner M, et al. Treatment of complex arteriosclerotic lesions with nitinol stents in the superficial femoral and popliteal arteries: a midterm follow-up. Radiology 2002;222(1):37–43.

[22] Jahnke T, Voshage G, Muller-Hulsbeck S, et al. Endovascular placement of self-expanding nitinol coil stents for the treatment of femoropopliteal obstructive disease. J Vasc Interv Radiol 2002;13(3):257–66.

[23] Henry M, Henry I, Klonaris C, et al. Clinical experience with the OptiMed sinus stent in the peripheral arteries. J Endovasc Ther 2003;10(4):772–9.

[24] Vogel TR, Shindelman LE, Nackman GB, et al. Efficacious use of nitinol stents in the femoral and popliteal arteries. J Vasc Surg 2003;38(6):1178–84.

[25] Mewissen MW. Self-expanding nitinol stents in the femoropopliteal segment: technique and mid-term results. Tech Vasc Interv Radiol 2004;7(1):2–5.

[26] Duda SH, Bosiers M, Lammer J, et al. Drug-eluting and bare nitinol stents for the treatment of atherosclerotic lesions in the superficial femoral artery: long-term results from the SIROCCO trial. J Endovasc Ther 2006;13(6):701–10.

[27] Duda SH, Bosiers M, Lammer J, et al. Sirolimus-eluting versus bare nitinol stent for obstructive superficial femoral artery disease: the SIROCCO II trial. J Vasc Interv Radiol 2005; 16(3):331–8.

[28] Surowiec SM, Davies MG, Eberly SW, et al. Percutaneous angioplasty and stenting of the superficial femoral artery. J Vasc Surg 2005;41(2):269–78.

[29] Scheinert D, Scheinert S, Sax J, et al. Prevalence and clinical impact of stent fractures after femoropopliteal stenting. J Am Coll Cardiol 2005;45(2):312–5.

[30] Adam DJ, Beard JD, Cleveland T, et al. Bypass versus angioplasty in severe ischaemia of the leg (BASIL): multicentre, randomised controlled trial. Lancet 2005;366(9501):1925–34.

[31] Lammer J, Dake MD, Bleyn J, et al. Peripheral arterial obstruction: prospective study of treatment with a transluminally placed self-expanding stent-graft. International Trial Study Group. Radiology 2000;217(1):95–104.

[32] Jahnke T, Andresen R, Muller-Hulsbeck S, et al. Hemobahn stent-grafts for treatment of femoropopliteal arterial obstructions: midterm results of a prospective trial. J Vasc Interv Radiol 2003;14(1):41–51.

[33] Saxon RR, Coffman JM, Gooding JM, et al. Long-term results of ePTFE stent-graft versus angioplasty in the femoropopliteal artery: single center experience from a prospective, randomized trial. J Vasc Interv Radiol 2003;14(3):303–11.

[34] Kedora J, Hohmann S, Garrett W, et al. Randomized comparison of percutaneous Viabahn stent grafts vs prosthetic femoral-popliteal bypass in the treatment of superficial femoral arterial occlusive disease. J Vasc Surg 2007;45(1):10–6 [discussion: 16].

[35] Zeller T, Rastan A, Schwarzwalder U, et al. Percutaneous peripheral atherectomy of femoropopliteal stenoses using a new-generation device: six-month results from a single-center experience. J Endovasc Ther 2004;11(6):676–85.

[36] Ramaiah V, Gammon R, Kiesz S, et al. Midterm outcomes from the TALON registry: treating peripherals with SilverHawk: outcomes collection. J Endovasc Ther 2006;13(5): 592–602.

[37] Yancey AE, Minion DJ, Rodriguez C, et al. Peripheral atherectomy in TransAtlantic InterSociety Consensus type C femoropopliteal lesions for limb salvage. J Vasc Surg 2006; 44(3):503–9.

[38] Scheinert D, Laird JR Jr, Schroder M, et al. Excimer laser-assisted recanalization of long, chronic superficial femoral artery occlusions. J Endovasc Ther 2001;8(2):156–66.

[39] Laird JR Jr, Reiser C, Biamino G, et al. Excimer laser assisted angioplasty for the treatment of critical limb ischemia. J Cardiovasc Surg (Torino) 2004;45(3):239–48.

[40] Bosiers M, Peeters P, Elst FV, et al. Excimer laser assisted angioplasty for critical limb ischemia: results of the LACI Belgium Study. Eur J Vasc Endovasc Surg 2005;29(6):613–9.

ELSEVIER
SAUNDERS

Surg Clin N Am 87 (2007) 1149–1177

SURGICAL
CLINICS OF
NORTH AMERICA

The Diabetic Foot

Charles A. Andersen, MD, FACS[a],*,
Thomas S. Roukis, DPM, FACFAS[b]

[a]*Vascular/Endovascular Surgery Service, Department of Surgery, Madigan Army Medical
Center, 9040-A Fitzsimmons Avenue, MCHJ-SV, Tacoma, WA 98431, USA*
[b]*Limb Preservation Service, Vascular/Endovascular Surgery Service, Department of Surgery,
Madigan Army Medical Center, 9040-A Fitzsimmons Avenue, MCHJ-SV,
Tacoma, WA 98431, USA*

The prevalence of diabetes mellitus is increasing at epidemic proportions. The worldwide prevalence of diabetes now exceeds 200 million and is expected to rise to more than 300 million in the next 20 years. It is estimated that 7% of the American population has diabetes. There is also an epidemic of obesity in the United States associated with an increased incidence of type II diabetes. With increasing longevity of the population, the incidence of diabetic-related complications is also increasing. These complications include specific diabetic foot problems as well as those resulting from peripheral arterial disease (PAD). Patients with diabetes have a 12% to 25% risk of developing a foot ulcer during their lifetime, and these are the most common risk factor for subsequent amputation. There are over 1 million amputations performed per year for diabetes-related foot problems, and diabetes is the most common cause of amputations in the United States [1–3].

The feet of diabetic patients can be affected with neuropathy, peripheral arterial disease, foot deformity, infections, ulcerations, and gangrene, and diabetic foot problems are a major source of morbidity and mortality. Knowledge of the pathophysiology, diagnosis, and treatment of problems in the diabetic foot is important for the general surgeon and is often neglected in surgical education. Diabetic foot infections represent a medical emergency: a delay in their diagnosis and management increases morbidity and mortality and contributes to a higher amputation rate [4,5].

* Corresponding author.
E-mail address: charles.andersen@us.army.mil (C.A. Andersen).

0039-6109/07/$ - see front matter © 2007 Elsevier Inc. All rights reserved.
doi:10.1016/j.suc.2007.08.001

Etiology of diabetic foot problems

The most important underlying condition leading to diabetic foot problems is neuropathy. Diabetic neuropathy involves sensory, motor, and autonomic nerves. Sensory neuropathy leads to a loss of protective sensation [4]. With the loss of protective sensation, foot trauma is unrecognized and leads to ulceration. The ulceration is often the portal of entry for bacteria, leading to cellulitis and/or abscess formation. Motor neuropathy can lead to muscle atrophy, foot deformity, and altered biomechanics. This leads to areas of high pressure during standing or walking and repeated trauma that may go unrecognized because of sensory deficit. Autonomic neuropathy results in a loss of sweating and dry skin that leads to cracks and fissures and a portal of entry for bacteria. Autonomic neuropathy also leads to an alteration of the neurogenic regulation of cutaneous blood supply that can contribute to ulceration and altered response to infection [6–8].

Diabetes is also associated with an increased risk of PAD. PAD is generally not the primary etiology of diabetic foot problems; however, it can be a major factor in an altered response to foot infections and nonhealing of foot ulcerations. Once an infection and/or ulceration is present, it increases the demand for blood supply to the foot. With PAD there may be an inability to meet that demand, leading to further tissue breakdown and progressive infection. The presence of PAD in a diabetic patient with foot ulceration or foot infection increases the risk of amputation. It is therefore of paramount importance to identify and treat coexisting PAD [6,9].

Diabetic foot infections

Any breach of the cutaneous integument of the foot in a person with diabetes can lead to a severe soft-tissue and/or osseous infection [4,6,7,10–13]. If medical attention is delayed as a result of dense sensory neuropathy or the patient's lack of a response to the infection by mounting constitutional symptoms, more invasive treatment, including amputation of the limb, may be required [13]. As the interaction of most general surgeons with patients with diabetic foot infections will occur in the emergency room (ER), the decision of whether the patient can be treated as an outpatient and referred for ongoing care or whether the patient requires admission and surgical intervention is paramount. Unfortunately, this is frequently not a clear process. The initial evaluation begins with a detailed history and physical examination.

A history of any type of foot trauma such as those previously mentioned should raise the suspicion for possible adjacent soft-tissue or osseous infection [14–16]. Persistently elevated or widely shifting blood glucose levels; constitutional symptoms, including nausea, emesis, tachycardia, fever with chills, lethargy, and pain; along with physical findings such as cellulitis, lymphangitis, ulceration, or purulent discharge are noteworthy findings.

Diabetic patients can have a significant foot infection and lack pain and not mount a systemic inflammatory response. A high index of suspicion is therefore required to diagnose foot infections in the patient with diabetes. Pain in a neuropathic foot is usually related to an underlying infection [8]. After a thorough surgical preparation in the ER to remove debris and allow proper evaluation of the patient's integument (Fig. 1), all open wounds should be counted, their locations documented, and they should be palpated and probed to determine the depth of the wound and the tissues involved [17,18]. This is followed by either admission for surgical decompression or outpatient follow-up using specific patient care instructions and close follow-up with the primary care physician, who may further refer the patient to a specialist in management of the diabetic foot.

A multidisciplinary team that includes a general surgeon, vascular surgeon, cardiologist, endocrinologist, infectious disease specialist, primary care physician, and an experienced podiatric foot and ankle surgeon or orthopaedic surgeon is necessary and vital to the patient's treatment. A nutritionist, psychologist, social worker, and certified prosthetist and/or

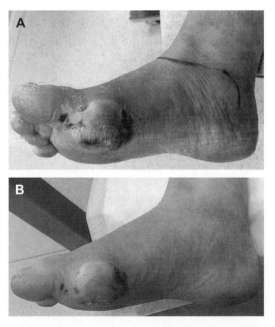

Fig. 1. Photograph of a diabetic foot ulcer with surrounding cellulitis plantar to the first metatarsal head upon first evaluation by the surgical staff but after being evaluated by emergency room personnel. Note the poor pedal hygiene and permanent marker application at the ankle level intended to demarcate the proximal extent of cellulitis. The initial appearance is consistent with a limb-threatening infection (*A*). Photograph taken after surgical scrub revealing much improved pedal hygiene and the actual extent of the cellulitis, which is contained to the medial forefoot. The appearance is therefore most consistent with a non–limb-threatening infection (compare with Fig. 1A) (*B*).

orthotist will also play a significant role in the patient's treatment and recovery [19,20].

Laboratory evaluation

Laboratory evaluation begins with a complete blood count and white blood cell (WBC) differential. Determination of anemia is important, as this should be addressed before any surgical intervention about the foot where a tourniquet is not routinely used for the reasons discussed later and blood loss can be substantial. An elevated WBC count with a left shift suggests a severe infection; however, the absence of an elevated WBC count does not preclude a severe infection [7]. A random glucose level and glycosolated hemoglobin (Hg A-1C) should be obtained to evaluate for acute severe hypo- or hyperglycemia as well as to gauge the patient's overall glycemic control throughout the previous 120 days [7]. The patient's acute nutritional status should be evaluated by obtaining a pre-albumin level, and general nutritional status should be evaluated by obtaining an albumin level. Hepatic and renal function tests are also necessary for monitoring the patient's metabolic status as well as for adjusting the chosen antibiotic regimen. Elevated inflammatory markers, such as an erythrocyte sedimentation rate (ESR) above 70 mm/hour, are highly suggestive of osteomyelitis [8,21]. Following the progression of the ESR over the course of the patient's hospitalization is an inexpensive way to monitor the effectiveness of antibiotic therapy. C-reactive protein is another marker that is more sensitive than ESR but is more costly. Electrolyte and coagulation lab studies should also be obtained. Blood cultures, urinalysis, radiographs of both feet, and further imaging studies such as MRI or bone scintigraphy should also be considered, depending on the severity of the infection and the course of intervention entertained. Most patients with diabetes who present to the ER with a severe foot infection have chronically poor glycemic control, chronic anemia, poor nutrition, and infrequent physician visits [8]. Therefore, it is paramount that ER personnel obtain the above laboratory studies on each patient with diabetes who presents with a foot infection before contacting the general surgeon for evaluation of the patient.

Microbiological diagnosis should start with a gram stain, which helps the surgeon select the most appropriate empiric antibiotic therapy. Specimens for cultures should be processed for aerobic, anaerobic, and fungal organisms. Antibiotic therapy should be reassessed and modified when cultures and sensitivities are available. Reliable deep-tissue or bone specimens are necessary for the appropriate antibiotic therapy. Superficial cultures taken by swab of an ulcer bed, especially while in the ER, are usually contaminated with colonizing bacteria and often do not identify the infected organism(s). Therefore, deep-tissue samples or osseous scrapings are more reliable specimens for cultures and for monitoring isolates with antibiotic resistance [22].

Diagnosing osteomyelitis

Osteomyelitis should be considered in any patient with a chronic non-healing wound, especially if it is deeper than the dermis layer. One bedside clinical test for osteomyelitis underlying an open wound is the "probe to bone test." In one study of patients with a limb-threatening infection, the ability to probe bone at the base of an ulcer with a sterile blunt steel probe had a positive predictive value of 89% and a negative predictive value of 56% [23].

Bone biopsy is the gold standard test for diagnosing osteomyelitis [24–26]. Osseous specimens can be taken percutaneously using a trephine or at the time of surgical intervention, preferably before antibiotic therapy being initiated. False-negative bone cultures can result from either an inadequate specimen or previous antibiotic therapy. In these situations, histopathological analysis is useful to determine whether there is an acute or chronic inflammatory response. In cases handled by delayed primary closure, consider deep soft-tissue and/or osseous cultures to identify any residual organisms. Imaging techniques commonly employed to diagnose osteomyelitis include plain radiographs of both feet, bone scintigraphy, MRI, CT, and diagnostic ultrasound. Each method has advantages and limitations; careful patient evaluation is necessary before obtaining an expensive and possibly unnecessary test.

Plain radiographs of both feet, with the contralateral uninvolved foot serving as a control, should be obtained at the initial visit to provide the baseline by which to monitor any progressive destruction of bone [27]. Developing radiolucency in bone as a result of osteomyelitis typically requires 5–7 days, and it takes at least 10–14 days for the first signs of sequestrum and involucrum to be noticeable [28]. Osseous focal demineralization, periosteal elevation, and cortical irregularity evidenced on plain radiographs are usually not detected until there has been between 35% and 50% reduction in bone mineral density compared with the adjacent normal bone [28]. In addition to information on osseous abnormalities, radiographs can be used to determine the presence of soft-tissue edema, gas within the soft-tissue planes, or foreign bodies. Consider repeating radiographs after 10–14 days, especially after surgical procedures, to assess the osseous quality and monitor for progression of osteomyelitis or healing [29,30].

A variety of nuclear medicine procedures has been used in suspected foot infection. Bone scintigraphy can both confirm the diagnosis of osteomyelitis and determine its extent. These scans are more sensitive than radiographs in early infection. Technesium-99 MDP bone scans can, however, show increased uptake in conditions other than osteomyelitis, including Charcot neuropathic osteoarthropathy, acute and chronic fractures, and tumors, as well as postsurgical changes [31–33]. Thus, this test is quite sensitive but not very specific for diagnosing osteomyelitis. Other scintigraphic procedures, including Gallium-67, leukocyte scans using Indium-111 or

Technesium-99 HMPAO, and sulfur colloid scans, may be more specific for diagnosing osteomyelitis [31–39]. The difficulties with bone scintigraphy include the lengthy nature of the procedure, user variability, and frequent difficulty in definitive evaluation owing to the small size and predominantly cortical nature of bone in the foot, especially the forefoot and toes.

Over the past decade, MRI has emerged as the most accurate imaging modality for the diagnosis of osteomyelitis and allows for superb detail of the surrounding soft-tissue structures [40–44]. However, postsurgical changes, Charcot neuropathic osteoarthropathy, acute and chronic fractures, and avascular necrosis may generate false-positive results. MRI is most appropriately employed in the face of a non–limb- or life-threatening infection to allow proper surgical planning and to identify the extent of any sinus tracts or abscess formation. Limitations of MRI include retained metallic implants, claustrophobia, the increased cost relative to plain radiographs, and availability of MRI scanning in the evenings and over weekends, when patients with diabetes and foot infections tend to present to the ER.

CT scans and ultrasound imaging have shown promise in the diagnosis of osteomyelitis, but each has certain limitations. CT scans are the imaging modality of choice for detecting sequestra and cortical changes in chronic osteomyelitis [45,46]. Ultrasound imaging, although user dependent and not usually readily available, represents a rapid, painless, and inexpensive tool to help define any soft-tissue inflammation or abscess and perhaps detect chronic osteomyelitis [47,48].

On the basis of the above discussion, it is apparent that myriad imaging modalities are available to detect osteomyelitis and to assist in surgical intervention. Selecting an imaging modality will often be based on local availability, cost, and expertise. Although MRI has emerged as the best of the imaging tests, the value of all depends on the pretest probability of osteomyelitis [49], and bone biopsy is still recommended to confirm the diagnosis.

Antibiotic therapy

One of the main determinants of the type of antibiotic therapy necessary for the treatment of a diabetic foot infection is its severity [50–74]. Diabetic foot infections are classified as non-limb threatening or limb threatening. Initial antibiotic therapy is selected based on the most commonly involved bacteria and the degree of infection. Non–limb-threatening infections are characterized by the presence of superficial ulcer that does not probe deep to bone and has less than 2 cm of surrounding cellulitis, in a patient with no signs of systemic toxicity and an absence of leukocytosis. Limb-threatening infections are characterized by the presence of an edematous foot with a full-thickness ulcer that probes to bone or communicates with the compartments of the foot, frequently with gangrene adjacent to the ulcer and purulence expressed upon compression, and has more than 2 cm of surrounding cellulitis or lymphangitis, in a patient that has systemic signs of toxicity (ie, fever, leukocytosis, tachycardia, hyperglycemia) or metabolic instability. Limb-threatening infections require hospitalization, surgical débridement, and prolonged intravenous antibiotic therapy, whereas non–limb-threatening infections can usually be treated in the outpatient setting with appropriate minor surgical débridement and oral antibiotic therapy. In all situations, adequate management of the wound through the use of well-padded and properly applied dressings, along with proper and continuous off-loading of the wound as well as treatment of the of patient's comorbidities, is necessary for a successful outcome. Antibiotic prophylaxis in non-infected chronic wounds can result in drug-related toxicity, can be expensive, and can drive the emergence of resistant organisms, and are therefore not warranted [7].

Most diabetic foot infections are treated with an empirically selected antibiotic regimen until cultures and sensitivities are available [4,6,7,10–13]. This initial therapy can usually be narrow-spectrum agents that cover aerobic gram-positive cocci for superficial and mild infections. Broader-spectrum agents are appropriate for deep or limb-threatening infections. Empiric antibiotic therapy should always include an agent active against the *Staphylococcus* and *Streptococcus* species, which represent the predominant pathogens. Therapy aimed at aerobic gram-negative and anaerobic bacteria should also be considered for gangrenous, ischemic, or malodorous wounds. Methicillin-resistant *Staphylococcus aureus* (MRSA) as a true pathogen in diabetic foot infections has become more common, especially in those patients treated haphazardly with extended courses of oral antibiotics and those who have been repeatedly hospitalized or placed in a skilled nursing facility for an extended period of time.

The dosage and duration of intravenous and oral antibiotic therapy in diabetic foot infections are not completely clear. Oral antibiotic therapy is less expensive and with fewer side effects. In limb-threatening diabetic foot infections or osteomyelitis, intravenous therapy and aggressive surgical débridement should be initiated and followed, if possible, by oral agents. The use of topical antibiotics in isolation has a limited place in the treatment of diabetic foot infections [50,51] and may produce the development of resistant strains of colonized surface bacteria.

Diabetic foot ulcers

Patients may present with ulceration without evidence of infection. Conservative treatment of diabetic foot ulcerations revolves around providing the proper wound-healing environment and stopping the repetitive trauma by off-loading the foot. The vascular status of a patient is obviously a critical element for wound healing because without sufficient arterial flow, antibiotics cannot be delivered and the critical elements associated with wound healing cannot reach the wound site. Any patient who does not have palpable pulses should have a formal evaluation of the vascular status as discussed in a following section. Edema is a significant negative healing factor. Edema may be due to venous insufficiency or secondary to other medical conditions such as congestive heart failure. Differentiation of the etiology and treatment of the edema is an important factor in wound healing. These topics are discussed in a future section below.

After arterial inflow and venous outflow are assessed, the wound itself should be thoroughly evaluated. The location of a diabetic foot wound will usually lead the surgeon to the underlying cause and therefore the most appropriate treatment modalities. An ulcer about the posterior border of the heel is usually the result of chronic pressure from prolonged contact with bedding, friction from rubbing against rough bed sheets, and lack of heel elevation [75]. This is most easily treated through prevention; diligence in maintaining pressure reduction about the heels; and education of the patient, his or her family members, and the nursing staff involved in the patient's care [75]. At the Madigan Army Medical Center, "heel boots," whether firm or soft, routinely are not used for several reasons. First, these devices are difficult to maintain in proper position because patients frequently move their lower limbs and the devices rotate about despite being secured with straps. Second, they limit air flow, which enhances growth of bacteria on skin and inhibits proper hygiene. Third, most if not all patients with diabetes posses an equinus contracture (ie, inability to dorsiflex the foot past 90° relative to the lower leg), which results from non-enzymatic glycosylation of the tendons, joint capsules, and ligaments about the lower extremity while the boots are universally fixed at 90°. This physiologic mismatch pushes the posterior heel out of the aperture present in the boots, negating the off-loading effect and resulting in excessive pressure about the forefoot—especially laterally—as well as the lateral ankle, which can rapidly result in ulceration (Fig. 2A). This is why the authors employ a "heel suspension pillow cocoon" that continuously suspends the heels off of the bed, even with patient movements, and disperses pressure throughout the entire posterior aspect of the lower legs, thereby limiting pressure ulceration (Fig. 2B). An added benefit is the slight elevation of both limbs that occurs and helps to reduce lower extremity edema.

An ulcer about the plantar foot is almost always the result of (1) excessive pressure and time between the foot and contact surface; (2) dense neuropathy; and (3) deformity of the foot, most commonly a prominent osseous segment (ie, metatarsal head) and rigid joint contracture (ie, equinus contracture) [4,6,7,10–13]. Understanding this process allows the surgeon to not only address the wound but also the underlying cause(s) that are usually responsible for the development of the wound in the first place. By understanding and addressing the underlying cause(s), the surgeon will allow wound care to more effectively heal the wound and maintain it closed once healed. Obviously, the single best means of reducing pressure on the sole of the foot is to employ strict non–weight-bearing of the involved limb through the use of gait aides (eg, crutches, walker, etc). Although ideal,

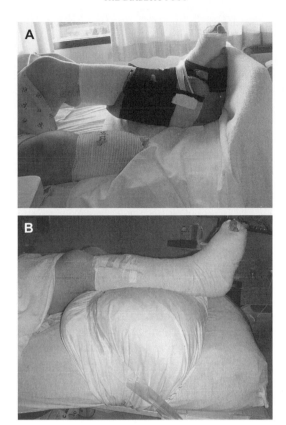

Fig. 2. Photograph of a padded heel boot applied to the left foot of a patient with a heel ulcer and equinus contracture and contralateral transtibial amputation preceded by foot ulceration (*A*). Note: (1) the posterior heel pushed out of the aperture present in the boot; (2) the direct contact of the forefoot with the foot board on the bed; (3) the forefoot extending out of the boot due to the inability of the boot, which is fixed at 90°, to accommodate an equinus contracture; and (4) the straps excessively tightened about the anterior ankle and foot in an attempt to hold the boot in place. Photograph demonstrating the "heel suspension pillow cocoon" from a side (*B*) that consists of three pillows encased in a bed sheet that has been secured to the sides of the bed either with tape or by tying the ends of the sheet to bed rails or to each other underneath the bed.

this is not always practical and in some cases dangerous, as the patient increases his or her likelihood of falling and being injured especially while maneuvering stairs. However, the authors inform every patient that a high concentration of weight-bearing is detrimental and, therefore, when the patient presents for the outpatient office visit, he or she is instructed to be dropped off at the entrance to the facility by a family member and then is brought into the clinic in a wheelchair. This saves many hundreds of steps concentrated in a brief time period and also increases the patient's understanding of just how detrimental excessive ambulation is when trying to heal a plantar foot wound. When a patient states that he or she is staying off the foot "as much as possible," a formal discussion of the accepted weight-bearing parameters ensues. These parameters include rising from a seated position, such as off of a recliner or toilet, and transferring in and out of a vehicle for transportation to and from office visits only. Any weight-bearing beyond this is unacceptable and re-emphasized to the patient and the family to enhance compliance. If any special circumstances exists that limit compliance, social work, physical therapy, and occupational therapy are involved to assess obstacles to compliance that can then be addressed. In addition to the above, excessive pressure and time can be reduced with the use of a properly applied and well-padded dressing that extends from the toes to the knee for the reasons described previously. This would be followed with a specialized postoperative shoe and multilayered insole [76,77]. The Med-Surg postoperative shoe (Darco International, Inc., Huntington, WV) has a stable and low-profile rocker sole that has been shown to reduce pressure about the forefoot and heel by more than 25% compared with a traditional postoperative shoe. Additionally, the Peg-Assist orthotic system (Darco International, Inc., Huntington, WV) consists of several layers of varying density and heat-moldable liners with a series of removable pegs that enhance shock absorption and off-loading, respectively. Modalities such as wedged postoperative shoes, removable walking boots, and total contact casting are also available [78]. Wedged postoperative shoes and removable walking boots are usually not well tolerated due to the presence of underlying osseous deformities that make application of an "off-the-shelf" device impractical and, frankly, dangerous. Although total contact casting has largely been considered the gold standard when trying to provide a measure of mechanical protection, the technique is expensive because of the length of time they take to apply, the number of supplies required, and the difficulty of use in practice, requiring significant knowledge of the application process. Additionally, the total contact cast must be changed as edema subsides—usually twice a week or more; cannot be used with draining or infected wounds; and frequently leads to complications, including new ulcerations about the osseous prominences of the foot, ankle, and lower leg [79].

Three types of neuropathy are commonly associated with the development of diabetic foot ulcerations [80–82]. Sensory neuropathy is most commonly associated with ulcer formation. Usually, a loss of protective sensation results in repetitive injury to the skin, ultimately leading to blister formation and breakdown. Motor neuropathy may produce asymmetric muscle weakness. Anterior and lateral compartment muscle weakness can result in clawing of the toes, foot drop, and apropulsive gait patterns. These abnormalities produce bony prominences, prolonged loads, and aberrant pressures, which increase the risk of repetitive stress injuries to the skin. Sympathetic neuropathy changes the flow of blood to the skin and may result in diminished healing capacity. In addition, this type of neuropathy may be responsible for persistent coldness or erythema, in the absence of other types of vascular disease. Dense neuropathy is usually irreversible, but tight glycemic control over a prolonged period can help prevent progression; therefore, referral to an endocrinologist and diabetic nurse educator is required [82]. Custom-molded insoles, extra-depth shoes, and various types of braces are all designed to eliminate repetitive mechanical forces and negate the aberrant mechanical forces created by muscle imbalances. These devices are frequently supplemented by insole modifications and reduced activity levels as described above [77]. Although beyond the scope of this article, any underlying deformities should be corrected, especially if the wound recurs. If this occurs, the patient should be referred to a podiatric foot and ankle surgeon or orthopaedic surgeon who specializes in the management of diabetic foot and ankle disorders [83].

Finally, ulceration about the dorsal aspect of the toes, at the insertion of the Achilles tendon, and at osseous prominences about the borders of the foot (ie, first and fifth metatarsal heads, fifth metatarsal base) is usually the result of improperly fitting shoe gear and requires referral to a knowledgeable pedorthist or orthotist, who should fit the patient with properly sized shoe gear and provide oral and written education for proper use [84].

Once the location of the wound and the underlying etiology have been determined, attention is then directed toward the characteristics of the wound itself. Wounds should neither be too wet nor too dry, should not contain any necrotic tissue, and must have adequate blood flow to heal. The length, width, and depth of the wound should be measured and recorded to monitor healing over time. When properly treated, wounds should first become filled with granulation tissue and then epithelialize. The presence of hyperkeratotic tissue surrounding the ulceration is a result of excessive pressure and is detrimental to successful closure of the wound because this tissue acts like a splint preventing contracture, increases pressure to the underlying deep tissues causing undermining and necrosis, and harbors bacteria that promote colonization [85]. This tissue should therefore be fully débrided down to the level of native healthy underlying tissue to properly evaluate the full dimensions of the ulceration and remove the diseased tissue. Although several classification systems exist for diabetic foot ulceration, the most widely employed system amongst specialists in the diabetic foot is the "University of Texas at San Antonio Ulcer Classification System," which has been validated (Table 1). As the stage and grade increase, the likelihood of requiring surgical intervention increases exponentially [86,87]. Use of this classification system will help the general surgeon to determine which patients require admission for more extensive surgical débridement and which ones can be managed as an outpatient.

All wounds present on the foot of a patient with diabetes should be considered colonized with bacteria. This is because people with diabetes frequently have diminished eyesight (ie, diabetic retinopathy), making it difficult for them to visually evaluate the foot and assess its hygiene.

Table 1
University of Texas at San Antonio Ulcer Classification System

| Stage | Grade | | | |
	0	I	II	III
A	Pre- or postulcerative lesions completely epithelized	Superficial wound not involving tendon, capsule, or bone	Wound penetrating to tendon or capsule	Wound penetrating to bone of joint
B	Infected	Infected	Infected	Infected
C	Ischemic	Ischemic	Ischemic	Ischemic
D	Infected and ischemic	Infected and ischemic	Infected and ischemic	Infected and ischemic

Mobility issues are common, and therefore the patient with diabetes is usually unable to readily inspect his or her feet and hand-wash them. Finally, the feet are easily concealed inside of socks and shoe gear, which often harbor bacteria and fungus, especially in shoe gear that is worn daily but infrequently—if ever—cleaned or replaced. The authors recommend that patients with diabetes cleane their feet daily for 3–5 minutes with a washcloth and liquid soap to improve pedal hygiene. A family member may need to be recruited to help with this if the patient is unable to reach the feet. Their shoe gear should consist of a pair of shoes dedicated to outdoor use only and that has been fitted by a pedorthist, as well as a separate pair of shoes that is worn only indoors and most commonly consists of a rubber clog. Rubber clogs (Crocs Footwear, Niwot, CO; www.crocs.com) are ideal in that they can easily be cleaned, are easy to put on and take off without having to bend over to apply them; are supportive; and, owing to their thick material, protect against mild trauma such as stubbing injuries to the toes. These measures are for daily use once the wound heals—not during the actual healing process on the affected limb. They are useful in protecting the uninvolved limb, which is at risk for ulceration owing to the extra weight-bearing demands placed on it [4,6,10,12].

Wound-cleaning compounds such as soaps, cleansers, and rinses will reduce the bacterial load dramatically when dressing is changed and are a good means of maximizing hygiene of the involved limb during outpatient clinical visits [88]. At the Madigan Army Medical Center, a "débridement pack" has been created that includes a topical antibiotic soap (Techni-Care Antiseptic Surgical Scrub Solution, Care-Tech Laboratories, Inc., St. Louis, MO) that is used to clean the foot, ankle, and lower leg of the patient as well as the wound through the use of sterile gauze. Techni-Care is a broad-spectrum microbicide effective against gram-positive and gram-negative bacteria, including MRSA, VRE, and Candida. Sterile instrumentation for sharp débridement of the wound is included, as are the dressings necessary to apply a well-padded dressing from the toes to knee (Fig. 3). This procedure is essential to maintain integrity of the dressing between

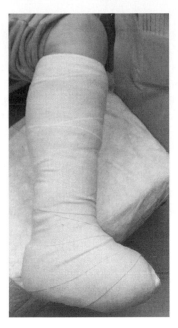

Fig. 3. Photograph demonstrating proper application of a well-padded lower extremity dressing extending from the toes to the knee.

outpatient office visits, pad osseous prominences, and control lower extremity edema.

Wound dressings are no longer simply gauze. The bandages available today are specifically designed to address various problems associated with the wound environment, and several options are available for controlling the fluid content of the wound. Occlusive or absorptive dressings can be selected to prevent desiccation or maceration as necessary. Products are now available that safely and effectively reduce bacterial count. Silver-impregnated bandages and bandages with antibiotic coating are readily available. Ultimately, the selection of a wound dressing should be based on an assessment of the wound and the perceived problems associated with the wound environment [89]. Regardless of what type of dressing is applied to the wound, the entire foot, ankle, and lower limb should be covered by a well-padded dressing for the reasons described previously.

Surgical management of diabetic foot infections: vascular anatomy of the foot

A thorough understanding of the vascular anatomy of the foot is essential before performing surgical intervention on the foot, as an improperly placed incision will frequently lead to necrosis of the adjacent tissues and also make subsequent closure of the wound more difficult.

Hidalgo and Shaw [90] performed polymer corrosion cast studies of the plantar vasculature in 15 fresh cadaveric specimens in an attempt to improve on flap design for soft-tissue coverage of the plantar aspect of the foot. Four zones of regional arterial anatomy were described: (1) the proximal plantar area, (2) the midplantar area, (3) the lateral foot, and (4) the distal foot. The proximal plantar area extends from the posterior aspect of the calcaneus to approximately half the length of the plantar aspect of the foot, and is supplied by "wrap-around" branches of the dorsalis pedis artery that inosculate with the lateral plantar artery. The midplantar area overlies the distal two thirds of the plantar aponeurosis. It is commonly referred to as the "watershed area" because its blood supply arises from multiple sources being supplied to a variable degree by the medial plantar, lateral plantar, and deep plantar arteries without significant musculocutaneous or fasciocutaneous arterial supply. The lateral foot area encompasses the region lateral to the plantar aponeurosis in the middle third of the plantar aspect of the foot and is supplied by the dorsalis pedis and lateral plantar arteries. The distal foot area includes that portion of the plantar aspect of the foot distal to the midplantar area and is supplied by inosculation of the deep plantar branch of the dorsalis pedis artery and the deep transverse component of the lateral plantar artery, with a small contribution from the medial plantar artery.

Attinger and colleagues [91,92] further expanded on the work of Hidalgo and Shaw [90] and described distinct angiosome boundaries that supplied the plantar foot. These angiosomes were defined by the (1) dorsalis pedis/first dorsal metatarsal artery, (2) calcaneal branch of the posterior tibial artery, (3) calcaneal branch of the peroneal artery, (4) medial plantar artery, and (5) lateral plantar artery. It was concluded that the superficial branch of the medial plantar artery, the deep medial plantar artery, and the lateral plantar artery supply the medial, central, and lateral portions of the plantar aspect of the foot, respectively. In addition, the plantar common digital and individual digital arteries supply the plantar aspect of the forefoot, and the calcaneal branches of the posterior tibial and peroneal arteries supply the heel.

Surgical management of diabetic foot infections: foot compartments

The number of foot compartments has not been universally accepted; however, 10 compartments have been identified that can require decompression with a surgical incision [93,94]: (1) the skin, (2) medial, (3) superficial central, (4) deep central, (5) lateral, (6–9) interosseoi, and (10) calcaneal compartments [93]. The skin of the foot is a highly specialized organ. The plantar skin consists of a complex array of fascia, fibrous septae, and columnar adipose that permits protection from vertical compressive and tangential shearing forces that occur during gait. The dorsal skin is bound to the underlying extensor retinaculum and intimately associated with the extensor digitorum brevis and hallucis muscles that are in close proximity to the dorsalis pedis and deep peroneal nerve. The medial compartment contains the abductor hallucis and flexor hallucis brevis muscles, the superficial medial plantar artery, and nerve, and communicates with the deep posterior compartment of the lower leg through continuation of the flexor hallucis longus tendon. The superficial central compartment contains the flexor digitorum brevis and attached lumbricale muscles, and the deep central compartment contains the transverse and oblique heads of the adductor hallucis muscles. The lateral compartment contains the abductor and flexor digiti minimi along with the lateral plantar artery and nerve after passing through the calcaneal compartment, which also contains the quatratus plantae muscle and nerve to the abductor digiti minimi muscle. The four interosseous compartments contain the dorsal and plantar interosseous muscles within the intermetatarsal spaces.

Surgical management of diabetic foot infections: incision placement

With the above anatomy in mind, the safest placement for foot incisions and drainage of a deep-space abscess within the various compartments of the foot [93,94] will now be described based on easily palpated osseous structures and topography of the foot. Regardless of where the incision is placed, the surgical knife should extend through the skin, dermis, superficial fascia, and adipose to maintain the resultant skin edges as thick as possible [18]. Note, however, that the incisions should not be placed "down to bone"; instead, controlled dissection with a combination of sharp and blunt instrumentation should be employed in line with the initial skin incisions to maintain thick skin flaps, prevent undermining of the tissues, and maintain cutaneous vascularity to promote delayed primary closure.

For the medial border of the foot, first the surgeon marks the center of the first metatarsal head medially, which can easily be identified by palpation and also by identifying the junction between the plantar and dorsal skin at this level. Next, the inferior aspect of the navicular tuberosity at the high point of the medial arch is identified through palpation and marked. Finally, the midpoint between the junction of the posterior and plantar heel and inferior aspect of the medial malleolus is identified and marked. Connecting the marks creates a curved incision along the medial border of the foot (Fig. 4A) that respects the junction between the dorsal and plantar vascular supply and courses along the dorsal aspect of the abductor hallucis muscle belly, which can be used as a muscle flap [95] that can easily be skin grafted and will not result in a noticeable functional deficit should delayed primary closure be impossible to perform. After reflecting the abductor hallucis muscle inferiorly, the deep fascia should be incised in line with the skin incision to limit potential damage to the underlying neurovascular structures while allowing for complete decompression of the medial, superficial central, deep central, and calcaneal compartments of the foot as well as the tarsal tunnel. Additionally, evaluation of the long flexor tendons coursing the full length of the foot can be inspected. The flexor tendons are a frequent conduit for bacteria to spread from the forefoot and toes into the lower leg, [44] at which point the incision can be extended proximally to explore the medial compartments of the lower leg.

For the lateral border of the foot, first the surgeon marks the center of the fifth metatarsal head using the same criteria as for the first metatarsal head described above. Next, the inferior aspect of the fifth metatarsal base is identified through palpation and marked. A line connecting these two marks is created and extended to the posterior aspect of the foot. Next, the midpoint between the Achilles tendon and the posterior border of the fibula is identified at the level of the ankle joint, and a line from this point is drawn distally to intersect the previous line drawn on the lateral border of the foot. This creates a linear incision about the lateral border of the foot (Fig. 4B) that respects the junction between the lateral and plantar blood supply and courses along the dorsal aspect of the abductor digiti minimi muscle belly, which can also be used as a muscle flap [95] as described above. After reflecting the abductor digiti minimi muscle inferiorly, the deep fascia should be incised in line with the skin incision for the reasons mentioned above. This incision allows for decompression of the lateral, superficial central, deep central, and calcaneal compartments of the foot as well as the peroneal tendons. The incision can be extended proximally if infection has tracked along the peroneal tendons into the lateral compartment of the lower leg.

For the dorsal aspect of the forefoot, two incisions are necessary to adequately decompress the inter-osseous compartments. The first incision should be placed overlying the medial border of the second metatarsal, and the second incision should be placed overlying the lateral border of the fourth metatarsal (Fig. 4C). The placement of these incisions is critical because a full-thickness skin bridge of at least 2 cm must be maintained to limit vascular compromise to the resultant skin bridge [94]. Both incisions should extend from the metatarsal head to the base. The medial incision will allow decompression of the first interosseous space between the first and second metatarsals, and the second interosseous space between the second and third metatarsals. The lateral incision will allow decompression of the third interosseous space between the third and fourth metatarsals, and the fourth metatarsal space between the fourth and fifth metatarsals. Decompression of the dorsal and plantar interosseoi within the interosseous spaces is aided by the used of a long, blunt, curved instrument that is first inserted until contact is made with the plantar structures and then fully opened. For the dorsal aspect of the midfoot and hindfoot, the forefoot incisions can be extended proximally, with the medial one coursing along the lateral border of the anterior tibial tendon and the lateral one along the lateral border of the extensor digitorum longus tendon (Fig. 4C).

Finally, for the plantar aspect of the foot, a single longitudinal incision that extends from just proximal to the weight-bearing surface of the forefoot and culminates just distal to the weight-bearing surface of the heel along an imaginary line drawn between the second toe and center of the heel (Fig. 4D) will allow full exposure of every compartment of the foot except the dorsal aspect once the plantar fascia has been incised. The main drawback is the need for prolonged non–weight-bearing to limit the potential for cicatrix formation and the potential to disrupt important anatomical structures necessary for normal foot function [96].

If a deep-space abscess is not present, the incisions employed should fully excise any ulceration present and extend proximal and distal to this site to expose the underlying tendinous and osseous structures while respecting the vascular supply.

Surgical management of the diabetic foot: débridement

The most important initial step in treating limb-threatening diabetic foot infections is to perform a timely and complete surgical débridement [97–100]. This entails the surgical excision of all nonviable and/or infected soft tissue and/or bone so that the margins and base of the defect are healthy and viable [98–100]. Gentle retraction and meticulous soft-tissue handling should be employed to preserve the viable tissue adjacent to the defect. Deep tissues obtained intra-operatively under aseptic technique should be cultured to ensure that the patient is placed on appropriate culture-specific, targeted antibiotics as described previously. Surgical débridement should be performed without the use of a tourniquet in order to appropriately evaluate the viability of the regional soft tissue and underlying structures. If there is exposed bone or suspicion for underlying osteomyelitis, bone cultures are obtained at this time, most commonly through the use of a bone trephine followed by application of polymethylmethacrylate–antibiotic-loaded cement [PMMA–ALC]. PMMA–ALC is used to fill the defect until the final surgery is performed, at which point the cement is removed and an allogenic bone graft inserted [18]. After adequate surgical débridement, the wound is irrigated with copious amounts of saline to reduce the number of bacteria present in the wound [101]. The authors' technique involves several steps. First, the limb is placed inside a sterile radiograph cassette cover with a suction tube placed to remove the irrigation. Next, the wound is irrigated with 3 L of sterile saline using a pulse lavage system (Interpulse System, Stryker Instruments, Kalamazoo, MI). Gram stain, aerobic, and anaerobic cultures are then obtained from the depths of the wound to identify any bacterial species remaining to further aid in medical and surgical decision making. Finally, either Bacitracin or Neosporin is infiltrated into the remaining 3 L of sterile saline and the wound is again irrigated using the pulse lavage system to afford regional asepsis. At this point, the outer gloves of the operative team are changed, and all instruments used in the initial débridement are removed from the surgical field to reduce the potential for further wound contamination. Meticulous hemostasis is then achieved through a combination of electrocautery with a bipolar hand piece and ligation using metallic ligation clips. These clips represent the least reactive foreign substance available and do not require the protracted series of steps necessary to perform suture ligation that can entrap vital structures beyond the vessel

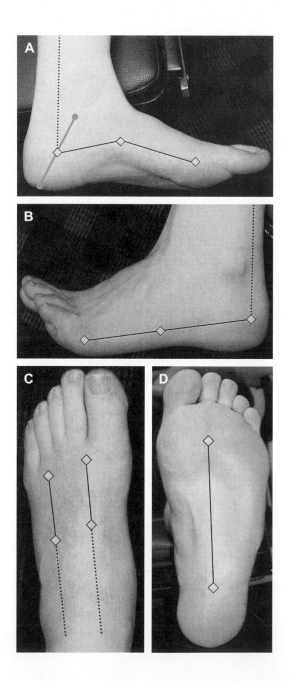

intended for ligation. The authors' have found the use of PMMA–ALC beads to be a simple means of promoting regional asepsis, filling dead spaces, preventing peri-articular soft-tissue contraction that makes subsequent osseous reconstruction more difficult, and maintaining a moist environment within the wound, as the antibiotics readily leach from the beads over several days into the blood coagulum. The use of PMMA–ALC in the treatment of foot-and-ankle osteomyelitis has been well described [102–104]. Because the polymerization process of PMMA–ALC is highly exothermic, with a mean heat of reaction at 94°C, the antibiotic chosen must be heat stable and should exist in a powder form for even distribution throughout the PMMA–ALC [105,106]. A number of antibiotics are available that are heat stable, exist in powdered form, and are compatible with PMMA–ALC [107]. The most commonly added antibiotics to PMMA–ALC are vancomycin, gentamycin, and tobramycin [108,109]. It is interesting to note that PMMA–ALC has also been shown to stimulate platelet activation [110] and thereby release growth factors from within the wound itself that may enhance soft-tissue and osseous healing adjacent to its implantation.

Fig. 4. Photograph of the medial border of the foot with the center of the first metatarsal head, inferior surface of the navicular tuberosity, and midpoint of a line (*gray line with round endpoints*) between the junction of the posterior and plantar heel and inferior surface of the medial malleolus as marked by white diamonds. The solid black lines connect these points and represent the proper location for an incision to expose the medial, superficial central, deep central, and calcaneal compartments of the foot as well as the tarsal tunnel. The dashed black line represents the proper incision location to explore the medial compartments of the lower leg (*A*). Photograph of the lateral border of the foot with the center of the fifth metatarsal head, inferior surface of the fifth metatarsal base, and intersection point between a horizontal line extending proximally from the first two points and a vertical line between the posterior aspect of the fibula and the anterior aspect of the Achilles tendon as marked by white diamonds. The solid black lines connect these points and represent the proper location for an incision to explore the lateral, superficial central, deep central, and calcaneal compartments of the foot as well as the peroneal tendons. The dashed black line represents the proper location for an incision to expose the entire length of the peroneal tendons and lateral compartment of the lower leg (*B*). Photograph of the dorsal surface of the foot with the medial aspect of the second metatarsal head and base and lateral aspect of the fourth metatarsal head and base as marked by white diamonds. The solid black lines connect these points and represent the proper location for an incision to expose the interosseous compartments. The dashed black line represents the proper location for an incision to expose the dorsal aspect of the midfoot, hindfoot, and anterior ankle region. Note that the medial incision courses along the lateral border of the anterior tibial tendon and the lateral incision courses along the lateral border of the extensor digitorum longus tendon (*C*). Photograph of the plantar aspect of the foot with the area just proximal to the weight-bearing surface of the forefoot and just distal to the weight-bearing surface of the heel marked with white diamonds. The solid black line connects these points and represents the proper location for an incision that will allow full exposure to every compartment of the foot except for the dorsal aspect once the plantar fascia has been incised. Note that this incision is placed along an imaginary line between the second toe and center of the heel pad (*D*).

PMMA–ALC beads (Fig. 5A) are most commonly fashioned by one of the surgical members at the time the wound is being irrigated, as at that point the final defect is appreciated, which allows for "economy of motion" in the operating theater thereby saving time. The PMMA–ALC beads should be between 5 and 10 mm in diameter for optimum elution characteristics and are strung by hand onto a No. 2 nylon suture. The PMMA–ALC beads are placed into the defect to cover all vital structures—including bone—and covered by either gently approximating the skin edges (Fig. 5B), covering them with petroleum-impregnated gauze, or with either an adhesive barrier alone or negative pressure therapy.

After the surgical débridement is completed and during subsequent evaluations of the wound, a well-padded bulky dressing should be applied that extends from the toes to the knee for the reasons discussed previously. The addition of a "sugar-tong" plaster splint will effectively immobilize the foot and ankle, thus decreasing pain associated with motion and limiting motion-induced disruption of the wounds. Occasionally, the authors have employed a spanning external fixation device to allow for sounder immobilization and easier dressing changes, as the limb does not require manipulation during the dressing removal, cleaning, and dressing reapplication

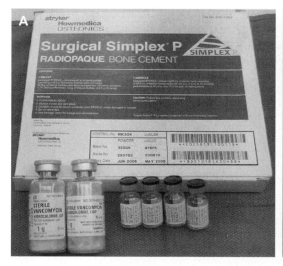
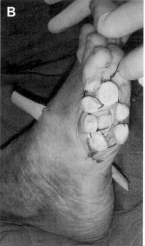

Fig. 5. Components used to create PMMA–ALC consisting of one pack of PMMA cement; two, 1-g vials of Vancomycin powder; and four, 80-mg vials of Gentamycin solution. Not shown is the No. 2 nylon required to string the resultant beads created (*A*). PMMA–ALC beads measuring between 5 and 10 mm in diameter have been applied to a No. 2 nylon suture that allows for postoperative MRI if needed, which would not be possible if metallic wire is used. Additionally, the nylon material is a monofilament and much less likely to harbor bacteria compared with umbilical tape, which is commonly used by some surgeons. The beads are gently placed within the wound and then covered with a petroleum-impregnated gauze, antibacterial impervious adhesive barrier, or negative pressure therapy (*B*).

process [111]. Another benefit of the use of external fixation is the ability to suspend the foot and lower leg, which prevents development of pressure ulceration about the heel [111]. The wound is inspected within 24 hours to evaluate the response to surgical débridement and evaluate the skin edges for necrosis or maceration. If the wound has stabilized and does not require a repeat débridement in the operating room (OR), the PMMA–ALC is left undisturbed for 72 hours to maximize the antibiotic dilution within the blood coagulum. After the initial bedside dressing is changed and the wound inspected under clean conditions, serial débridement in the operating theater is performed as needed to obtain a stable wound free of necrotic tissue and cardinal signs of infection. At each dressing change, the skin about the foot, ankle, and lower leg is cleaned with the previously mentioned surgical preparation from the authors' "débridement pack," and the wound is irrigated with 1 L of sterile saline. A useful technique is to use a 1-L intravenous (IV) bag of sterile saline for irrigation. This is performed by cutting off one of the IV access ports, that is then partially closed by pinching the index finger and thumb together. This is followed by squeezing the IV bag to create a fairly forceful stream of sterile saline. It is not uncommon for a patient to be brought back to the OR several times for débridement before the wound is optimized for definitive closure. The authors typically use a power hydro-dissection tool (Versajet Hydrosurgery System, Smith & Nephew, Inc., Memphis, TN) during serial débridement to remove any remaining nonviable tissue or granulation tissue where bacterial colonization may be evident. This device creates a localized vacuum effect (ie, Venturi effect) that allows for irrigation, hydration of the wound, and precise débridement, which prevents excessive soft tissue loss. After appropriate preparation of the wound bed, negative pressure [112] can be used to facilitate granulation tissue until definitive wound closure is performed. Its mechanism of action of negative-pressure therapy includes minimizing localized edema by removing interstitial fluid, increasing blood flow to the wound bed, and promoting granulation tissue through cell proliferation [113].

Before closing a wound, the surgeon must make certain that the wound is ready for closure by ensuring that the wound possesses no necrotic or fibrotic tissue, bleeds freely when débrided, and is free of localized edema and cardinal signs of infection. As mentioned above, it is not uncommon for a patient who has undergone an emergent extensive débridement or partial foot amputation to return to the OR several times for repeat débridement before the wound is considered adequately prepared for closure.

Peripheral arterial disease

Diabetes is associated with an increased risk of PAD. PAD is generally not the primary etiology of diabetic foot problems; however, it can be a major factor in an altered response to foot infections and nonhealing of foot ulcerations. An infection and/or ulceration, once present, increases the demand for blood supply to the foot. With PAD there may be an inability to meet that demand, leading to further tissue breakdown and progressive infection. The presence of PAD in a diabetic patient with foot ulceration or foot infection increases the risk of amputation. It is therefore very important to identify and treat coexisting PAD [9].

Assessment of peripheral arterial disease in the patient with diabetes

The patient with diabetes may not give the typical history of claudication because of associated neuropathy or lack of activity. It is therefore important to evaluate for PAD even in the absence of symptoms. The routine exam of the diabetic patient should include a complete foot examination and a vascular examination. If pedal pulses are not clearly palpable, further vascular studies are indicated. An ankle-brachial index (ABI) should be obtained, although there may be a false elevation of the ABI because of calcification of the pedal vessels. Toe pressures are a more accurate measure of perfusion in the diabetic foot. The indications for a vascular consultation include an ABI less that 0.7, toe pressures less than 40 mmHg, or transcutaneous oxygen tension (TcPO2) less than 30 mmHg. A nonhealing foot ulcer is an additional indication for a vascular evaluation looking for regional malperfusion in the diabetic foot.

The non-invasive vascular laboratory can be very helpful in the diagnosis, quantitation, and localization of PAD. An ABI of greater than 1.0 generally means the number is not accurate. Normal ABIs in the face of monophasic Doppler signals also indicate that the ABIs are falsely elevated. Toe pressures are a more accurate measure of perfusion in the diabetic foot.

Segmental pressures can be obtained by placing four cuffs on the leg. There is a cuff on the high thigh, above the knee, below the knee, and at the ankle. Documentation of gradients between the cuffs can help localize the location of PAD [114].

Treatment of peripheral arterial disease in the patient with diabetes

PAD is associated with the systemic disease process of atherosclerosis [114–116]. There is a close association between PAD and coronary arterial disease. Patients with severe limb-threatening PAD often have severe coronary arterial disease, making them high risk for traditional open bypass procedures [115,116].

Because the patients are at a high risk for systemic complications and wound problems, many centers, including the Madigan Army Medical Center, have developed an endovascular first philosophy for re-establishing adequate perfusion to the diabetic foot in the face of limb-threatening ischemia [117,118]. The endovascular options include percutaneous angioplasty with or without a stent, cryoplasty, or resectional or laser atherectomy. These procedures can be performed under local anesthesia or sedation and as an outpatient. The procedures result in minimal physiologic insult to the patient. The procedures can be repeated, and the saphenous vein is saved for other uses. The procedures can be performed with very low morbidity and mortality [117].

Over the 12-month period of 1 March 2006–1 March 2007, 30 patients with limb-threatening ischemia were treated at the Madigan Army Medical Center. Eight distal bypasses were performed; all resulted in limb salvage. Six procedures were performed because of surgeon preference or a long segment of total occlusion. Twenty-four endovascular procedures were performed. Eighteen had atherectomy alone; 4 had atherectomy plus angioplasty. One had cryoplasty alone and 1 had a cutting balloon angioplasty plus stenting. Of 24 endovascular procedures 22 were technically successful (92%). One procedure was unsuccessful in reestablishing in-line flow to the foot, and a distal bypass to the dorsalis pedis artery was performed. This patient had successful limb salvage. One patient had a cardiac arrest during the endovascular procedure. The procedure was aborted and the patient subsequently had a trans-femoral amputation performed. One patient had early thrombosis of an endovascular procedure that resulted in amputation. The limb salvage rate in patients receiving endovascular procedures was 92%.

If vascular insufficiency is identified before significant tissue loss, revascularization can be accomplished in a high percentage of patients, resulting in limb salvage. Even in patients with significant comorbid disease, endovascular procedures can be performed with high rates of limb salvage.

Edema and venous insufficiency

Edema from any etiology is a detriment to healing of foot ulcers or surgical incisions. Edema may be due to venous insufficiency or secondary to other medical illnesses. In the vascular laboratory of the Madigan Army Medical Center, 30% of patients referred with a diagnosis of venous insufficiency had a completely normal venous duplex scan, and it was determined that the edema was due to cardiac dysfunction. It is important to distinguish between the two types of edema. Edema secondary to venous insufficiency can be selectively treated surgically, although the main stay of treatment is external compression. Edema secondary to cardiac dysfunction is treated by improving cardiac performance and diuresis. Management of extremity edema is critical to wound healing in the diabetic patient with a foot wound.

Summary

The incidence of diabetes is increasing. Lower extremity complications of diabetes, such as neuropathy, ulceration, infection, and PAD, are common and can lead to significant morbidity, including major amputation. The recognition and treatment of these complications are discussed. The general surgeon should have a good understanding of the pathophysiology and treatment of complications associated with the diabetic foot.

References

[1] Boulton AJ, Vileikyte L, Ragnarson-Tennvall G, et al. The global burden of diabetic foot disease. Lancet 2005;366(9498):1719–24.

[2] Centers for Disease Control and Prevention. National diabetes fact sheet: general information and national estimates on diabetes in the United States. Atlanta (GA): Centers for Disease Control and Prevention; 2005.

[3] Wild S, Roglic G, Green A, et al. Global prevalence of diabetes: estimates for the year 2000 and projections for 2030. Diabetes Care 2004;27:1047–53.

[4] Reiber GE, Vileikyte L, Boyko EJ, et al. Causal pathways for incident lower-extremity ulcers in patients with diabetes from two settings. Diabetes Care 1999;22(1):157–62.

[5] Mills JL, Beckett WC, Taylor SM. The diabetic foot: consequences of delayed treatment and referral. South Med J 1991;84(8):970–4.

[6] Pecoraro RE, Reiber GE, Burgess EM. Pathways to diabetic limb amputation. Basis for prevention. Diabetes Care 1990;13(5):513–21.

[7] Lipsky BA. A report from the international consensus on diagnosing and treating the infected diabetic foot. Diabetes Metab Res Rev 2004;20(Suppl 1):S68–77.

[8] Lipsky BA, Berendt AR, Embil J, et al. Diagnosing and treating diabetic foot infections. Diabetes Metab Res Rev 2004;20(Suppl):S56–64.

[9] Akbari CM, Macsata R, Smith BM, et al. Overview of the diabetic foot. Semin Vasc Surg 2003;16(1):3–11.

[10] Jeffcoate WJ, Harding KG. Diabetic foot ulcers. Lancet 2003;361(9368):1545–51.

[11] Ramsey SD, Newton K, Blough D, et al. Incidence, outcomes, and cost of foot ulcers in patients with diabetes. Diabetes Care 1999;22(3):382–7.

[12] Reiber GE. The epidemiology of diabetic foot problems. Diabet Med 1996;13(Suppl 1): S6–11.

[13] Tennvall GR, Apelqvist J, Eneroth M. Costs of deep foot infections in patients with diabetes mellitus. Pharmacoeconomics 2000;18(3):225–38.

[14] Lipsky BA. Medical treatment of diabetic foot infections. Clin Infect Dis 2004;39(Suppl): S104–14.

[15] Armstrong DG, Lipsky BA. Advances in the treatment of diabetic foot infections. Diabetes Technol Ther 2004;6(2):167–77.

[16] Lipsky BA, Berendt AR. Principles and practice of antibiotic therapy of diabetic foot infections. Diabetes Metab Res Rev 2000;16(Suppl):S42–6.

[17] Zgonis T, Roukis TS. A systematic approach to diabetic foot infections. Adv Ther 2005; 22(3):244–62.

[18] Roukis TS. Radical solutions: bold débridement techniques can work for both chronic and acute wounds. OrthoKinetic Rev 2004;4(1):20–3.

[19] Tan JS, Fiedman NM, Hazelton-Miller C, et al. Can aggressive treatment of diabetic foot infections reduce the need for above-ankle amputation? Clin Infect Dis 1996;23(2):286–91.

[20] Zgonis T, Jolly GP, Buren BJ, et al. Diabetic foot infections and antibiotic therapy. Clin Podiatr Med Surg 2003;20(4):655–69.

[21] Kaleta JL, Fleischli JW, Reilly CH. The diagnosis of osteomyelitis in diabetes using the erythrocyte sedimentation rate: a pilot study. J Am Podiatr Med Assoc 2001;91(9):445–50.

[22] Pellizzer G, Strazzabosco M, Presi S, et al. Deep tissue biopsy vs. superficial swab culture monitoring in the microbiological assessment of limb-threatening diabetic foot infection. Diabetes Med 2001;18(10):822–7.

[23] Grayson ML, Gibbons GW, Balogh K, et al. Probing to bone in infected pedal ulcers: a clinical sign of underlying osteomyelitis in diabetic patients. J Am Med Assoc 1995;273(9): 721–3.

[24] Howard CB, Einhorn M, Dagan R, et al. Fine-needle bone biopsy to diagnose osteomyelitis. J Bone Joint Surg Br 1994;76(2):311–4.

[25] Khatri G, Wagner DK, Sohnle PG. Effect of bone biopsy in guiding antimicrobial therapy for osteomyelitis complicating open wounds. Am J Med Sci 2001;321(6):367–71.

[26] Zuluaga AF, Galvis W, Jaimes F, et al. Lack of microbiological concordance between bone and non-bone specimens in chronic osteomyelitis: an observational study. BMC Infect Dis 2002;2:8–12.

[27] Sella EJ, Grosser DM. Imaging modalities of the diabetic foot. Clin Podiatr Med Surg 2003; 20(4):729–40.

[28] Bonakdar-pour A, Gaines VD. The radiology of osteomyelitis. Orthop Clin North Am 1983;14(1):21–37.

[29] Tomas MB, Patel M, Marwin SE, et al. The diabetic foot. Br J Radiol 2000;73(868): 443–50.

[30] Gold RH, Tong DJ, Crim JR, et al. Imaging the diabetic foot. Skeletal Radiol 1995;24(8): 563–71.

[31] Poirier JY, Garin E, Derrien C, et al. Diagnosis of osteomyelitis in the diabetic foot with a 99mTc-HMPAO leucocyte scintigraphy combined with a 99mTc-MDP bone scintigraphy. Diabetes Metab 2002;28(6):485–90.

[32] Devillers A, Moisan A, Hennion F, et al. Contribution of technetium-99m hexamethylpropylene amine oxime labelled leucocyte scintigraphy to the diagnosis of diabetic foot infection. Eur J Nucl Med 1998;25(2).132–8.

[33] Sarikaya A, Aygit AC, Pekindil G. Utility of 99mTc dextran scintigraphy in diabetic patients with suspected osteomyelitis of the foot. Ann Nucl Med 2003;17(8):669–76.

[34] Schauwecker DS, Park HM, Burt RW, et al. Combined bone scintigraphy and indium-111 leukocyte scans in neuropathic foot disease. J Nucl Med 1988;29(10):1651–5.

[35] Johnson JE, Kennedy EJ, Shereff MJ, et al. Prospective study of bone, indium-111-labeled white blood cell, and gallium-67 scanning for the evaluation of osteomyelitis in the diabetic foot. Foot Ankle Int 1996;17(1):10–6.

[36] Becker W. Imaging osteomyelitis and the diabetic foot. Q J Nucl Med 1999;43(1):9–20.

[37] Palestro CJ, Caprioli R, Love C, et al. Rapid diagnosis of pedal osteomyelitis in diabetics with a technetium-99m-labeled monoclonal antigranulocyte antibody. J Foot Ankle Surg 2003;42(1):2–8.

[38] Devillers A, Garin E, Polard JL, et al. Comparison of Tc-99m-labelled antileukocyte fragment Fab' and Tc-99m-HMPAO leukocyte scintigraphy in the diagnosis of bone and joint infections: a prospective study. Nucl Med Commun 2000;21(8):747–53.

[39] Palestro CJ, Kipper SL, Weiland FL, et al. Osteomyelitis: diagnosis with (99m) Tc-labeled antigranulocyte antibodies compared with diagnosis with (111) In-labeled leukocytes—initial experience. Radiology 2002;223(3):758–64.

[40] Morrison WB, Schweitzer ME, Wapner KL, et al. Osteomyelitis in feet of diabetics: clinical accuracy, surgical utility, and cost-effectiveness of MR imaging. Radiology 1995;196(2): 557–64.

[41] Croll SD, Nicholas GG, Osborne MA, et al. Role of magnetic resonance imaging in the diagnosis of osteomyelitis in diabetic foot infections. J Vasc Surg 1996;24(2):266–70.

[42] Weinstein D, Wang A, Chambers R, et al. Evaluation of magnetic resonance imaging in the diagnosis of osteomyelitis in diabetic foot infections. Foot Ankle 1993;14(1):18–22.

[43] Cook TA, Rahim N, Sompson HCR, et al. Magnetic resonance imaging in the management of diabetic foot infection. Br J Surg 1996;83(2):245–8.

[44] Ledermann HP, Morrision WB, Schweitzer ME, et al. Tendon involvement in pedal infection: MR analysis of frequency, distribution, and spread of infection. AJR Am J Roentgenol 2002;179(4):939–47.

[45] Gold RH, Hawkins RA, Katz RD. Bacterial osteomyelitis: findings on plain radiography, CT, MR, and scintigraphy. AJR Am J Roentgenol 1991;157(2):365–70.

[46] Tehranzadeh J, Wong E, Wang F, et al. Imaging of osteomyelitis in the mature skeleton. Radiol Clin North Am 2001;39(2):223–50.

[47] Enderle MD, Coerper S, Schweizer HP, et al. Correlation of imaging techniques to histopathology in patients with diabetic foot syndrome and clinical suspicion of chronic osteomyelitis. The role of high-resolution ultrasound. Diabetes Care 1999;22(2):294–9.

[48] Sammak B, Abd El Bagi M, Al Shahed M, et al. Osteomyelitis: a review of currently used imaging techniques. Eur Radiol 1999;9(5):894–900.

[49] Wrobel JS, Connolly JE. Making the diagnosis of osteomyelitis. The role of prevalence. J Am Podiatr Med Assoc 1998;88(7):337–43.

[50] O'Meara SM, Cullum NA, Majid M, et al. Systemic review of antimicrobial agents used for chronic wounds. Br J Surg 2001;88(1):4–21.

[51] Lipsky BA. Evidence-based antibiotic therapy of diabetic foot infections. FEMS Immunol Med Microbiol 1999;26(3):267–76.

[52] Lipsky BA, Pecoraro RE, Larson SA, et al. Outpatient management of uncomplicated lower-extremity infections in diabetic patients. Arch Intern Med 1990;150(4):790–7.

[53] Frykberg RG, Zgonis T, Armstrong DG, et al. Diabetic foot disorders: a clinical practice guideline. J Foot Ankle Surg 2006;45(Suppl):2–66.

[54] Lipsky BA, Baker PD, Landon GC, et al. Antibiotic therapy for diabetic foot infections: comparison of two parenteral-to-oral regimens. Clin Infect Dis 1997;24(4):643–8.

[55] Peterson LR, Lissack LM, Canter K, et al. Therapy of lower extremity infections with ciprofloxacin in patients with diabetes mellitus, peripheral vascular disease, or both. Am J Med 1989;86(6):801–8.

[56] Gerding DN. Foot infections in diabetic patients: the role of anaerobes. Clin Infect Dis 1995;20(3):S283–8.

[57] Lipsky BA. Osteomyelitis of the foot in diabetic patients. Clin Infect Dis 1997;25(6): 1318–26.

[58] Akova M, Ozcebe O, Gullu I, et al. Efficacy of sulbactam-ampicillin for the treatment of severe diabetic foot infections. J Chemother 1996;8(4):284–9.

[59] Zeillemaker AM, Veldkamp KE, van Kraaij MG, et al. Piperacillin/tazobactam therapy for diabetic foot infection. Foot Ankle Int 1998;19(3):169–72.

[60] Hughes CE, Johnson CC, Bamberger DM, et al. Treatment and long-term follow-up of foot infections in patients with diabetes or ischemia: a randomized, prospective, double-blind comparison of cefoxitin and ceftizoxime. Clin Ther 1987;10(Suppl A):36–49.

[61] Lobmann R, Ambrosch A, Seewald M, et al. Antibiotic therapy for diabetic foot infections: comparison of cephalosporins with chinolones. Diabetes Nutr Metab 2004;17(3): 156–62.

[62] Raymakers JT, Houben AJ, Heyden JJ, et al. The effect of diabetes and severe ischaemia on the penetration of ceftazidime into tissue of the limb. Diabetes Med 2001;18(3): 229–34.

[63] Raymakers JT, Schaper NC, van der Heyden JJ, et al. Penetration of ceftazidime into bone from severely ischaemic limbs. J Antimicrob Chemother 1998;42(4):543–5.

[64] Grayson ML, Gibbons GW, Habershaw GM, et al. Use of ampicillin/sulbactam versus imipenem/cilastatin in the treatment of limb-threatening foot infections in diabetic patients. Clin Infect Dis 1994;18(5):683–93.

[65] McKinnon PS, Paladino JA, Grayson ML, et al. Cost-effectiveness of ampicillin/sulbactam versus imipenem/cilastatin in the treatment of limb-threatening foot infections in diabetic patients. Clin Infect Dis 1997;24(1):57–63.

[66] Torres A, Ramirez-Ronda CH. Aztreonam in the treatment of soft tissue infections including diabetic foot infections. Bol Asoc Med P R 1985;77(5):191–4.

[67] Boyce JM, Havill NL, Kohan C, et al. Do infection control measures work for methicillin-resistant *Staphylococcus aureus*? Infect Control Hosp Epidemiol 2004;25(5):395–401.

[68] Herwaldt LA. Control of methicillin-resistant *Staphylococcus aureus* in the hospital setting. Am J Med 1999;106(5-A):S11–8.

[69] Karchmer TB, Durbin LJ, Simonton BM, et al. Cost-effectiveness of active surveillance cultures and contact/droplet precautions for control of methicillin-resistant *Staphylococcus aureus*. J Hosp Infect 2002;51(2):126–32.

[70] Bernard L, Vaudaux P, Vuagnat A, et al, Osteomyelitis Study Group. Effect of vancomycin therapy for osteomyelitis on colonization by methicillin-resistant *Staphylococcus aureus*: lack of emergence of glycopeptide resistance. Infect Control Hosp Epidemiol 2003;24(9): 650–4.

[71] Turco TF, Melko GP, Williams JR. Vancomycin intermediate-resistant *Staphylococcus aureus*. Ann Pharmacother 1998;32(7):758–60.

[72] Linares J. The VISA/GISA problem: therapeutic implications. Clin Microbiol Infect 2001; 7(Suppl 4):S8–15.

[73] Lipsky BA, Itani K, Norden C. Treating foot infections in diabetic patients: a randomized, multicenter, open-label trial of linezolid versus ampicillin-sulbactam/amoxicillin-clavulanate. Clin Infect Dis 2004;38(1):17–24.

[74] Carpenter CF, Chambers HF. Daptomycin: another novel agent for treating infections due to drug-resistant gram-positive pathogens. Clin Infect Dis 2004;38(7):994–1000.

[75] Kerstein MD. Heel ulcerations in the diabetic patient. Wounds 2002;14(5):212–6.

[76] Lavery LA, Vela SA, Fleischli JG, et al. Reducing plantar pressure in the neuropathic foot. A comparison of footwear. Diabetes Care 1997;20(11):1706–10.

[77] Boulton AJ. Pressure and the diabetic foot: clinical science and offloading techniques. Am J Surg 2004;187(5-A):S17–24.

[78] Armstrong DG, Stacpoole-Shea S. Total contact casts and removable cast walkers: mitigation of plantar pressure. J Am Podiatr Med Assoc 1999;89(1):50–3.

[79] Wukich DK, Motko J. Safety of total contact casting in high-risk patients with neuropathic foot ulcers. Foot Ankle Int 2004;25(8):556–60.

[80] Little AA, Edwards JL, Feldman EL. Diabetic neuropathies. Pract Neurol 2007;7(2): 82–92.

[81] Bloomgarden ZT. Diabetic neuropathy. Diabetes Care 2007;30(4):1027–32.

[82] Boucek P. Advanced diabetic neuropathy: a point of no return? Rev Diabet Stud 2006;3(3): 143–50.

[83] Frigg A, Pagenstert G, Schaffer D, et al. Recurrence and prevention of diabetic foot ulcers after total contact casting. Foot Ankle Int 2007;28(1):64–9.

[84] Nixon BP, Armstrong DG, Wendell C, et al. Do US veterans wear appropriately sized shoes? The Veterans Affairs shoe size selection study. J Am Podiatr Med Assoc 2006; 96(4):290–2.

[85] Steed DL, , The Diabetic Ulcer Study Group. Clinical evaluation of recombinant human platelet-derived growth factor for the treatment of lower extremity diabetic ulcers. J Vasc Surg 1995;21(1):71–81.

[86] Armstrong DG. The University of Texas Diabetic Foot Classification System. Ostomy Wound Manage 1996;42(8):60–1.

[87] Armstrong DG, Lavery LA, Harkless LB. Validation of a diabetic wound classification system. The contribution of depth, infection, and ischemia to risk of amputation. Diabetes Care 1998;21(5):855–9.

[88] Kirsner RS, Froelich CW. Soaps and detergents: understanding their composition and effect. Ostomy Wound Manage 1998;44(Suppl-3A):S62–9.

[89] Hilton JR, Williams DT, Beuker B, et al. Wound dressings in diabetic foot disease. Clin Infect Dis 2004;39(Suppl 2):S100–3.

[90] Hidalgo DA, Shaw WW. Anatomic basis of plantar flap design. Plast Reconstr Surg 1986; 78(5):627–36.

[91] Attinger C, Cooper P, Blume P. Vascular anatomy of the foot and ankle. Oper Techn Plast Recontstr Surg 1997;4(4):183–98.

[92] Attinger C, Cooper P, Blume P, et al. The safest surgical incisions and amputations applying the angiosome principles and using the Doppler to assess the arterial-arterial connections of the foot and ankle. Foot Ankle Clin 2001;6(4):745–99.

[93] Reach JS Jr, Amrami KK, Felmlee JP, et al. The compartments of the foot: a 3-tesla magnetic resonance imaging study with clinical correlates for needle pressure testing. Foot Ankle Int 2007;28(5):584–94.

[94] Myerson MS. Experimental decompression of the fascial compartments of the foot: the basis for fasciotomy in acute compartment syndromes. Foot Ankle 1988;8(6):308–14.

[95] Attinger CE, Ducic I, Cooper P, et al. The role of intrinsic muscle flaps of the foot for bone coverage in foot and ankle defects in diabetic and nondiabetic patients. Plast Reconstr Surg 2002;110(4):1047–54.

[96] Levin LS, Serafin D. Plantar skin coverage. Prob Plast Reconstr Surg 1991;1(2):156–84.

[97] Levin LS. Personality of soft-tissue injury. Tech Orthop 1995;10(1):65–72.

[98] Levin LS. Débridement. Tech Orthop 1995;10(2):104–8.

[99] Attinger CE, Bulan E, Blume PA. Surgical débridement: the key to successful wound healing and reconstruction. Clin Podiatr Med Surg 2000;17(4):599–630.

[100] Attinger CE, Bulan EJ. Débridement: the key initial first step in wound healing. Foot Ankle Clin 2001;6(4):627–60.

[101] Bahrs C, Schnabel M, Frank T, et al. Lavage of contaminated surfaces: an in vitro evaluation of the effectiveness of different systems. J Surg Res 2003;112(1):26–30.

[102] Stabile DE, Jacobs AM. Local antibiotic treatment of soft tissue and bone infections of the foot. J Am Podiatr Med Assoc 1990;80(7):345–53.

[103] Jacobs AM, Siefert AM, Kirisits TJ, et al. Use of antibiotic-loaded bone cement in the management of common infections of the foot and ankle. Clin Podiatr Med Surg 1990;7(3): 523–44.

[104] Roeder B, Van Gils CC, Mailing S. Antibiotic beads in the treatment of diabetic pedal osteomyelitis. J Foot Ankle Surg 2000;39(2):124–30.

[105] Bertazzoni-Minelli E, Caveiari C, Benini A. Release of antibiotics from polymethylmethacrylate cement. J Chemother 2002;14(5):492–500.

[106] Baker AS, Greenham LW. Release of gentamycin from acrylic bone cement. J Bone Joint Surg Am 1988;70(10):1551–7.

[107] Bibbo C. Treatment of the infected extended ankle arthrodesis after tibiotalocalcaneal retrograde nailing. Tech Foot Ankle Surg 2002;1(1):74–86.

[108] Mader JT, Calhoun J, Cobos J. In vitro evaluation of antibiotic diffusion from antibiotic-impregnated biodegradable beads and polymethylmethacrylate beads. Antimicrob Agents Chemother 1997;41(2):415–8.

[109] Ethell MT, Benett RA, Brown MP, et al. In vitro elution of gentamycin, amikacin, and ceftiofur from polymethylmethacrylate and hydroxyapatite. Vet Surg 2000;29(5):375–82.

[110] Cenni E, Granchi D, Pizzoferrato A. Platelet activation after in vitro contact with seven acrylic bone cements. J Biomater Sci Polym Ed 2002;13:17–25.

[111] Roukis TS, Landsman AS, Weinberg SA, et al. Use of a hybrid "kickstand" external fixator for pressure relief following soft-tissue reconstruction of heel defects. J Foot Ankle Surg 2003;42(4):240–3.

[112] Paul JC. Vacuum assisted closure therapy: a must in plastic surgery. Plast Surg Nurs 2005; 25(2):61–5.

[113] Saxena V, Hwang CW, Huang S, et al. Vacuum-assisted closure: microdeformations of wounds and cell proliferation. Plast Reconstr Surg 2004;114(5):1086–96.

[114] Sumpio BE, Lee T, Blume PA. Vascular evaluation and arterial reconstruction of the diabetic foot. Clin Podiatr Med Surg 2003;20(4):689–708.

[115] Criqui MH, Denenberg JO, Langer RD, et al. The epidemiology of peripheral arterial disease: importance of identifying the population at risk. Vasc Med 1997;2(3):221–6.

[116] Ness J, Aronow WS. Prevalence of coexistence of coronary artery disease, ischemic stroke, and peripheral arterial disease in older persons, mean age 80 years, in an academic hospital-based geriatrics practice. J Am Geriatr Soc 1999;47(6):1255–6.

[117] Wilson SE, Wolf GL, Cross AP. Percutaneous transluminal angioplasty versus operation for peripheral arteriosclerosis: report of a prospective randomized trial in a selected group of patients. J Vasc Surg 1989;9(1):1–9.

[118] Tehrani H, Otero C, Arosemena M, et al. Endovascular-first strategy in patients with critical limb ischemia. Vasc Dis Manage 2006;3(6):380–3.

ELSEVIER
SAUNDERS

Surg Clin N Am 87 (2007) 1179–1192

SURGICAL
CLINICS OF
NORTH AMERICA

Vascular Trauma: Endovascular Management and Techniques

CPT Zachary M. Arthurs, MD[a],*,
CPT Vance Y. Sohn, MD[a],
Benjamin W. Starnes, MD, FACS[b]

[a]Department of Surgery, Madigan Army Medical Center, Fitzsimmons Drive, Building 9040,
Tacoma, WA 98431, USA
[b]Division of Vascular Surgery, University of Washington, Harborview Medical Center,
325 Ninth Avenue, Seattle, WA 98104, USA

Catheter-based therapy has evolved from a diagnostic modality to primary treatment for various vascular disease processes. Over the past 2 decades, vascular surgeons have embraced this technology and have altered their approach to aneurysmal and peripheral vascular disease. This modality has become commonplace in the operative theater, and it is not uncommon for endoluminal techniques to be performed in conjunction with open surgery (hybrid procedures). The early mortality benefit of endoluminal therapy for elective vascular procedures has led centers of excellence to adopt these techniques for emergent aortic pathology.

In addition, the same benefits from endovascular therapies can be applied in the management of severely injured trauma patients. Whether remote aortic occlusion is performed to avoid a second cavitary incision or an endovascular stent is placed to cover a lacerated vessel, these techniques can minimize the physiologic burden placed on patients who have very little physiologic reserve. This article reviews the endovascular treatment of vascular trauma by anatomic regions: neck, thoracic, abdominal, and extremities.

Endovascular management of cervical vascular trauma

Penetrating carotid injury

Following penetrating neck trauma, cervical blood vessels are the most commonly injured structures [1], and their location relative to anatomic

* Corresponding author.
E-mail address: arthursz@mac.com (Z.M. Arthurs).

0039-6109/07/$ - see front matter © 2007 Elsevier Inc. All rights reserved.
doi:10.1016/j.suc.2007.07.006   surgical.theclinics.com

landmarks dictates the diagnostic evaluation and therapeutic approach of these injuries. Monson and colleagues [2] originally described three zones: Zone I (below the cricoid cartilage), Zone II (between the cricoid cartilage and the angle of the mandible), and Zone III (above the angle of the mandible). Ongoing controversy remains with regard to the diagnostic evaluation and approach within each zone, but an endoluminal approach in this region could potentially avoid the morbidity of median sternotomy, a high thoracic incision, or difficult dissection at the base of the skull. In addition, endoluminal therapy can be performed under local anesthesia, allowing the provider direct assessment of the patient's neurologic status.

Unstable patients who have Zone I injuries may be approached through a cervical incision, but obtaining proximal control most likely requires a median sternotomy. Depending on the patient's clinical course and the availability of a vascular surgeon, proximal control of the great vessels may be performed from a femoral approach with balloon occlusion. Alternatively, if the proximal vessel can be visualized from a cervical approach but not secured with a vascular clamp, a compliant balloon or Fogarty catheter can be passed retrograde for temporary proximal control. Once the vessel is properly exposed, the balloon can be replaced with a vascular clamp.

An overt injury in Zone II can be readily approached through a cervical incision, and repair performed under direct visualization. The operative feasibility, ability to examine the aerodigestive tract, and relatively low risk to exploration in this region favor open exploration over endovascular techniques in emergent situations. Hemorrhage from a Zone III injury can be devastating, and an immediate operative approach through a cervical incision can be used to first control inflow and assess the injury pattern. If the vessel is transected with inadequate length for clamp application, distal control can be performed by placing a compliant balloon or Fogarty balloon within the vessel lumen. If the vessel is lacerated, a sheath can be placed in the common carotid artery and a Fogarty catheter (size 4–8) can be passed to control back bleeding. Once the Fogarty is inflated, an arteriogram can be performed through the side arm of the sheath to delineate the injury and further guide operative exposure. After hemorrhage is arrested, further maneuvers can be performed to gain exposure, such as dividing the digastric muscles or subluxation of the mandible. Remote occlusion of the vessel affords a bloodless field and allows time for a difficult dissection at the base of the skull.

Alternatively, patients who present with suspected penetrating cervical injury or with soft signs of vascular injury (stable hematoma, history of blood-loss at the scene, or penetration below the platysma) are typically hemodynamically stable, allowing time for detailed evaluation. In this group of patients, controversy still exists on how to best manage Zone II injuries. Classically, these injuries have mandated operative exploration of the carotid vessels and aerodigestive tracts [3]; however, some authors have recommended selective management of this region based on imaging modalities and physical examination [4]. Using multiplanar CT with arterial enhanced imaging, vessels can be assessed for pseudoaneurysm, complete or partial transection, thrombosis, or arterio-venous fistula. The majority of Zone II lesions should be treated with standard open-repair. For Zone I and III, endovascular exclusion of the pseudoaneurysm, partial transection, or arterio-venous fistula remains a viable option. Self-expanding covered stents can be safely delivered to these locations with limited morbidity [5–8].

It is important to note that hard signs of vascular injury, to include overt hemorrhage, expanding hematoma, or loss of pulse with a neurologic deficit, demand operative exploration regardless of location, and endovascular techniques should not be used as the first line of therapy; however, endovascular techniques may assist classical operative approaches and can allow for temporary control of the great vessels or to arrest back bleeding at the base of the skull.

Blunt carotid injury

Delayed recognition of occult carotid injuries carries an increased mortality [9], and compared with penetrating carotid injuries, patients have an overall decrease in functional outcome measures [10]. Although routine four-vessel angiography was formerly recommended for patients who have a cervical seatbelt sign or mechanism suggestive of blunt carotid injury [11], computed tomographic angiography (CTA) now offers accurate screening without the embolic risk associated with selective angiography of the carotid and vertebral vessels [12]. Blunt carotid injuries are caused by rotational and hyperflexion forces placed on the carotid vessels, and typically occur in Zone III at the base of the skull. Potential intra luminal lesions include an intimal flap, nonocclusive or occlusive dissection, and thrombosis. Although operative intervention has been shown to reduce the mortality and stroke rate associated with these lesions [13], Fabian and colleagues [14] have reported that the majority of these lesions have limited embolic potential with early anticoagulation. Unfortunately, patients who sustain blunt carotid injuries typically have associated closed-head injuries, solid organ injuries, or pelvic fractures that prevent the use of early anticoagulation. Depending on the patient's clinical status, the severity of the intimal lesion, and the ability to assess neurologic status, treatment may range from observation with or without antiplatelet therapy to endovascular stent placement to operative intervention.

Small intimal-based flaps with minimal or no dissection are best managed with antiplatelet therapy or observation with transcranial Doppler examination for embolic potential. Similarly, nonocclusive dissections typically resolve in approximately 70% of patients with anticoagulation therapy, with the remaining 30% developing a pseudoaneurysm of the carotid artery. Once a pseudoaneurysm has developed, it is unlikely to spontaneously resolve with continued anticoagulation therapy, and these lesions tend to be the source of embolic events or thrombosis [15,16]. Although a consensus does not exist on the management of these conditions, several case series exist with acceptable outcomes with endovascular therapy.

The primary treatment for nonocclusive dissections of the carotid artery should be anticoagulation therapy, but when anticoagulation is not feasible, endoluminal treatment with either a bare or covered stent is an alternative to open repair [17,18]. Balloon expandable and self-expanding stents have been used in this location, and in all cases, apposition of the dissection to the wall was achieved with no neurologic events reported [18,19]. Bejjani and colleagues [18] treated four symptomatic carotid dissections with endovascular bare stents, and all patients had improvement in their neurologic examination. Unlike dissections, once a pseudoaneurysm has developed after blunt carotid trauma, it should be excluded from the circulation to eliminate embolic potential. Initial reports from Parodi and colleagues [20] relied on balloon expandable bare Palmaz stents (Cordis, Johnson and Johnson, Miami Lakes, Florida) to cover the orifice of the pseudoaneurysm. Covering the orifice will typically promote thrombosis of the pseudoaneurysm, but if the sac fails to thrombose, an option has been to coil embolize the sac through the interstices of the bare stent [21].

In these series, the mean follow-up was 3.5 years without neurologic sequelae, but thrombosis and embolic potential, as well as the potential for restenosis, remain concerns after endovascular placement of devices in the carotid artery. Post-stent therapy is variable, but extrapolating data from carotid artery stenting for atherosclerotic disease, a regimen of dual antiplatelet therapy (aspirin and clopidogrel) appears adequate to prevent stent thrombosis and embolic ischemic events [22]. In the presented series, patients were treated with anticoagulation for 8 weeks if tolerated, or dual-antiplatelet therapy without any events; however, Duane and colleagues [6] managed a patient who was unable to comply with antiplatelet therapy because of cost and returned with a thrombosed stent. Fortunately, the patient did not experience a neurologic event, but compliance should be considered when planning appropriate therapy for this population of patients.

Vertebral artery injury

Injuries to the vertebral vessels, typically from penetrating trauma, are a rare occurrence and account for only 0.5% of vascular trauma [23]. Although the first portion of the vertebral artery is readily accessible, the second portion (within the bony foramen of the cervical canal) and the third portion (as the vessel exits the bony foramen and enters the base of the skull) can be extremely difficult to control. Mwipatayi and colleagues [24] reported their experience with 101 traumatic vertebral artery injuries managed with both open and endovascular techniques. In their series, only 6 of the injuries were secondary to blunt trauma. Sixty-five percent of patients were treated primarily with endovascular means, and half of the patients revealed a thrombosed vessel that required no further treatment. The remaining patients were treated with embolization to arrest hemorrhage. When possible, both proximal and distal ends of the vertebral artery were embolized with coils or balloons [24]. Of the patients approached with open exploration, 50% required postoperative endoluminal embolization to arrest bleeding or control arterio-venous fistulae [24], illustrating the difficulty in controlling hemorrhage with open techniques.

Endovascular management of thoracic vascular trauma

Thoracic vascular trauma carries a high mortality rate. The utility of endovascular techniques in the management of penetrating thoracic trauma is limited to patients presenting with hemodynamic stability, and the foundation for repair of these injuries should rely on standard open surgical approaches. Although there have been isolated case reports describing patients with penetrating aortic injuries managed with stent-grafts [25], these patients were hemodynamically stable and had contained hematomas. The delayed manifestations of penetrating trauma such as pseudoaneurysms and arterio-venous fistulas can easily be excluded with stent-grafts in the descending thoracic aorta.

Blunt aortic injury (BAI) is associated with nearly 85% mortality at the scene of injury. The patients that survive the initial injury most likely have containment of their rupture, but still 50% of patients die within 24 hours of admission to a trauma center [26]. If the patient's contained rupture converts to free rupture while awaiting therapy, the mortality is 100% [27]. Of the patients that survive, 90% of injuries occur in the region of the aortic isthmus (Fig. 1). Conventional operative repair has been associated with mortality rates of 15% to 25% and paraplegia rates of 8% to 20% [28]. The impact of an operative repair in a patient who has simultaneous head injury, severe pulmonary contusions, and abdominal injuries cannot be

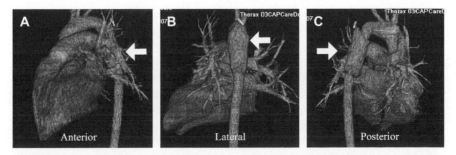

Fig. 1. Three-dimensional reconstruction of BAI. The white arrows denote the injury. (A) From the anterior view, the injury is covered by the pulmonary vasculature. (B) On the lateral image, the extent of the injury can be seen down to normal caliber aorta. (C) From the posterior view, the length of the injury can be appreciated as well as its relationship to the left subclavian artery.

overstated [29,30], and endovascular therapy can potentially afford the patient repair without the physiologic stress of general anesthesia and single-lung ventilation.

As endovascular technology has evolved over the last decade to treat aortic pathology, the use of endografts has been extended to patients who have BAI. For elective thoracic aneurysm repairs, thoracic endografts have been associated with mortality and paraplegia rates of 8.7% and 3.6% respectively [31,32]. The first cases of an endograft used to treat BAI were reported by Dake and colleagues [33] in three patients who all survived without paraplegia. Since those cases in 1997, endovascular treatment of BAI has been performed at several centers, and the average reported mortality is 7% and paraplegia rate is less than 1% [34]. Although there is significant reporting and selection bias within these cohorts, the results are promising for improving the outcome of this devastating injury. Single-institution comparative studies exist, and all afford patients a survival benefit and reduction in paraplegia with endovascular therapy over open repair [34,35]. Without randomized data to support using endovascular approaches in all patients, it is appropriate to reserve open operative repair for patients who have low risk, adequate pulmonary function, and other injuries precluding an open repair. Patients who have moderate polytrauma (Injury Severity Score >25) who may not tolerate an open repair should be treated with an endovascular approach.

Challenges to performing an endovascular repair for BAI revolve around the patient's anatomy and stent-related complications. Trauma patients are often younger than patients treated with thoracic stent grafts for aortic aneurysmal disease; hence their aortic diameters are markedly smaller caliber. Currently, the smallest US Food and Drug Administration (FDA)-approved device available for the thoracic aorta is the 26 mm TAG (W.L. Gore, Flagstaff, Arizona). The manufacturer and experts recommend that these devices be sized 10% to 15% over the targeted landing zones in the patient; therefore the 26 mm graft should be placed in a 22 to 24 mm aorta; however, the mean aortic diameter for patients who have blunt aortic injury is 20 mm [35]. Oversizing the graft more than 15% results in pleating of the graft, resultant endoleak, and potential for graft compression and collapse [35,36]. Several authors have now reported graft compression [36,37], and it is felt that this is largely caused by graft separation at the proximal landing zone that acts as a lead point for collapse (Fig. 2). When this is recognized, the proximal seal zone has been reinforced with various cuffs, extenders, or relined with another TAG device extending the proximal seal zone [38].

Obtaining a proximal seal zone (recommended 2 cm) in this location can be difficult secondary to the injury's location in relation to the left subclavian orifice. Borsa and colleagues [35] reported a mean proximal landing zone of 6 mm in a cohort of BAI patients. Initial efforts were made to abut the subclavian artery, but often proximal endoleaks developed with limited seal zones in this location [38]. Although an endoleak can be

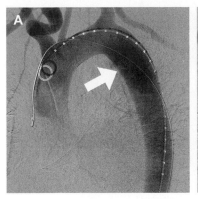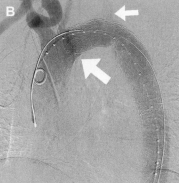

Fig. 2. Aortogram of BAI and stent graft. In (*A*) the white arrow marks the aortic injury distal to the left subclavian artery. In (*B*) the large white arrow marks the proximal landing zone of the stent graft. Note the small lip where the stent does not oppose the inside wall of the aorta. The small white arrow marks the left subclavian artery, which has been partially covered with the stent graft.

asymptomatic, it can also lead to rupture, graft occlusion, or graft migration. Depending on the severity of the leak and ability to interrogate the lumen of the graft with endovascular techniques, the leak may progress, cause aneurysmal expansion, and lead to mandatory operative repair. In an attempt to avoid this complication, some authors have recommended intentional coverage of the left subclavian vessel to obtain an adequate landing zone in the proximal aorta [39]. This has proven to be a fairly innocuous maneuver in selected patients, with few patients developing malperfusion symptoms to the arm or vertebrobasilar insufficiency. If symptoms do arise, they can be treated with a carotid to subclavian artery bypass; however, caution is warranted in patients who have an occluded right vertebral artery (ie, dominant or indispensable left vertebral artery) or those who have prior coronary artery bypass grafts based off the left internal mammary artery.

Complications of thoracic stent grafts occur infrequently and experience thus far reveals promising results for BAI patients. As smaller caliber commercial devices become available, this procedure will be performed with increasing frequency in trauma centers. Providers should become familiar with evaluating stent grafts on daily chest radiographs and monitoring for graft malformation (Fig. 3). It is imperative that patients treated with stent grafts be managed with a high index of suspicion for stent graft collapse with early recognition of resultant malperfusion. Although the majority of these complications can be treated with endovascular techniques, if the patient's physiologic reserve has improved to tolerate general anesthesia and single lung ventilation, graft explantation and open repair remain a viable option.

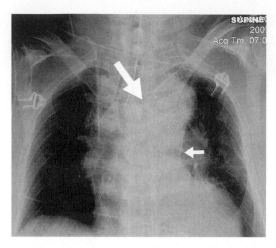

Fig. 3. Chest radiograph illustrating a thoracic stent graft. The large white arrow marks the proximal landing zone of the stent graft in the aortic arch. The small white arrow marks the distal landing zone in the thoracic aorta.

Axillo-subclavian trauma

Injuries to the thoracic outlet can be difficult to expose in an acute setting. Proximal control requires either a median sternotomy for the innominate and right subclavian arteries or a high left anterolateral thoracotomy with potential clavicular resection for the left subclavian artery. Although the upper extremities rarely suffer from ischemia caused by intense collaterals at the level of the shoulder, the long-term morbidity of these injuries is secondary to brachial plexus injuries. Plexus injuries can be caused by penetrating injuries that directly transect nerve roots, blunt injuries that result in shear or traction forces, and operative exposure that can result in iatrogenic injury.

In the unstable patient, there are few options other than immediate exploration, but because of the fibrous attachments surrounding the subclavian vessels, injuries will frequently result in a contained extrapleural hematoma that may extend into the supraclavicular fossa. If time allows, CTA can be invaluable for identifying the location of injury and evaluating the mediastinum. Rather than directly exploring the hematoma, a remote occlusion balloon can be placed either from the groin or retrograde from the brachial artery. In doing so, the surgeon can perform an arteriogram, and with proximal control, the operative tempo changes from emergent to semi-urgent. Either an endovascular treatment can ensue or the surgeon can proceed with a meticulous dissection at the base of the neck. Covered stent grafts have been used in this location, with several authors reporting immediate technical success for treating iatrogenic pseudoaneurysm, lacerations, and even complete transactions [40]. Undoubtedly, endovascular techniques reduce the morbidity of operative exposure and potential nerve injury in a blood-stained field.

There should be concern about the unknown long-term outcome of covered stents in this location. The mobility and compression between the first rib and clavicle raise concern about long-term patency in the young trauma population; it is imperative to follow these patients for late complications. Alternatively, at a later date when the hematoma and edema have resolved, the stent can be explanted with a formal open repair; this approach would ideally reduce the potential for iatrogenic nerve injury in the acute setting and delay open repair. Finally, patients can be longitudinally followed and complications addressed as they arise. Endovascular therapy in the thoracic outlet offers a less invasive, rapid treatment, and has the added benefit of avoiding injury to the brachial plexus, which has long-term implications for a functional recovery.

Endovascular management of abdominal vascular trauma

Vascular injuries in the abdomen are the most frequently encountered, and remain the leading cause of death after penetrating abdominal trauma [41]. When a patient is in extremis with a suspected penetrating or blunt abdominal injury, emergent operative exploration is required to arrest hemorrhage. When the abdomen is explored, immediate four-quadrant packing of the abdomen ensues, with careful examination of each quadrant until all sites of injury are identified. Concomitant solid organ and gastrointestinal injuries are common with both penetrating and blunt mechanisms. The abdomen has classically been divided into four zones: Zone I (central retroperitoneum), Zone II (lateral retroperitoneum), Zone III (pelvis), and Zone IV (portal structures and retrohepatic vena cava).

Typically any zone with hematoma formation should demand exploration for penetrating trauma, whereas a more selective approach is used for blunt trauma. It is unquestionable that unstable patients who have rapidly expanding hematomas should be directly explored. In this situation, remote aortic occlusion can be particularly useful in the acute setting if the patient has had prior foregut surgery or cardiac surgery that could potentially complicate supraceliac control.

With endovascular technology, the patient that has a contained hematoma in the retroperitoneum may have more options other than mandatory exploration. If the patient has a perforated viscous, small bowel anastomosis, partial colectomy, or ostomy, endoluminal treatment avoids opening the retroperitoneum and placing prosthetic conduit in a contaminated field. If the patient is prepared for intraoperative imaging, the surgeon can perform an intraoperative arteriogram, delineate the injury, and then determine if the injury can be temporized or treated with an endovascular technique. By not violating the retroperitoneum, the operative approach is preserved for a delayed reconstruction when the patient's physiologic status has returned to baseline and the infectious risk is lower. Other advantages include avoidance

of aortic cross-clamping, which can lead to varying periods of visceral ischemia, hepatic hypoperfusion, and the resultant fibrinolytic state [42].

Commercial stent grafts are readily available in most centers for the treatment of aortic pathology, and covered stents have been used for traumatic
aortic injuries. These case reports have included both acute injuries (dissection and hemorrhage) and delayed manifestations of trauma (pseudoaneurysms and arterio-venous fistulas) [41,43,44]. The morbidity and mortality
for these delayed interventions are dramatically lower compared with those
in the acute setting.

Iliac and femoral vessel trauma

Iliac and femoral vessel injuries often require intra-abdominal proximal
control and infrainguinal distal control, depending on the extent of hematoma formation. If the abdomen is being explored for other injuries, the
groin should be directly explored; however, if the groin is an isolated injury,
guide wire and sheath access can be obtained in the contralateral groin.
Remote occlusion can be performed in the distal aorta, and an arteriogram
performed. If injured, the hypogastric artery can be embolized for ongoing
extravasation. Common iliac and external iliac artery dissections, lacerations, and pseudoaneurysms can easily be treated with covered stents
[40,45,46].

White and colleagues [40] performed a prospective multi-institutional
trial to evaluate covered stents in vascular trauma. Compared with historical
controls, they found that endovascular treatments have a high rate of technical success (94%), an early mortality benefit, and a reduction in adverse
events. In addition, they found that devastating complications associated
with surgical repair (enteric fistula, coagulopathy, evisceration, visceral ischemia, and evisceration) did not occur in patients treated with endovascular techniques; the most common complication was stenosis, which was
treated by minimally invasive reintervention.

Extremity vascular trauma

The majority of extremity vascular trauma can be controlled with directed tamponade, and the extremities tolerate longer ischemia times of
4 to 6 hours, thus allowing time to address other life-threatening injuries
[47]. This also allows time for radiographic evaluation of associated fractures and arteriographic evaluation of the vascular injury. Complete transections of proximal vessels are better served by open repair, but vessel
thrombosis, intimal disruptions, and partial lacerations may be addressed
with endovascular techniques.

In the upper extremity, intimal disruptions of the brachial artery are classically associated with shoulder or elbow dislocations and fractures of the

humerus. After a blunt injury with either soft or hard signs of vascular injury, the upper extremity should be evaluated with either duplex ultrasound or arteriogram. If thrombus is identified, this can be managed with thrombectomy catheters or with catheter-directed lytic therapy. Once the vessel lumen is opened, intimal flaps can be treated with prolonged angioplasty, which apposes the intima to the vessel wall. Partial transections can be treated with covered stents [47,48]. Covered stents in this location should be reserved for patients who have life-threatening injuries that do not allow time for a formal vascular repair. Treatment for radial or ulnar artery injuries should generally be limited except when associated with hand ischemia. Most of these injuries can simply be ligated or coil embolized.

Lower extremity vascular injuries can be approached in a similar manner as upper extremity injuries. Proximally, both penetrating and blunt traumatic lesions have been successfully treated with covered stents in the common or superficial femoral arteries [20,49]. More distally, injuries to the tibial and peroneal vessels can be embolized when associated with active bleeding, pseudoaneurysm, or arterio-venous fistula formation. If pseudoaneurysms are superficial, ultrasound guided thrombin injection has been used. Otherwise, catheter-directed embolization can usually easily be performed. Arterio-venous fistulas can also be treated with transcatheter coils or balloons, and this technique avoids having to re-explore an extremity through a healed traumatic wound, which may lead to healing complications.

Both blunt and penetrating trauma to the popliteal artery have been associated with significant morbidity and high amputation rates [50]. Vascular surgeons have approached the popliteal artery with caution regarding the use of endovascular techniques because of the instability of a rigid stent across the motion of the knee joint [51]. Hutto and Reed [52] reported treatment of an ischemic limb secondary to blunt popliteal trauma in which they performed a thrombectomy and identified a proximal popliteal intimal disruption. A 5 mm angioplasty balloon was used to tack the intima, and with dual antiplatelet therapy, the patient's limb was salvaged with good function. In addition, there are case reports of covered stents in the popliteal artery for iatrogenic pseudoaneurysms with good outcomes [53].

Summary

Endovascular techniques for the management of vascular trauma represent a significant advancement in the care of the traumatically injured patient. Previously, only stable patients could be transferred to an imaging suite for diagnosis and potential therapeutic intervention. Vascular surgeons using endovascular techniques in an operative theater now provide the trauma specialist with options that previously involved transferring an unstable patient. The benefit to the patient is readily apparent as either a "damage-control" approach or as definitive primary treatment. As endovascular therapy becomes increasingly used for trauma, trauma specialists will need to become facile with basic access techniques and guide wire skills, and master the technique of remote aortic balloon occlusion. The burden of education lies on the vascular surgeon to train fellow general and trauma surgeons and surgical residents.

References

[1] Beitsch P, Weigelt JA, Flynn E, et al. Physical examination and arteriography in patients with penetrating zone II neck wounds. Arch Surg 1994;129(6):577–81.

[2] Monson DO, Saletta JD, Freeark RJ. Carotid vertebral trauma. J Trauma 1969;9(12): 987–99.

[3] Feliciano DV. Management of penetrating injuries to carotid artery. World J Surg 2001; 25(8):1028–35.

[4] Sekharan J, Dennis JW, Veldenz HC, et al. Continued experience with physical examination alone for evaluation and management of penetrating zone 2 neck injuries: results of 145 cases. J Vasc Surg 2000;32(3):483–9.

[5] Coldwell DM, Novak Z, Ryu RK, et al. Treatment of posttraumatic internal carotid arterial pseudoaneurysms with endovascular stents. J Trauma 2000;48(3):470–2.

[6] Duane TM, Parker F, Stokes GK, et al. Endovascular carotid stenting after trauma. J Trauma 2002;52(1):149–53.

[7] Ellis PK, Kennedy PT, Barros D'Sa AA. Successful exclusion of a high internal carotid pseudoaneurysm using the Wallgraft endoprosthesis. Cardiovasc Intervent Radiol 2002;25(1): 68–9.

[8] McNeil JD, Chiou AC, Gunlock MG, et al. Successful endovascular therapy of a penetrating zone III internal carotid injury. J Vasc Surg 2002;36(1):187–90.

[9] Rozycki GS, Tremblay L, Feliciano DV, et al. A prospective study for the detection of vascular injury in adult and pediatric patients with cervicothoracic seat belt signs. J Trauma 2002;52(4):618–23 [discussion: 623–4].

[10] Martin MJ, Mullenix PS, Steele SR, et al. Functional outcome after blunt and penetrating carotid artery injuries: analysis of the National Trauma Data Bank. J Trauma 2005;59(4):860–4.

[11] Biffl WL, Moore EE, Ryu RK, et al. The unrecognized epidemic of blunt carotid arterial injuries: early diagnosis improves neurologic outcome. Ann Surg 1998;228(4):462–70.

[12] Ofer A, Nitecki SS, Braun J, et al. CT angiography of the carotid arteries in trauma to the neck. Eur J Vasc Endovasc Surg 2001;21(5):401–7.

[13] Ramadan F, Rutledge R, Oller D, et al. Carotid artery trauma: a review of contemporary trauma center experiences. J Vasc Surg 1995;21(1):46–55 [discussion: 55–6].

[14] Fabian TC, Patton JH Jr, Croce MA, et al. Blunt carotid injury. Importance of early diagnosis and anticoagulant therapy. Ann Surg 1996;223(5):513–22 [discussion: 522–5].

[15] Duke BJ, Ryu RK, Coldwell DM, et al. Treatment of blunt injury to the carotid artery by using endovascular stents: an early experience. J Neurosurg 1997;87(6):825–9.

[16] Pretre R, Kursteiner K, Reverdin A, et al. Blunt carotid artery injury: devastating consequences of undetected pseudoaneurysm. J Trauma 1995;39(5):1012–4.

[17] Cohen JE, Ben-Hur T, Rajz G, et al. Endovascular stent-assisted angioplasty in the management of traumatic internal carotid artery dissections. Stroke 2005;36(4):e45–7.

[18] Bejjani GK, Monsein LH, Laird JR, et al. Treatment of symptomatic cervical carotid dissections with endovascular stents. Neurosurgery 1999;44(4):755–60 [discussion: 760–1].

[19] Liu AY, Paulsen RD, Marcellus ML, et al. Long-term outcomes after carotid stent placement treatment of carotid artery dissection. Neurosurgery 1999;45(6):1368–73 [discussion 1373–4].

[20] Parodi JC, Schonholz C, Ferreira LM, et al. Endovascular stent-graft treatment of traumatic arterial lesions. Ann Vasc Surg 1999;13(2):121–9.

[21] Horowitz MB, Miller G 3rd, Meyer Y, et al. Use of intravascular stents in the treatment of internal carotid and extracranial vertebral artery pseudoaneurysms. AJNR Am J Neuroradiol 1996;17(4):693–6.

[22] Bhatt DL, Kapadia SR, Bajzer CT, et al. Dual antiplatelet therapy with clopidogrel and aspirin after carotid artery stenting. J Invasive Cardiol 2001;13(12):767–71.

[23] Goaley TJ, Dente CJ, Feliciano DV. Torso vascular trauma at an urban level I trauma center. Perspect Vasc Surg Endovasc Ther 2006;18(2):102–12.

[24] Mwipatayi BP, Jeffery P, Beningfield SJ, et al. Management of extra-cranial vertebral artery injuries. Eur J Vasc Endovasc Surg 2004;27(2):157–62.

[25] Fang TD, Peterson DA, Kirilcuk NN, et al. Endovascular management of a gunshot wound to the thoracic aorta. J Trauma 2006;60(1):204–8.

[26] Jamieson WR, Janusz MT, Gudas VM, et al. Traumatic rupture of the thoracic aorta: third decade of experience. Am J Surg 2002;183(5):571–5.

[27] Fabian TC, Richardson JD, Croce MA, et al. Prospective study of blunt aortic injury: Multicenter Trial of the American Association for the Surgery of Trauma. J Trauma 1997;42(3): 374–80 [discussion: 380–3].

[28] von Oppell UO, Dunne TT, De Groot MK, et al. Traumatic aortic rupture: twenty-year metaanalysis of mortality and risk of paraplegia. Ann Thorac Surg 1994;58(2):585–93.

[29] Kasirajan K, Heffernan D, Langsfeld M. Acute thoracic aortic trauma: a comparison of endoluminal stent grafts with open repair and nonoperative management. Ann Vasc Surg 2003;17(6):589–95.

[30] Cowley RA, Turney SZ, Hankins JR, et al. Rupture of thoracic aorta caused by blunt trauma. A fifteen-year experience. J Thorac Cardiovasc Surg 1990;100(5):652–60 [discussion: 660–1].

[31] Mitchell RS, Miller DC, Dake MD, et al. Thoracic aortic aneurysm repair with an endovascular stent graft: the "first generation." Ann Thorac Surg 1999;67(6):1971–4 [discussion: 1979–80].

[32] Makaroun MS, Dillavou ED, Kee ST, et al. Endovascular treatment of thoracic aortic aneurysms: results of the phase II multicenter trial of the GORE TAG thoracic endoprosthesis. J Vasc Surg 2005;41(1):1–9.

[33] Dake MD, Miller DC, Mitchell RS, et al. The "first generation" of endovascular stent-grafts for patients with aneurysms of the descending thoracic aorta. J Thorac Cardiovasc Surg 1998;116(5):689–703 [discussion: 703–4].

[34] Starnes BW, Arthurs ZM. Endovascular management of vascular trauma. Perspect Vasc Surg Endovasc Ther 2006;18(2):114–29.

[35] Borsa JJ, Hoffer EK, Karmy-Jones R, et al. Angiographic description of blunt traumatic injuries to the thoracic aorta with specific relevance to endograft repair. J Endovasc Ther 2002;9(Suppl 2):I184–91.

[36] Lin PH, Bush RL, Zhou W, et al. Endovascular treatment of traumatic thoracic aortic injury—should this be the new standard of treatment? J Vasc Surg 2006;43(Suppl A): 22A–9A.

[37] Mestres G, Maeso J, Fernandez V, et al. Symptomatic collapse of a thoracic aorta endoprosthesis. J Vasc Surg 2006;43(6):1270–3.

[38] Karmy-Jones R, Hoffer E, Meissner MH, et al. Endovascular stent grafts and aortic rupture: a case series. J Trauma 2003;55(5):805–10.

[39] Mattison R, Hamilton IN Jr, Ciraulo DL, et al. Stent-graft repair of acute traumatic thoracic aortic transection with intentional occlusion of the left subclavian artery: case report. J Trauma 2001;51(2):326–8.

[40] White R, Krajcer Z, Johnson M, et al. Results of a multicenter trial for the treatment of traumatic vascular injury with a covered stent. J Trauma 2006;60(6):1189–95 [discussion: 1195–6].

[41] Mattox KL, Feliciano DV, Burch J, et al. Five thousand seven hundred sixty cardiovascular injuries in 4459 patients. Epidemiologic evolution 1958 to 1987. Ann Surg 1989;209(6): 698–705 [discussion: 706–7].

[42] Illig KA, Green RM, Ouriel K, et al. Primary fibrinolysis during supraceliac aortic clamping. J Vasc Surg 1997;25(2):244–51 [discussion: 252–4].

[43] Picard E, Marty-Ane CH, Vernhet H, et al. Endovascular management of traumatic infrarenal abdominal aortic dissection. Ann Vasc Surg 1998;12(6):515–21.

[44] Scharrer-Pamler R, Gorich J, Orend KH, et al. Emergent endoluminal repair of delayed abdominal aortic rupture after blunt trauma. J Endovasc Surg 1998;5(2):134–7.

[45] Lyden SP, Srivastava SD, Waldman DL, et al. Common iliac artery dissection after blunt trauma: case report of endovascular repair and literature review. J Trauma 2001;50(2): 339–42.

[46] Tsai FC, Wang CC, Fang JF, et al. Isolated common iliac artery occlusion secondary to atherosclerotic plaque rupture from blunt abdominal trauma: case report and review of the literature. J Trauma 1997;42(1):133–6.

[47] Wolma FJ, Larrieu AJ, Alsop GC. Arterial injuries of the legs associated with fractures and dislocations. Am J Surg 1980;140(6):806–9.

[48] Lonn L, Delle M, Karlstrom L, et al. Should blunt arterial trauma to the extremities be treated with endovascular techniques? J Trauma 2005;59(5):1224–7.

[49] Risberg B, Lonn L. Management of vascular injuries using endovascular techniques. Eur J Surg 2000;166(3):196–201.

[50] Frykberg ER. Popliteal vascular injuries. Surg Clin North Am 2002;82(1):67–89.

[51] Arena FJ. Arterial kink and damage in normal segments of the superficial femoral and popliteal arteries abutting nitinol stents—a common cause of late occlusion and restenosis? A single-center experience. J Invasive Cardiol 2005;17(9):482–6.

[52] Hutto JD, Reed AB. Endovascular repair of an acute blunt popliteal artery injury. J Vasc Surg 2007;45(1):188–90.

[53] D'Angelo F, Carrafiello GP, Lagana D, et al. Popliteal artery pseudoaneurysm after a revision of total knee arthroplasty: endovascular treatment with a stent graft. Emerg Radiol 2007;13(6):323–7.

SURGICAL
CLINICS OF
NORTH AMERICA

Surg Clin N Am 87 (2007) 1193–1211

Vascular Surgery on the Modern Battlefield

LTC Charles J. Fox, MD[a,b,*],
LTC Benjamin W. Starnes, MD, FACS[c]

[a]Walter Reed Army Medical Center, Vascular Surgery, Bldg 2, Ward 64,
6900 Georgia Avenue NW, Washington, DC 20307, USA
[b]Department of Surgery, Uniformed Services University of the Health Sciences,
Bethesda, MD 20814, USA
[c]Madigan Army Medical Center, Fitzsimmons Drive, Building 9040, Fort Lewis,
Tacoma, WA 98431, USA

Management of traumatic vascular injuries can offer special challenges to experienced surgeons in peacetime and in combat. Lessons from past conflicts have advanced practice of vascular trauma surgery through the twentieth century. Original contributions from DeBakey, Hughes, Rich, and others have taught the impact of and have defined the standards for vessel ligation, or repair of arterial and venous injuries in resource-limited situations. Moreover, the presence of forward surgical support, aeromedical evacuation, and novel resuscitation strategies has influenced the evolution of vascular trauma surgery on the battlefield [1–8]. Since the Vietnam War there has been substantial modernization of the battlefield environment that has translated into a measurable survival advantage [9,10]. These technologic advancements have not only expanded our capabilities but have changed the contemporary practice of vascular surgery during wartime. The present situations and capabilities trauma surgeons are currently confronted with in treating vascular injuries on the modern battlefield serve as the focus for this review.

The opinions or assertions contained herein are the private views of the authors and are not to be construed as official or as reflecting the views of the Department of the Army or the Department of Defense. The authors are employees of the US government. This work was prepared as part of their official duties and, as such, there is no copyright to be transferred.

* Corresponding author. Walter Reed Army Medical Center, Vascular Surgery, Bldg 2, Ward 64, 6900 Georgia Avenue NW, Washington, DC 20307.
E-mail address: charles.fox@us.army.mil (C.J. Fox).

0039-6109/07/$ - see front matter. Published by Elsevier Inc.
doi:10.1016/j.suc.2007.07.015

Historical perspective

Extremity injuries account for most wounds on the battlefield, and hemorrhage from extremity wounds remains a leading cause of potentially preventable death [11,12]. Historically most military injuries are the result of blast-mediated fragmentation and the current conflict is consistent with past experience [13–15].

During World War II, time lags, practical difficulties, and poor physiologic conditions led DeBakey to conclude after an analysis of nearly 2500 cases that vessel ligation, although not the "procedure of choice, is one of necessity" [1]. During the Korean War, a surgical research team was established to study this problem in an effort to improve on the management of combat-related vascular injury [4]. Since the spring of 1952, several reports on successful arterial repairs performed under austere conditions without the benefit of proper instruments gained the attention of the Office of the Surgeon General [2,16,17]. Hughes demonstrated among 269 repairs an impressive reduction in the amputation rate from 36% in World War II to 13% during the Korean War. Time lags and ongoing resuscitation needs remained the ultimate Achilles heel of successful vascular surgery during the Korean War [4]. Battlefield environments became more favorable for difficult vascular reconstructions during the Vietnam War. Forward surgical positioning to minimize ischemic time, along with modern resuscitation practices, permitted the widespread application and success of arterial reconstruction. The management of complex injuries such as those involving the popliteal artery and vein, or large cavitary wounds that threaten graft viability, and those associated with severe open contaminated fractures became the focus of attention during this era [18]. The Vietnam Vascular Registry details a careful analysis with completed follow-up of more than 1000 cases and now serves as a reference standard for the application of vascular surgery during the modern conflicts of the twenty-first century [8]. The application of lessons learned in prior conflicts and the use of new technologies are partially responsible for the significant reduction in mortality observed during the wars in Iraq and Afghanistan [19]. Moreover, advances in hemorrhage control, wound care, and orthopedic surgery during this war have allowed greater attention to shift toward limb salvage efforts. The expectation to reconstruct vascular injuries during this conflict has therefore allowed the practice of vascular surgery on the modern battlefield to become increasingly sophisticated.

Modern advancements

The battlefield is a noisy, contaminated, and dynamic environment, full of extremes and uncertainties that underscore the need for preparation. Resource-limited situations in combat are common and these unique differences are eloquently expressed by others [10,20]. These external forces serve as a predictable constant that can influence the type and quality of surgical care provided depending on the tactical situation. Vascular surgery in this setting is obviously taxing and is a technically exacting practice that must be perfected and rehearsed frequently to achieve a successful outcome [21]. There is no substitute for the experience gained and the pattern recognition that is learned from managing wartime vascular injuries. Modern advances and evolving surgical practices all serve to increase the number of vascular injuries that reach a combat support hospital and subsequently undergo complex or prolonged vascular reconstruction [22,23]. Advancements in hemorrhage control and resuscitation strategies have reduced potentially survivable deaths from extremity injury and may represent the greatest contribution toward the advance of vascular trauma surgery during the current conflict [24–37].

Prehospital hemorrhage control

Surgical doctrine in prior conflicts taught that tourniquet application was a plan of last resort only performed when necessary to save life over limb [38]. In an effort to reduce potentially survivable deaths from hemorrhage, the role of early tourniquet use has been recently reviewed. The US Army implemented a rapid design, testing, training, and fielding program for battlefield tourniquets [39–41]. Laboratory testing in human volunteers demonstrated 100% efficacy of the three most commonly used tourniquets in current military distribution. These are the Combat Application Tourniquet (CAT; North American Rescue Products, Greenville, SC), the Special Operations Forces Tactical Tourniquet (SOFTT; Tactical Medical Solutions, Anderson, SC), and the Emergency Medical Tourniquet (EMT; Delfi Medical, Vancouver, Canada) [39,41]. As a result, tourniquets have now become familiar items on the battlefields of Iraq and Afghanistan and have enhanced hemorrhage control over similar casualties without tourniquets [22,42,43]. They are widely disseminated to the combat maneuver and forward surgical units with more than 275,000 in distribution as of the summer of 2005 [42]. Preliminary reports have demonstrated that early and liberal tourniquet use is saving lives and has led to changes in prehospital trauma life support (PHTLS) teaching for military wounds (John F. Kragh, Jr, MD, COL, personal communication, 2007). This improvement in prehospital hemorrhage control has led to substantial numbers of patients arriving at combat hospitals with extremity injuries and may amplify the opportunities for trauma surgeons to reconstruct injured vessels (Fig. 1).

Damage control resuscitation

The essence of damage control is to achieve and conclude an operative procedure before the physiologic "point of no return" is reached. Original

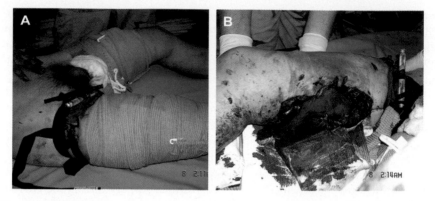

Fig. 1. Prehospital hemorrhage control is optimized with an Israeli dressing and two tourniquets (*A*) for a soldier who had deep cavitary fragment wounds of the lower extremities and transected femoral artery (*B*). The SOF Tactical Tourniquet is shown more inferiorly with the aluminum windless.

descriptions of staged abdominal approaches in patients who are coagulopathic led to the term "damage control" as an approach to improve survival in critically injured patients [44–47]. Hirshberg and others expanded this approach to regions beyond the abdomen and as a result have advanced the practice of vascular trauma surgery by using damage control principles [21,48]. Because of wounding patterns seen in combat casualties, these techniques are particularly important in the care of military trauma patients [19]. This approach facilitates the movement of casualties through the battlefield healthcare system and minimizes their exposure to the traditionally physiologically hostile environment of the operating room [31,49–51].

Developing an early advanced resuscitation strategy for vascular trauma patients is a key component for successful limb salvage in massively injured casualties. The soft-tissue destruction associated with high-energy munitions results in early and profound coagulopathy associated with death [52,53]. Traditional resuscitation techniques using liberal amounts of crystalloid and packed red blood cells (PRBCs) can exacerbate this coagulopathy and render a patient unfit for anything more than a hasty operative procedure [34]. Combining the concepts of damage control surgery with a resuscitation strategy that quickly restores physiology may allow preservation of limbs that previously would have been amputated early to avoid exacerbating the lethality of coagulopathy, acidosis, and hypothermia. Surgical doctrine is not easily changed, however, and this is supported by the recently published Emergency War Surgery textbook strongly recommending extremity amputation in situations in which a poor physiologic condition may preclude a safe vascular reconstruction. This practice remains a widely accepted surgical teaching that has emerged from prior conflicts [1,4,10,21,51].

As experience with these injuries has evolved, so has the philosophy on the benefits of early rapid infusion of blood products, high plasma ratios, recombinant VIIa, and minimal crystalloid use in trauma [26,27,29,30,35,37]. This new way of thinking known as damage control resuscitation (DCR) is a necessary concept when considering simultaneous limb salvage efforts in combat casualties and should be combined with other traditional damage control maneuvers. In essence this practice serves to customize a vascular surgical plan based on the wounds, physiologic condition, and response to resuscitation efforts.

During the spring of 2006, the 10th Combat Support Hospital, located in Baghdad, Iraq, embraced the concept of DCR, and the early experience with this strategy has been recently reported [54]. The general guidelines called for early transfusion of blood products, warmed and infused rapidly, when the patients arrived in the admitting area (Fig. 2). An emergency release consisted of 4 units of type O PRBCs and 4 units of AB plasma, but could include fresh whole blood if the situation dictated. The 1:1 ratio of fresh frozen plasma (FFP) to red blood cell units, was intentionally high, and this has been recently shown to reduce mortality [27].Three vials of rFVIIa (2.4 mg ×3) were typically given in the emergency department (ED), operating room (OR), and intensive care unit (ICU). The goal of these interventions was a normal INR. In particular, crystalloid fluids were kept to an absolute minimum to avoid further iatrogenic physiologic derangement [26]. Heparin was not used in all cases and was often limited to a locally injected half dose when used. For isolated extremity trauma, rFVIIa was used sparingly and reserved for cases in which hemorrhage was not surgically treatable or controlled with hemostatic dressings. Trometamol;

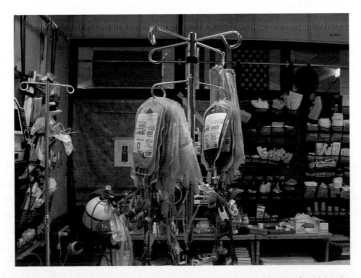

Fig. 2. Emergency release of blood products is initiated early and transfused in the admitting area. Equal ratios of plasma to red blood cell units, or fresh whole blood are advocated. Only a single bag of crystalloid is noted in the photograph.

tris-hydroxymethyl aminomethane (THAM) is a biologically inert amino alcohol of low toxicity that buffers carbon dioxide and acids in vitro and in vivo. In trauma, THAM is a potent and effective buffering agent that can be used to counter the coagulopathic effects of a progressive lactic acidosis [55,56]. THAM was routinely given when the admission base deficit was less than −10 or a massive transfusion was required. Calcium chloride was also supplemented based on transfusion requirements and ionized calcium levels that were obtained frequently and treated accordingly.

Based on this experience, the authors continue to advocate for the early implementation of blood products, with equal ratios of plasma to packed cells, fresh whole blood, selective use of rFVIIa, and minimal crystalloid use when planning for vascular reconstructions in severely injured casualties. These principles represent an evolution in current traditional damage control philosophy in which amputation was previously favored over elaborate vascular surgery. Modern advancements in DCR during this conflict may have expanded the opportunity for battlefield surgeons to provide definitive procedures at the initial operative setting.

Temporary shunting

The modern battlefield is organized to provide surgical care that is divided into echelons based on size, capability, and proximity to the front line (Fig. 3). A forward surgical team (FST) is a level II facility that can perform limited lifesaving procedures close to the lines of battle. Current capabilities of the FST and combat support hospital (CSH) are well described in other recent publications [10,22,28]. Resource limitations at the FST do not allow for prolonged vascular procedures. In particular, blood product availability may be highly variable because of storage constraints, although walking donor pools affect the ability to provide fresh whole blood when needed emergently [10].

Because shunts allow for perfusion during temporary delays needed for extremity fixation or patient transport, their use has gained some popularity during the current conflict [10,13,57]. Eger championed the notion of temporary shunting of combat-related arterial injuries in 1971 [58]. Since that report, this practice has been supported by several small series from civilian trauma centers and is well summarized by Rasmussen and colleagues [23]. The potential for dislodgment, thrombosis, or reduced limb viability are obvious drawbacks and require good surgical judgment for effective use. Military operations in Iraq have produced the largest series of combat casualties since Vietnam and provide an opportunity to examine the patterns of temporary shunt use and effectiveness. Data from the Balad Vascular Registry demonstrated that shunts placed in proximal vascular injuries have acceptable (86%) patency, and failure of distal shunts did not decrease limb viability [23]. Rasmussen concluded from this data analysis that the use of shunts

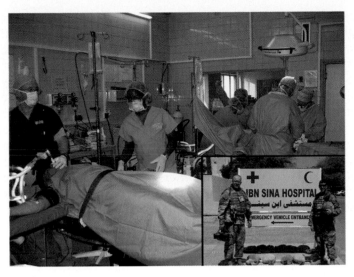

Fig. 3. The 10th Combat Support Hospital, located within the international zone of Baghdad, Iraq during 2005–2006, is an example of an echelon level III facility. The 772nd Forward Surgical Team augmentation enabled this unit to function like a regional trauma center. This Army hospital operated out of Ibn Sina Hospital, a former three-story private hospital for Saddam Hussein. The photograph depicts one of the two operating theaters that accommodated two tables with modern anesthesia apparatus. CPT Tom Chenowith, CRNA, and CPT Annette Conley, RN, are shown with members of the trauma team. (*Insert*) Major Chistopher W. Swicckim a general surgeon from the Forward Surgical Team, is with the author (Fox) at the emergency entrance.

was an effective technique to facilitate immediate evacuation and was preferable to prolonged reconstruction efforts in remote austere locations. The authors advocate for the use of temporary shunting as a damage control adjunct when patients who have vascular injuries can be transported to a level III CSH that is capable of providing the expertise and typical resuscitation necessary for a lengthy limb salvage effort.

Imaging and endovascular therapies

The diagnosis and management of vascular injury has rapidly evolved with innovative imaging technology. Catheter-based applications have been used frequently in trauma patients, mostly by surgeons previously familiar with basic access techniques and static film arteriography [14,59]. Specialized training in the last decade has integrated catheter skills to the point that the modern management of traumatic vascular injuries can often incorporate sophisticated endovascular therapies. These concepts were originally promoted in urban trauma centers by visionary vascular surgeons and this process has continued to evolve considerably over time [60–62]. Although arteriography remains the gold standard for guiding surgical reconstruction, static film arteriography has largely been replaced in this war by a portable C-arm and digital subtraction angiography [10]. At the 10th CSH, a portable unit shared with orthopedic surgery was adequate when a road map was necessary to localize a point of injury in pulseless patients who had multiple levels of fragmentation and the effectiveness of this has been previously reported [10]. Typically, serial hand-injected retrograde imaging is preferred to "up and over" techniques, because ordinary OR tables do not allow for patient repositioning or tracking wire location. Alternative imaging modalities currently exist at level III facilities and in the authors' experience are gaining value as important screening studies that may improve preoperative planning for exploration in trauma patients. For example, color flow duplex examinations are helpful to identify and direct the treatment of arteriovenous fistulae and false aneurysms. CT angiography has been invaluable in cervical and thoracic trauma in which negative nontherapeutic explorations may be avoided or the surgical approach improved when the location of injury is identified preoperatively. Embolization with gel foam pledgets or stainless steel coils has been helpful in controlling pelvic hemorrhage and in treating false aneurysms that are difficult to expose. Equipment shortages are not uncommon, and surgical expectations have to be adjusted to comply with the mission of a mobile hospital unit. Acquisition of a modern endovascular trauma inventory allowed the 332nd Expeditionary Medical Group, the first Air Force Theater Hospital since the Vietnam War, to promote a liberal use of arteriography for diagnosis and endovascular intervention. The experience described by Clouse and colleagues has been the most advanced wartime application of this technology to date. A 16-slice multidetector CT capable of high-resolution arteriography and a mobile OEC 9800 with a floating fluoroscopy table permitted the use of their endovascular skills in the acute management of several cerebrovascular, lower extremity, and abdominal aortic or iliac wounds [13]. Covered stent grafts have expanded the possible treatment options for vessel injury, and potential roles are well described by Starnes and others in current civilian trauma literature [59,63,64]. Use of stent grafts does raise a question regarding long-term durability and potential infectivity. For example, during the Vietnam experience and also in the current conflict, the preferred conduit remains the saphenous vein. This practice has been based on the poor historical results of prosthetic material when used in contaminated war wounds [65]. Several reports have suggested that a prosthetic conduit yields satisfactory results, yet inferior long-term patency and the real potential for infection in war wounds validate the controversy and illustrate a similar concern regarding the indication and use of covered stents [66–68]. Alternatively, temporary balloon occlusion for immediate hemostasis and transcatheter embolization may prove invaluable for surgically inaccessible vessels and may provide a novel endovascular alternative to reducing potentially survivable hemorrhagic deaths [14,69,70].

Early decision making for vascular trauma

Combat wounded patients should be immediately evaluated and resuscitated in a treatment area by an emergency medicine physician to allow the trauma surgeon to focus on the operative considerations. Immediate airway and hemorrhage control followed by intraosseous or intravenous access is the first priority. Patients in extremis from multiple fragment wounds often have several mangled extremities that may require inspection, adjustment, or exchange of tourniquets. In stable patients a tourniquet can be carefully released by the surgeon to establish the indication for placement. For unstable patients or situations in which arterial injury is obvious, the tourniquets are better "prepped-in" and manipulated in the OR.

Emergency release of blood products and activation of a massive transfusion protocol should be one of the earliest decisions made. This involves a standardized release and early transfusion of PRBCs, FFP, cryoprecipitate, and platelets when available. Vital signs and admission physiology predict mortality, and immediate resuscitation efforts should be directed at correcting the presenting base deficit and coagulopathy so that "life over limb" decisions become less of a concern [71–73].

When indicated, DCR maneuvers initiated in the ED are continued intraoperatively. Blood products should be transfused through a rapid infuser and warmer system (Belmont Instrument Corporation, Billerica, MA) reserved in the admitting area for instantaneous use. Fresh whole blood, used in every major United States military conflict since World War I, is safe and can be effective in certain situations [35,43]. Hesitancy to request blood may lead to lag times in resuscitation during surgery and force a change in the operative plan based the physiologic condition. The authors therefore favor fresh whole blood for vascular trauma when multiple simultaneous vascular reconstructions are planned or when a single extremity injury occurs with major thoracoabdominal trauma and hemorrhagic shock. Recombinant FVIIa can be given routinely for patients who meet the indications for DCR. The use and benefits of rFVIIa for trauma have been described previously [32,33,36,74–78]. Administration of a 90 to 120 ug/kg IV dose of rFVIIa given first in the ED, with additional doses given intraoperatively, is used to treat acquired coagulopathy and reduce hemorrhage.

Radiographs are carefully evaluated, because fracture patterns can offer reliable clues that predict the need for vessel reconstruction. Supracondylar femur and tibial plateau fractures in the authors' experience have a high association with popliteal and femoral arterial injury. Rapid surgical planning and effective communication with the OR personnel are essential and best accomplished when the orthopedic and trauma surgeon work together in the ED. This approach quickly relays information regarding the patient condition and urgency for an OR. Special instructions to the OR should consist of patient and table positioning, need for special or preferred instruments, the basic operative plan, body areas to prepare, and other details concerning arteriography or vein harvesting. These issues are often communicated late by inexperienced teams.

Early decisions for additional preoperative imaging are usually necessary for military trauma. Many patients also have maxillofacial and ophthalmologic injuries and benefit from a simultaneous multidisciplinary approach to their care [70]. For unstable patients who have severe thoracic or abdominal injuries, the descending thoracic aorta can be clamped and the patient immediately transported to the OR. Stable patients who have suspected head injury or those who have uncertain thoracoabdominal wounds may benefit from CT before operative exploration. In Baghdad in 2006, the authors used an 8-slice multidetector CT scanner. This was frequently helpful for neck or thoracic aortic injury but was never used for extremity vascular wounds.

Vascular assessment

Knowing early that a vascular procedure is necessary for limb salvage is crucial for a successful outcome, as indecision and progressive ischemic burden may ultimately result in graft failure. In the current conflict, surgeons generally attempted limb salvage unless the extremity was so mangled that salvage was pointless or the orthopedic surgeon discouraged reconstruction based on the degree of soft-tissue, nerve, and bony injury present. The ability to predict a vascular injury is gained from pattern recognition and cannot be overemphasized (Fig. 4). This skill is developed and polished in a combat environment and has been noted by others [43]. The Mangled Extremity Severity Score, or MESS, described by Johansen in 1990 has recently been validated in a combat setting and may be useful for determining limb

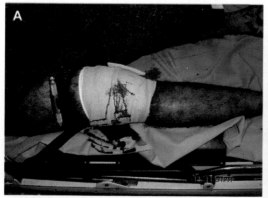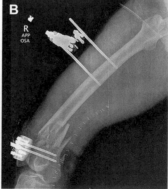

Fig. 4. Pattern recognition is an important skill to learn quickly. This casualty received a gunshot wound to the right knee. A Special Operations Forces Tactical Tourniquet (SOFTT) applied to control hemorrhage from a knee wound (*A*), coupled with a plain radiograph showing a fracture of the supracondylar femur (*B*) is highly suggestive of a vascular injury.

viability and the need for amputation. (CPT Randy J. Kjorstad, MD, LTC Benjamin W. Starnes, MD, personal communication, 2007) [79].

Arterial hemorrhage should be controlled with direct pressure, gauze packing, hemostatic dressings, and pneumatic tourniquets, in that order. Venous bleeding can usually be controlled by direct pressure or gauze packs, and can be made worse with an improperly applied tourniquet. In stable patients, prehospital tourniquets can be carefully loosened to determine the degree of vascular injury and immediately reapplied if active bleeding occurs (Fig. 5). The EMT pneumatic tourniquet may be applied above or exchanged with the narrow prehospital (CAT or SOFTT) tourniquets if additional control is necessary [39,40,80]. Once a deformed extremity is straightened, a pulse examination can be performed. A Doppler assessment is encouraged for added confirmation and to perform an ankle brachial index if possible. Pulseless extremities or other obvious signs of arterial injury should have an open exploration. Contrast arteriography may be necessary to evaluate an abnormal ankle brachial index (<0.9) and becomes especially useful for fragment injuries to guide the location for exploration [10]. The total time from injury on a Baghdad battlefield to operative intervention is approximately 45 to 60 minutes.

Management of vascular injury

For patients who have multiple injuries, a dedicated two-team approach should be used, especially for those who have extremity wounds needing simultaneous thoracic or abdominal explorations. To minimize ischemic time, additional surgeons are case accelerators and can be used to apply external fixation, perform fasciotomies, or harvest vein from a non-injured or amputated extremity.

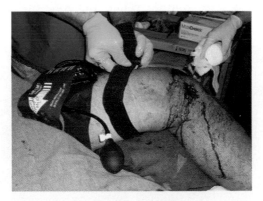

Fig. 5. The combat application tourniquet (CAT) is carefully loosened to evaluate a potential vascular injury. The Emergency Medical Tourniquet (EMT) is preferred for hospital use and is exchanged out or applied above the narrow field tourniquets. (*Courtesy of* Col. John F. Kragh, Jr, MD, San Antonio, TX.)

Initial control of hemorrhage is best accomplished by a hasty preparation using Betadine spray over a wide surgical field and digital occlusion within the wound bed. Tourniquets are loosened after anesthesia has been provided with sufficient resuscitation time. Very proximal lower extremity injuries can be easily managed by division of the inguinal ligament or by an oblique retroperitoneal approach and control of the iliac artery. For proximal axillosubclavian wounds, sternotomy or left anterior thoracotomy and clamping of the subclavian artery improves control and eliminates unwise dissection through an expanding hematoma. The concept of early, rapid proximal control should be encouraged for war injuries.

End-to-end or lateral suturing methods are the simplest and most expedient manner to repair injured vessels. When a primary repair is not feasible, the saphenous vein is the preferred conduit for extremity injuries based on durability and superior long-term patency. It is important to emphasize that amputated limbs can provide an important source of autologous conduit. Vein grafts are generally placed in the reversed configuration and tunneled around the zone of injury when the soft-tissue wound is particularly extensive (Fig. 6). All devitalized tissue should be excised and irrigated under low pressure, with careful evaluation of muscle tissue for viability. The temptation to perform a lengthy and meticulous debridement at the outset should be resisted, because these wounds look much better in a few days after subsequent washouts and vacuum dressing application. It is essential to cover interposition vein grafts with viable muscle tissue, and reversed saphenous vein bypass around the zone of injury may be preferred over interposition grafts when soft tissue defects are large. In military wounds, the regional damage is frequently so extensive that when the injury involves the calf, bone is destroyed and tibial vessels are transected by the fragments. The authors favor tibial bypass over below-knee amputation when the orthopedic surgeon is optimistic (Fig. 7). Vein grafts seem to be better protected when routed around the zone of injury through an

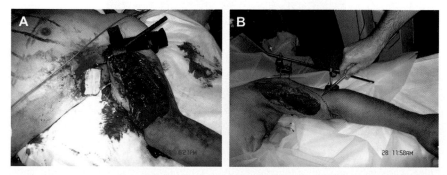

Fig. 6. High-energy military munitions produce fragment wounds associated with massive soft-tissue destruction (*A*). The surgical marking pen illustrates the path of an axillobrachial artery reconstruction using a reversed saphenous vein graft routed out of the zone of injury (*B*).

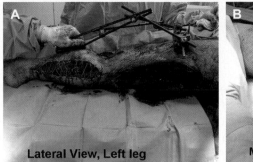
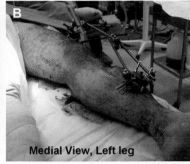

Fig. 7. A lower extremity fragment wound resulting in severe destruction of the popliteal and tibial vessels (*A*) was reconstructed with an above-knee popliteal to posterior tibial artery bypass using a reversed saphenous vein graft. The photograph shows how knee spanning external fixation for this tibial plateau fracture can be applied to stabilize the limb and permit excellent surgical exposure out of the injured region (*B*).

extra-anatomic tunnel. Progressive myonecrosis and expanding wounds result in early graft exposure when the effortless approach of laying the vascular conduit in the wound bed is taken initially. Regardless of the approach taken, the nondiseased distal posterior tibial artery often provides a suitable site for the distal anastomosis and retrograde thrombectomy when necessary. Typical anastomotic construction is taught using a four-quadrant heel to toe spatulated anastomosis with 6.0 sutures under 2.5× loupe magnification and use of a headlamp. Small Heifitz clips or atraumatic Bulldog clamps are preferred to minimize the chance of a clamp injury. The injured segment of the artery should be aggressively debrided back to normal tissue and any temptation to make compromises on this step should be avoided. After debridement, a Fogarty catheter can be advanced retrograde to remove any accumulated thrombus proximal to the injury and to confirm or re-establish the inflow. Retrograde passage of a thrombectomy catheter from an uninjured site can also be used as a technique to quickly identify the severed end of the artery in a severe wound. Because heparin is often limited to half dose or not used at all, precautions should be taken to liberally flush the graft and native artery free of fibrin strands and platelet debris. Use of rFVIIa does not seem to result in thrombus accumulation around construction of the anastomosis [54]. Papaverine, a smooth muscle relaxant, can be flushed into the graft or applied topically to treat spasm and should be readily available.

There has been sustained interest in repair of venous injuries to avoid the potential for early limb loss from venous hypertension or long-term disability from chronic edema. In the summer of 2006, 12 of 14 popliteal artery injuries that presented to a Baghdad Combat Support Hospital were successfully repaired. Ten were associated with a concomitant injury to the popliteal vein. Although one venous injury was ligated, nine of these underwent successful repair using a saphenous vein graft, end-to-end anastomosis, or lateral sutures. During the current conflicts, the routine has been to continue the practices and teachings learned from the Vietnam experience [81,82].

Postoperative considerations

Completion assessments following repair are performed using physical examination, handheld Doppler, or arteriography (Fig. 8). Palpable pulses with normal ankle brachial ratios (>0.9) should be confirmed in the ICU after an appropriate resuscitation period. Coagulopathic hemorrhage may persist from fasciotomy sites and should be medically supported in the ICU. Attempts to re-look should be discouraged, because removing Kerlix gauze and Ace bandages only exacerbates this bleeding. Most patients should be returned to the OR within 24 hours for wound inspection and adjustment of external fixation. Careful assessment of the pulse examination should be performed by the surgeon before and after these interventions, because this is a vulnerable period of graft viability. Determining the proper time for evacuation to the next echelon of care is a matter of good surgical judgment and experience. Airway issues, associated injuries, and the complexity of the vascular reconstruction are important factors to consider. A liberal policy on fasciotomy in the management of these wounds is encouraged. Vacuum dressings are helpful in wound stabilization; however, during transport, air leaks and equipment failures can lead to devastating wound complications.

Trauma system development

The development of a theater trauma system has enhanced communication and advanced the contemporary management of wartime vascular

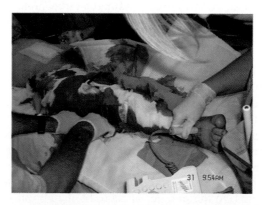

Fig. 8. Examinations are meticulously performed in the intensive care unit on all vascular reconstructions. Palpable pulses may be delayed for several hours in severe trauma; however, a normal ankle brachial index (>0.9) is confirmed after an appropriate resuscitation period. The temptation to take down dressings early should be resisted, because coagulopathic bleeding is best treated medically. All wounds are reinspected within 24 hours.

trauma. The impact of a formal, integrated trauma systems approach in caring for the injured patient has drastically improved surgical outcomes and reduced mortality in civilian trauma centers. The fundamental desire to "get the right patient to the right place at the right time" led to a joint initiative to form a similar trauma systems approach to military casualties in this conflict. In 2004, the formal military medical leadership in conjunction with the US Army Institute of Surgical Research and the American College of Surgeons Committee on Trauma established a trauma system in the theater of operations. This included a trauma system director, along with a team of trauma nurse coordinators and a data collection tool known as the Joint Theater Trauma Registry (JTTR). Data gathering from this registry has led to improvements in body armor, training, and battlefield care. The joint leadership has promoted the implementation of clinical practice guidelines and outcomes research using this robust registry to provide the best evidence-based practice for combat casualty care [28].

In all of these areas, the development of a Joint Theater Trauma System (JTTS) has closed knowledge gaps and improved the practice of vascular surgery. Data show that the rate of vascular injury seems to have increased compared to that seen in Vietnam [22]. Extremity injuries are prevalent and account for most of the vascular reconstructions performed [13,14]. A transition from a maneuver war to an insurgency characterized by ambush and explosions may be partly responsible for this observation, because an increase in fragment wounds tends to cause simultaneous injury to multiple vascular beds. Analysis of injury patterns has led to positive changes in training and equipment that has reduced the number of soldiers killed in combat and may have allowed for a greater percentage of patients who have vascular trauma to present at the doorsteps of a combat support hospital. For example, use of body armor has reduced the rate of thoracic injury and therefore amplified the ratio of potentially survivable vascular injuries. The application of these "lessons learned" is exemplified by the constant decline in total mortality observed during the last three major conflicts. In point of fact, a comparative analysis of United States combat casualty statistics shows that fewer soldiers are killed in action today and a larger majority are surviving the battle to reach a medical facility for surgical treatment [28]. Research initiatives aimed at hemorrhage control have led to the use of novel hemostatic dressings and widespread tourniquet distribution. Finally, redistribution of resources has led to the augmentation of the combat hospitals with forward surgical teams. This has synergized the capabilities of both elements and expanded the capacity of larger units that now function more like major regional trauma centers. Regarding vascular care, weekly video-teleconferencing is conducted across three continents to discuss the preferred management of vascular injury and provide feedback between level V centers and the front line. Additionally, a newly formed Joint Patient Tracking Application (JPTA) conveniently offers a Web-based electronic medical record to follow the vascular trauma patient through echelons of care back to the United States [42,43,83].

Summary

The management of combat-related vascular injuries in previous conflicts has advanced the practice of vascular surgery in military and urban trauma centers. Important differences in military wounding patterns offer a fresh opportunity to analyze recent trends on a modern military battlefield. The rate of vascular injury now seems higher than in past wars and may account for a greater percentage of the combat wounded. Surgeons must be prepared to handle the technical challenges of simultaneous vascular reconstruction and important tips are suggested. Technologic development in prehospital hemorrhage control, resuscitation, and a theater-wide trauma system have reduced the case fatality rate and evolved the practice of vascular surgery on the modern battlefield.

References

[1] DeBakey ME, Simeone MC. Battle injuries of the arteries in World War II: an analysis of 2,471 cases. Ann Surg 1946;123(4):534–79.
[2] Hughes CW. Acute vascular trauma in Korean War casualties; an analysis of 180 cases. Surg Gynecol Obstet 1954;99(1):91–100.
[3] Hughes CW. The primary repair of wounds of major arteries, an analysis of experience in Korea in 1953. Ann Surg 1955;141(3):297–303.
[4] Hughes CW. Arterial repair during the Korean war. Ann Surg 1958;147(4):555–61.
[5] Rich NM, Hughes CW. Vietnam vascular registry: a preliminary report. Surgery 1969;65(1): 218–26.
[6] Rich NM, Baugh JH, Hughes CW. Popliteal artery injuries in Vietnam. Am J Surg 1969; 118(4):531–4.
[7] Jahnke EJ Jr, Hughes CW, Howard JM. The rationale of arterial repair on the battlefield. Am J Surg 1954;87(3):396–401.
[8] Rich NM, Baugh JH, Hughes CW. Acute arterial injuries in Vietnam: 1,000 cases. J Trauma 1970;10(5):359–69.
[9] Gawande A. Casualties of war—military care for the wounded from Iraq and Afghanistan. N Engl J Med 2004;351(24):2471–5.
[10] Starnes BW, Beekley AC, Sebesta JA, et al. Extremity vascular injuries on the battlefield: tips for surgeons deploying to war. J Trauma 2006;60(2):432–42.
[11] Holcomb JB, McMullin NR, Pearse L, et al. Causes of death in US special operations forces in the global war on terrorism 2001–2004. Ann Surg 2007;(6):986–91.
[12] Wolf SE, Kauvar DS, Wade CE, et al. Comparison between civilian burns and combat burns from operation Iraqi freedom and operation enduring freedom. Ann Surg 2006;243(6): 786–92.
[13] Clouse WD, Rasmussen TE, Peck MA, et al. In-theater management of vascular injury: 2 years of the Balad vascular registry. J Am Coll Surg 2007;204(4):625–32.
[14] Fox CJ, Gillespie DL, O'Donnell SD, et al. Contemporary management of wartime vascular trauma. J Vasc Surg 2005;41(4):638–44.
[15] Rich NM. Vascular trauma in Vietnam. J Cardiovasc Surg (Torino) 1970;11(5):368–77.
[16] Jahnke EJ Jr, Howard JM. Primary repair of major arterial injuries; report of fifty-eight casualties. AMA Arch Surg 1953;66(5):646–9.
[17] Jahnke EJ Jr, Seeley SF. Acute vascular injuries in the Korean War. Ann Surg 1953;138(2): 158–77.

[18] Rich NM, Rhee P. An historical tour of vascular injury management: from its inception to the new millennium. Surg Clin North Am 2001;81(6):1199–215.

[19] Beekley AC, Watts DM. Combat trauma experience with the United States Army 102nd Forward Surgical Team in Afghanistan. Am J Surg 2004;187(5):652–4.

[20] Champion HR, Bellamy RF, Roberts CP, et al. A profile of combat injury. J Trauma 2003; 54(Suppl 5):S13–9.

[21] Porter JM, Ivatury RR, Nassoura ZE. Extending the horizons of "damage control" in unstable trauma patients beyond the abdomen and gastrointestinal tract. J Trauma 1997; 42(3):559–61.

[22] Rasmussen TE, Clouse WD, Jenkins DH, et al. Echelons of care and the management of wartime vascular injury: a report from the 332nd EMDG/Air Force Theater Hospital, Balad Air Base, Iraq. Perspect Vasc Surg Endovasc Ther 2006;18(2):91–9.

[23] Rasmussen TE, Clouse WD, Jenkins DH, et al. The use of temporary vascular shunts as a damage control adjunct in the management of wartime vascular injury. J Trauma 2006; 61(1):8–12.

[24] Alam HB, Koustova E, Rhee P. Combat casualty care research: from bench to the battlefield. World J Surg 2005;29(Suppl 1):S7–11.

[25] Alam HB, Burris D, DaCorta JA, et al. Hemorrhage control in the battlefield: role of new hemostatic agents. Mil Med 2005;170(1):63–9.

[26] Alam HB, Rhee P. New developments in fluid resuscitation. Surg Clin North Am 2007;87(1): 55–72, vi.

[27] Borgman MA, Spinella PC, Perkins J, et al. The ratio of blood products transfused affects mortality in patients receiving massive transfusions at a combat support hospital. J Trauma, in press.

[28] Eastridge BJ, Jenkins D, Flaherty S, et al. Trauma system development in a theater of war: experiences from operation Iraqi freedom and operation enduring freedom. J Trauma 2006; 61(6):1366–72.

[29] Gonzalez EA, Moore FA, Holcomb JB, et al. Fresh frozen plasma should be given earlier to patients requiring massive transfusion. J Trauma 2007;62(1):112–9.

[30] Hess JR, Holcomb JB, Hoyt DB. Damage control resuscitation: the need for specific blood products to treat the coagulopathy of trauma. Transfusion 2006;46(5):685–6.

[31] Holcomb JB, Champion HR. Military damage control. Arch Surg 2001;136(8):965–7.

[32] Holcomb JB. Methods for improved hemorrhage control. Crit Care 2004;8(Suppl 2):S57–60.

[33] Holcomb JB. Use of recombinant activated factor VII to treat the acquired coagulopathy of trauma. J Trauma 2005;58(6):1298–303.

[34] Holcomb JB, Jenkins D, Rhee P, et al. Damage control resuscitation: directly addressing the early coagulopathy of trauma. J Trauma 2007;62(2):307–10.

[35] Kauvar DS, Holcomb JB, Norris GC, et al. Fresh whole blood transfusion: a controversial military practice. J Trauma 2006;61(1):181–4.

[36] Mohr AM, Holcomb JB, Dutton RP, et al. Recombinant activated factor VIIa and hemostasis in critical care: a focus on trauma. Crit Care 2005;9(Suppl 5):S37–42.

[37] Perkins JG, Schreiber MA, Wade CE, et al. Early versus late recombinant factor VIIa in combat trauma patients requiring massive transfusion. J Trauma 2007;62(5): 1095–101.

[38] Welling DR, Burris DG, Hutton JE, et al. A balanced approach to tourniquet use: lessons learned and relearned. J Am Coll Surg 2006;203(1):106–15.

[39] Walters TJ, Wenke JC, Kauvar DS, et al. Effectiveness of self-applied tourniquets in human volunteers. Prehosp Emerg Care 2005;9(4):416–22.

[40] Walters TJ, Mabry RL. Issues related to the use of tourniquets on the battlefield. Mil Med 2005;170(9):770–5.

[41] Wenke JC, Walters TJ, Greydanus DJ, et al. Physiological evaluation of the U.S. Army one-handed tourniquet. Mil Med 2005;170(9):776–81.

[42] Beekley AC, Starnes BW, Sebesta JA. Lessons learned from modern military surgery. Surg Clin North Am 2007;87(1):157–84, vii.

[43] Sebesta J. Special lessons learned from Iraq. Surg Clin North Am 2006;86(3):711–26.

[44] Stone HH, Strom PR, Mullins RJ. Management of the major coagulopathy with onset during laparotomy. Ann Surg 1983;197(5):532–5.

[45] Feliciano DV, Mattox KL, Burch JM, et al. Packing for control of hepatic hemorrhage. J Trauma 1986;26(8):738–43.

[46] Kobayashi K. [Damage control surgery—a historical view]. Nippon Geka Gakkai Zasshi 2002;103(7):500–2 [in Japanese].

[47] Rotondo MF, Schwab CW, McGonigal MD, et al. 'Damage control': an approach for improved survival in exsanguinating penetrating abdominal injury. J Trauma 1993;35(3): 375–82.

[48] Aucar JA, Hirshberg A. Damage control for vascular injuries. Surg Clin North Am 1997; 77(4):853–62.

[49] Holcomb JB, Helling TS, Hirshberg A. Military, civilian, and rural application of the damage control philosophy. Mil Med 2001;166(6):490–3.

[50] Hirshberg A, Holcomb JB, Mattox KL. Hospital trauma care in multiple-casualty incidents: a critical view. Ann Emerg Med 2001;37(6):647–52.

[51] Damage control surgery. In: Burris D, Fitzharris JB, Holcomb JB, et al, editors. Emergency war surgery. Washington, DC: Borden Institute; 2004. p. 12.1–12.10.

[52] Brohi K, Singh J, Heron M, et al. Acute traumatic coagulopathy. J Trauma 2003;54(6): 1127–30.

[53] MacLeod JB, Lynn M, McKenney MG, et al. Early coagulopathy predicts mortality in trauma. J Trauma 2003;55(1):39–44.

[54] Fox CJ, Gillespie DL, Cox ED, et al. Damage control resuscitation for vascular surgery in a combat support hospital. Presented at the 37th Annual Meeting of the Western Trauma Association. Steamboat Springs (CO), March 2, 2007.

[55] Engstrom M, Schott U, Nordstrom CH, et al. Increased lactate levels impair the coagulation system—a potential contributing factor to progressive hemorrhage after traumatic brain injury. J Neurosurg Anesthesiol 2006;18(3):200–4.

[56] Nahas GG, Sutin KM, Fermon C, et al. Guidelines for the treatment of acidaemia with THAM. Drugs 1998;55(2):191–224.

[57] Dawson DL, Putnam AT, Light JT, et al. Temporary arterial shunts to maintain limb perfusion after arterial injury: an animal study. J Trauma 1999;47(1):64–71.

[58] Eger M, Golcman L, Goldstein A, et al. The use of a temporary shunt in the management of arterial vascular injuries. Surg Gynecol Obstet 1971;132(1):67–70.

[59] Starnes BW, Arthurs ZM. Endovascular management of vascular trauma. Perspect Vasc Surg Endovasc Ther 2006;18(2):114–29.

[60] Marin ML, Veith FJ, Panetta TF, et al. Transluminally placed endovascular stented graft repair for arterial trauma. J Vasc Surg 1994;20(3):466–72.

[61] Ohki T, Veith FJ, Marin ML, et al. Endovascular approaches for traumatic arterial lesions. Semin Vasc Surg 1997;10(4):272–85.

[62] Patel AV, Marin ML, Veith FJ, et al. Endovascular graft repair of penetrating subclavian artery injuries. J Endovasc Surg 1996;3(4):382–8.

[63] White R, Krajcer Z, Johnson M, et al. Results of a multicenter trial for the treatment of traumatic vascular injury with a covered stent. J Trauma 2006;60(6):1189–95.

[64] Lin PH, Bush RL, Zhou W, et al. Endovascular treatment of traumatic thoracic aortic injury—should this be the new standard of treatment? J Vasc Surg 2006;43(Suppl A):22A–9A.

[65] Rich NM, Hughes CW. The fate of prosthetic material used to repair vascular injuries in contaminated wounds. J Trauma 1972;12(6):459–67.

[66] Feliciano DV, Mattox KL, Graham JM, et al. Five-year experience with PTFE grafts in vascular wounds. J Trauma 1985;25(1):71–82.

[67] Vaughan GD, Mattox KL, Feliciano DV, et al. Surgical experience with expanded polytetra-fluoroethylene (PTFE) as a replacement graft for traumatized vessels. J Trauma 1979;19(6): 403–8.

[68] Martin TD, Mattox KL, Feliciano DV. Prosthetic grafts in vascular trauma: a controversy. Compr Ther 1985;11(2):41–5.

[69] Lin PH, Bush RL, Weiss VJ, et al. Subclavian artery disruption resulting from endovascular intervention: treatment options. J Vasc Surg 2000;32(3):607–11.

[70] Fox CJ, Gillespie DL, Weber MA, et al. Delayed evaluation of combat-related penetrating neck trauma. J Vasc Surg 2006;44(1):86–93.

[71] Holcomb JB, Salinas J, McManus JM, et al. Manual vital signs reliably predict need for life-saving interventions in trauma patients. J Trauma 2005;59(4):821–8.

[72] Davis JW, Shackford SR, Mackersie RC, et al. Base deficit as a guide to volume resuscitation. J Trauma 1988;28(10):1464–7.

[73] Eastridge BJ, Owsley J, Sebesta J, et al. Admission physiology criteria after injury on the battlefield predict medical resource utilization and patient mortality 5. J Trauma 2006;61(4): 820–3.

[74] Holcomb JB, Hoots K, Moore FA. Treatment of an acquired coagulopathy with recombinant activated factor VII in a damage-control patient. Mil Med 2005;170(4):287–90.

[75] Klemcke HG, Delgado A, Holcomb JB, et al. Effect of recombinant FVIIa in hypothermic, coagulopathic pigs with liver injuries. J Trauma 2005;59(1):155–61.

[76] McMullin NR, Kauvar DS, Currier HM, et al. The clinical and laboratory response to recombinant factor VIIA in trauma and surgical patients with acquired coagulopathy. Curr Surg 2006;63(4):246–51.

[77] Schreiber MA, Holcomb JB, Rojkjaer R. Preclinical trauma studies of recombinant factor VIIa. Crit Care 2005;9(Suppl 5):S25–8.

[78] White CE, Schrank AE, Baskin TW, et al. Effects of recombinant activated factor VII in traumatic nonsurgical intracranial hemorrhage. Curr Surg 2006;63(5):310–7.

[79] Johansen K, Daines M, Howey T, et al. Objective criteria accurately predict amputation following lower extremity trauma. J Trauma 1990;30(5):568–72.

[80] Walters TJ, Holcomb JB, Cancio LC, et al. Emergency tourniquets. J Am Coll Surg 2007; 204(1):185–6.

[81] Brigham RA, Eddleman WL, Clagett GP, et al. Isolated venous injury produced by penetrating trauma to the lower extremity. J Trauma 1983;23(3):255–7.

[82] Rich NM. Management of venous trauma. Surg Clin North Am 1988;68(4):809–21.

[83] Beekley AC. United States military surgical response to modern large-scale conflicts: the ongoing evolution of a trauma system. Surg Clin North Am 2006;86(3):689–709.

ELSEVIER
SAUNDERS

SURGICAL
CLINICS OF
NORTH AMERICA

Surg Clin N Am 87 (2007) 1213–1228

Successful Angioaccess

Niten Singh, MD[a],*, Benjamin W. Starnes, MD, FACS[b],
Charles Andersen, MD[a]

[a]Vascular and Endovascular Surgery Madigan Army Medical Center,
9040-A Fitzsimmons Avenue, Tacoma, WA 98431, USA
[b]Vascular and Endovascular Surgery, Harborview Medical Center,
University of Washington, Seattle, WA, USA

Surgery for hemodialysis (HD) access is the most commonly performed vascular surgical operation in the United States, predominantly because of a steady increase in the prevalence of end-stage renal disease (ESRD). Despite a concomitant increase in the mean age of these patients and more coexisting morbidities, advances in the management of renal failure and dialysis have allowed for a longer survival among patients on HD. The Achilles heel for these patients remains vascular access, however, with poor long-term patency rates resulting in multiple interventions for thrombosis and maintenance, and, in many patients, the eventual need for lifelong catheter placement. Access failure is the second leading cause of hospitalization among patients who have ESRD, and the annual cost of access maintenance is estimated to be $1 billion in the United States [1].

Multiple studies have confirmed the improved patency rate and lower infection rates for native arteriovenous fistulae (AVF) compared with prosthetic arteriovenous grafts (AVG). Although approximately 60% to 90% of nonautogenous grafts are functional at 1 year, the patency falls to 40% to 60% at 3 years [2]. Despite inferior patency rates, prosthetic grafts continue to be more common than native fistulae in the United States, accounting for 65% of all access procedures. In contrast, data from Canada and Europe demonstrate greater use of autogenous fistulae in those countries, with prosthetic grafts accounting for less than 35% of all access procedures in Canada and 10% in Europe [3].

In an effort to promote more standardized practice patterns and greater success with autogenous access placement, the National Kidney Foundation

* Corresponding author.
E-mail address: nhsingh@aol.com (N. Singh).

0039-6109/07/$ - see front matter. Published by Elsevier Inc.
doi:10.1016/j.suc.2007.08.004

introduced the Dialysis Outcome Quality Initiative (DOQI) [4]. In the past these guidelines set the goal of greater than 50% of all dialysis access being autogenous. The most recent recommendation is a prevalence of AVF of greater 65% by 2009 [5]. This performance metric is a goal that the Center for Medicare Services expects for reimbursement. Although it is a useful guideline, it does not take into account variations in patient populations. Many patients are not referred to a surgeon per DOQI guidelines when their creatinine clearance is less than 25 mL/min for access consideration before initiation of HD. Many patients present with a tunneled catheter in place that is malfunctioning and may not have time to wait for an autogenous access to mature. Usually it is between these two extremes that we, as surgeons, are asked to see these patients. Using a "fistula first" practice results in better long-term patency but must be tempered with the needs of the specific patient in question.

In formulating a strategy for successful dialysis access a comprehensive approach should be undertaken. This approach involves understanding this patient population and working with the nephrologist to create an environment that is beneficial to the patient. Surgeons who perform these procedures understand that the challenge is not the simple technical process of creating an AVF, but understanding the potential pitfalls that can be associated with access. The preoperative planning, as with any surgical procedure, is the most important aspect, followed by the postoperative maintenance of the access.

Preoperative strategy

The planning for HD access should ideally allow for adequate maturation time for an AVF, which is between 6 and 8 weeks (up to 12 weeks). This timing would optimize the use of autogenous access; however, this is often not possible and the patient requires access sooner. Every surgeon should adopt a standard algorithm for HD access. Our algorithm of access is as follows: nondominant upper extremity, the most distal site first, and autogenous access before prosthetic. Within every algorithm there exist variations. For example, women are more likely to undergo insertion of prosthetic grafts than men and have higher failure rates of AVF, which is likely a reflection of the larger caliber of superficial arm veins in men [6]. Maintaining a standard practice has been shown to increase the percentage of autogenous access, however [7].

History should include any prior access procedures or recent intravenous lines, particularly central lines, because subclavian lines are associated with an extremely high rate of stenosis [8]. Physical examination should focus on bilateral upper extremity blood pressure to detect a potential subclavian artery stenosis and palpation of the brachial and radial pulses. An Allen test should be performed to ensure there is adequate radial and ulnar flow to the hand (Fig. 1).

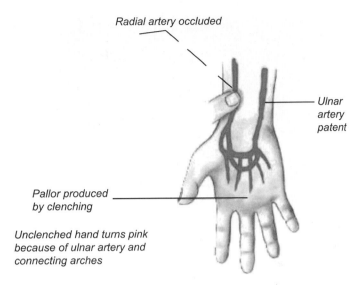

Radial artery occluded

Ulnar
artery
patent

Pallor produced
by clenching

Unclenched hand turns pink
because of ulnar artery and
connecting arches

Fig. 1. Allen test.

Ultrasound may be incorporated into preoperative planning, particularly for autogenous access placement. Duplex ultrasound (DU) has been used for preoperative planning in dialysis access, and studies have shown a proven benefit of ultrasound in predicting success in patients who have undergone a preoperative ultrasound [9]. Robbin and colleagues [10] noted an increase in autogenous arteriovenous access creation from 32% to 58% after a preoperative DU program was started. With preoperative ultrasonography, Silva and colleagues [11] were also able to demonstrate an increase in autogenous access placement from 14% to 63% and a decrease in failure of autogenous access from 38% to 8.3%. In that study, veins greater than 2.5 mm were required for autogenous access placement and greater than 4 mm for non-autogenous placement. Using the criteria of a 2-mm vein at the wrist and greater than 3 mm in the upper arm, Ascher and colleagues [12] reported a similar increase in autogenous access placement with preoperative DU.

Most preoperative ultrasound procedures can be performed in an office or vascular laboratory setting. The forearm venous network is superficial and easily imaged (Fig. 2). Superficial veins can be visualized longitudinally and in cross section. If these veins are compressible, greater than 2.5 mm, and patent throughout their course, then an autogenous access can likely be performed. Mendes and colleagues [13] studied the cephalic vein preoperatively with DU to determine whether a minimal cephalic vein size in the forearm could predict successful wrist autogenous access. They noted that patients who had a cephalic vein size of 2.0 mm or smaller were less likely to have a successful wrist autogenous access than if the cephalic vein was greater than 2.0 mm [13]. If the patient's history suggests previous central venous lines or arm swelling, the deep veins, such as the

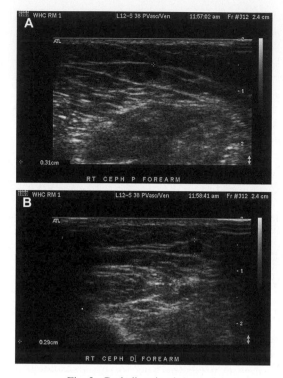

Fig. 2. Cephalic vein ultrasound.

axillary and distal subclavian, can also be interrogated (Fig. 3). The bony clavicle limits accurate assessment at the mid to proximal subclavian level. Color flow DU may also be used to assess the arterial inflow. Starting at the wrist the radial artery can be identified and followed proximally to the brachial artery. Using color flow in the longitudinal view, occlusive arterial disease can be identified. Unobstructed arterial inflow of 2.0 mm has been used as a predictor of success [14,15].

Arteriography and venography may be incorporated into the preoperative planning of patients. Iodinated contrast agents are nephrotoxic and carbon dioxide or gadolinium should be used instead in patients who have residual renal function. Arteriography is usually recommended in patients who have evidence of significant inflow disease as directed by physical examination or ultrasonography. If a short-segment subclavian stenosis is identified, it may be treated with angioplasty and stenting. Contrast venography should be incorporated in the preoperative planning in patients who have poor veins noted on duplex or if there is a history of prior central venous access, particularly in the subclavian vein [16,17].

After adequate preoperative planning the choice of access can be determined and can either be autogenous or prosthetic. Generally in our practice, when patients are referred relatively early we aggressively attempt

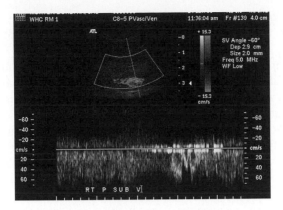

Fig. 3. Ultrasound of proximal subclavian vein.

autogenous access and attempt radiocephalic access with a smaller cephalic vein (ie, 1.6 mm). The reason for this is that it is a relatively benign procedure and potentially has the benefit of increasing the caliber of the more proximal veins if it does not mature itself.

Autogenous access

The first choice of autogenous access is the radial artery to cephalic vein fistula. First described in 1966, it is the most well-known autogenous access performed and is also referred to as the Brescia-Cimino fistula or the wrist fistula [18]. It is performed in various ways but the most common involves an end of the cephalic vein to the side of the radial artery. This procedure can be accomplished with one or two incisions. In general the vein is mobilized near the wrist, an adequate segment of the radial artery is identified, and the anastomosis is performed with 6-0 polypropylene suture in a running style (Fig. 4). This fistula is then given 6 to 8 weeks to mature before accessing it for HD. Many times this AVF is slow to mature because large tributaries in the forearm may shunt flow away from the cephalic vein.

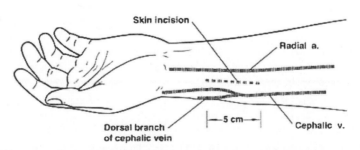

Fig. 4. Radiocephalic fistula.

Identification of these tributaries by physical examination, ultrasonography, or fistulogram and ligation usually allows the cephalic vein to subsequently mature.

Another variation of the Brescia-Cimino fistula is the "snuffbox" fistula [19]. It is an anastomosis between the distal cephalic vein and the thenar branch of the radial artery that can be found in the anatomic snuffbox of the hand (Fig. 5). It can generally be performed through one incision over the snuffbox and is the most distal autogenous fistula. It is an end of the cephalic vein to the side of the thenar branch of the radial artery anastomosis. It may require finer suture (7-0) because the vessels are smaller. This fistula affords the luxury of an extremely small incision and the potential of increasing the size of the more distal veins.

Another forearm autogenous access is the radial artery to forearm basilic vein transposition [20]. It involves an incision along the forearm portion of

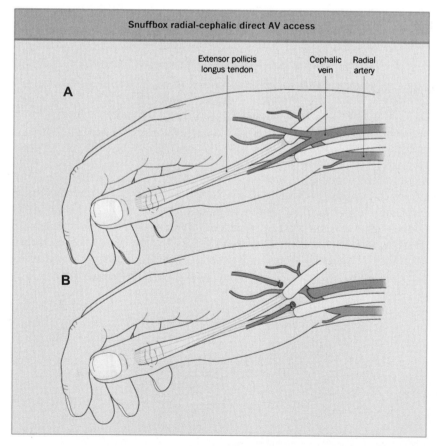

Fig. 5. Snuffbox fistula. (*From* Hallett JW Jr, Mills JL, Earnshaw JJ, et al, editors. Comprehensive vascular and endovascular surgery. St. Louis: Mosby; 2004; with permission.)

the basilic vein and mobilization toward the antecubital fossa. The radial artery is than exposed and a subcutaneous tunnel is created to allow the basilic vein to be transposed toward the proximal radial artery (Fig. 6). Using this fistula still preserves the upper arm access if it does not mature.

The brachial artery to cephalic vein fistula is the next higher-level autogenous fistula. It involves an anastomosis between the brachial artery and cephalic vein in the antecubital fossa. It is generally performed in an end of cephalic vein to side of brachial artery configuration. It has excellent flow

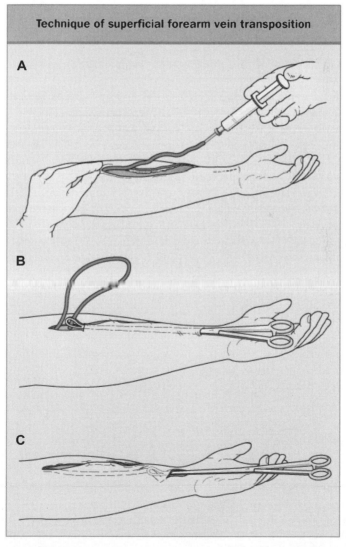

Fig. 6. Forearm basilic vein transposition. (*From* Hallett JW Jr, Mills JL, Earnshaw JJ, et al, editors. Comprehensive vascular and endovascular surgery. St. Louis: Mosby; 2004; with permission.)

and maturation rates but has been associated with higher rates of "steal" phenomenon [21]. It also eliminates the forearm for consideration of future access.

The brachial artery to basilic vein fistula is the last autogenous conduit in the upper arm. The operation is done under general anesthesia; it requires more extensive dissection because the basilic vein is deeper in the upper arm. The preoperatively marked basilic vein requires transposition to a more superficial location so it can be accessed. Results have varied with some reporting excellent patency and others reporting less favorable results [22,23].

Prosthetic access

AVGs are associated with poorer patency than an AVF; however, they do have the advantage of easier cannulation and a much shorter time to maturation requiring only 14 days before access can be achieved. Generally these grafts are made from expanded polytetrafluoroethylene (PTFE) and come in a variety of sizes. Most grafts are 6 mm but there are also tapered grafts with a 4-mm arterial end and a 7-mm venous end. The principle cause of failure in an AVG (80%) is neointimal hyperplasia at the venous anastomosis. Compared with AVF, however, the secondary patency rates may be higher because salvage procedures are more readily performed in prosthetic grafts.

The most distal forearm graft is the straight radial artery to cephalic or antecubital vein graft. Another forearm graft is the brachial to cephalic or basilic vein loop graft. These grafts are performed with end of graft to side of artery and vein anastomosis with 6-0 polypropylene sutures or CV6 Gore-Tex PTFE suture. Again these AVGs provide relatively simple access and may be used in the face of disadvantaged forearm veins (Figs. 7 and 8).

The next level of prosthetic is the brachial artery to axillary vein graft that provides the last level of access in the upper arm. It can be performed after a failed brachial-basilic AVF as long as the axillary vein is patent and it is an end of graft to side of artery and vein anastomosis. Other potential and less often used sites are the cross-chest axillary artery to axillary vein graft and lower extremity thigh loop grafts, which are not discussed here.

Complications

Failure of maturation of arteriovenous fistulae

AVFs may take up to 12 weeks to mature but in an access such as the radial-cephalic fistula the cause may be multiple tributaries of the cephalic vein that should be ligated. This ligation can be accomplished by identifying prominent vessels on physical examination, using duplex ultrasonography to mark these, or using fistulograms to identify and ligate these branches. Even if the radiocephalic AVF does not mature properly it may promote

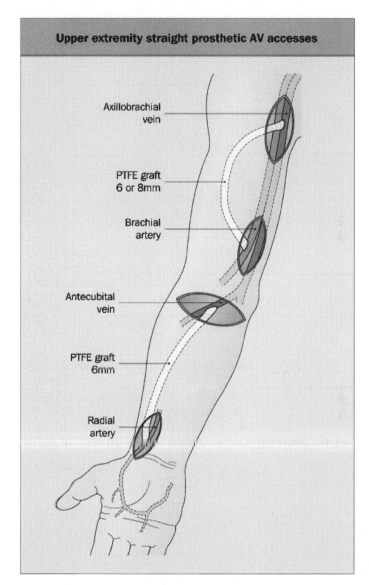

Fig. 7. Prosthetic straight arm grafts. (*From* Hallett JW Jr, Mills JL, Earnshaw JJ, et al, editors. Comprehensive vascular and endovascular surgery. St. Louis: Mosby; 2004; with permission.)

the enlargement of the more prominent veins to allow for a more durable proximal upper extremity fistula.

The failing or thrombosed access

Often a patient is referred back to the surgeon with a question of a poorly functioning AVF and AVG. Unlike AVGs, an AVF can remain patent with

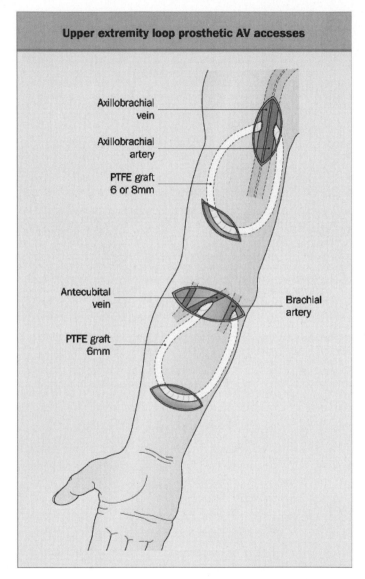

Upper extremity loop prosthetic AV accesses

Axillobrachial vein

Axillobrachial artery

PTFE graft 6 or 8mm

Antecubital vein

Brachial artery

PTFE graft 6mm

Fig. 8. Prosthetic loop grafts. (*From* Hallett JW Jr, Mills JL, Earnshaw JJ, et al, editors. Comprehensive vascular and endovascular surgery. St. Louis: Mosby; 2004; with permission.)

minimal flow, therefore Doppler or duplex interrogation of a suspected thrombosed AVF should be performed to confirm or exclude the diagnosis. High recirculation times, elevated venous pressures, and inability to achieve adequate urea clearance are signs of a venous outflow obstruction. The treatment of a thrombosed AVG has been described in several series and can range from endovascular thrombolysis to surgical thrombectomy with patch angioplasty of the venous outflow. Rescue of a failing or thrombosed AVF has been mixed with AVG studies but in general they are not as easily salvaged. These results are similar to a thrombosed autogenous lower extremity bypass [24,25].

Endovascular therapy involves assessing the venous outflow and dilating any stenosis noted along with a central venogram to rule out a central vein stenosis. One technique that is used for thrombosed AVGs is the "lyse and wait" technique. This technique involves cannulating the AVG with an 18-guage Angiocath and instilling 3 mg of tissue plasminogen factor (tPA) and 3000 units of heparin while compressing the arterial and venous ends of the graft. After waiting anywhere from 30 minutes to 2 hours a venogram is performed. Any outflow stenosis is angioplastied. Next a sheath, directed toward the arterial end, is placed and a Fogarty embolectomy catheter is used to dislodge the arterial plug. This technique is useful and can be repeated without having to perform surgical correction or revision and unidentified lesions can be found and treated from the venous outflow tract to the central veins [26].

Surgical thrombectomy is fairly standard with the incision placed over the venous outflow and the use of a Fogarty catheter to remove the arterial thrombus. The venous end then has a PTFE or Dacron patch placed. Completion venography should be performed to visualize the venous outflow and identify lesions that may require further treatment.

Venous hypertension

Mild arm swelling is a common finding in these patients; however, this can be a more devastating complication with some patients having severe swelling. This complication is usually the result of outflow vein or subclavian or central vein stenosis or occlusion. This problem can be treated by angioplasty of the central vein with good initial results; however, these are prone to recurrence and the need for reintervention [27]. If swelling is not controlled and the patient begins to have signs of venous ulceration, then ligation of the AVF or AVG is warranted.

Infection

AVGs are more prone to infection, particularly with *Staphylococcus aureus*. The very nature of a superficial graft, with repeated punctures in perhaps not the most sterile of environments, and the impaired immunity of these dialysis patients all play a role [28]. If a graft is suspected of infection without any signs of exposed graft than a trial of antibiotics should be initiated. If there is a tract or exposed graft then excision of this portion of the graft should be performed with removal of all of the unincorporated graft. If it is a short section, using another graft tunneled in a clean plane between the uninfected incorporated portions of the graft can be performed (Fig. 9) [29].

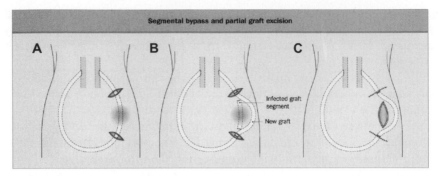

Fig. 9. Segmental excision and bypass of infected graft. (*From* Hallett JW Jr, Mills JL, Earnshaw JJ, et al, editors. Comprehensive vascular and endovascular surgery. St. Louis: Mosby; 2004; with permission.)

Pseudoaneurysm

Pseudoaneurysm (PSA) formation within an AVF does not necessarily imply infection, because repeated cannulation can cause this problem. A PSA of an AVG may be associated with infection because the scar tissue around the graft limits the formation of a PSA. If a PSA continues to enlarge and the overlying skin is threatened, it should be repaired. This repair can be done with segmental excision and bypass or with emerging endovascular techniques with a covered stent. There are case reports describing this technique and the results have been variable [30].

Steal

Creation of either an AVF or AVG may predispose a patient to ischemic steal symptoms. This phenomenon may manifest as cool digits or profound ischemic changes, such as tissue loss. A patient develops steal because of the reduced pressure just proximal to the fistula secondary to the large capacitance of the venous outflow and blood preferentially flowing in this direction. Generally this can be managed with a trial of observation if the symptoms are mild. To diagnose steal various techniques from physical examination to arteriography are required. If compression of the AVF results in restoration of a palpable radial pulse and resolution of symptoms, a confirmatory arteriogram to rule out an inflow stenosis or more distal native arterial stenosis is required. The brachial artery to cephalic vein fistula is the fistula most commonly associated with this complication. The treatment can involve revision of the anastomosis or operative banding, which has not been too successful. Another procedure that involves preservation of the access site is the distal revascularization with interval ligation (DRIL) procedure. Originally described by Shanzer and colleagues [31] it involves ligating the artery distal to the fistula and than constructing a bypass 3 to 5 cm above the AVF anastomosis (above the reduced pressure area) to the distal native artery (Fig. 10). The DRIL procedure is extremely effective

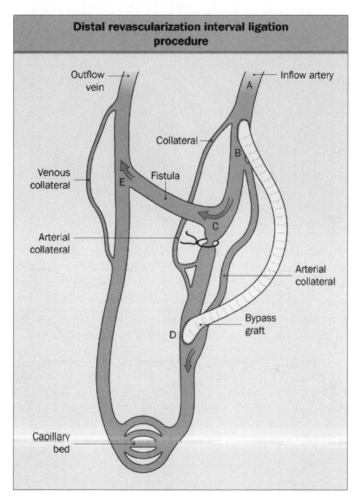

Fig. 10. DRIL procedure. (*From* Hallett JW Jr, Mills JL, Earnshaw JJ, et al, editors. Comprehensive vascular and endovascular surgery. St. Louis: Mosby; 2004; with permission.)

and should be used in patients who have a functioning native AVF and limited access availability. The decision to ligate an axial artery for preservation of a prosthetic fistula needs to be weighed carefully with consideration given to the lifespan of a prosthetic graft. Another technique is proximalization of the arterial anastomosis, which has recently been described with good results by Zanow and colleagues [32]. This technique involves dissecting the arterialized fistula vein near the AVF anastomosis and ligating and dividing it. The inflow artery (more proximal brachial or axillary artery) is then dissected and a 4-mm expanded PTFE graft is used between this artery and the efferent vein to construct a bypass (Fig. 11). In their series 84% of access-related ischemic symptoms resolved. The increasing use of endovascular procedures has led to novel approaches to difficulties with HD access. Recently

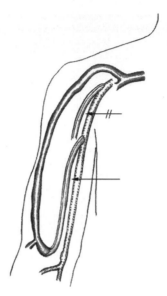

Fig. 11. Proximalization of arterial inflow. Arterial anastomosis divided and a tapered graft placed between the more proximal axillary artery and outflow (cephalic) vein. (*From* Zanow J, Kruger U, Scholz H. Proximalization of the arterial inflow: a new technique to treat access-related ischemia. J Vasc Surg 2006;43:1217; with permission.)

steal has been managed using minimally invasive techniques whereby the venous end of the AV anastomosis is accessed with a wire and a 4-mm angioplasty balloon inflated. A small incision is made over the vein and a single Prolene suture tied around the vein with the balloon inflated. The vein is thus banded with exacting fashion to relieve steal. With this technique, the authors have noted a 94% technical success rate for treating patients who have steal, thus avoiding an extensive DRIL procedure [33].

Summary

Creating effective dialysis access requires a comprehensive plan formulated between the nephrologist, the surgeon, and the patient. In this setting, HD access is the patient's lifeline and maintaining it requires a plan to deal with the aforementioned complications and sometimes low patency rates. To optimize success, the most important aspect, as with any other surgical procedure, is the preoperative planning. Understanding and dealing with the potential complications allows the surgeon the ability to optimize the practice of HD access.

References

[1] United States Renal Data System. The economic cost of ESRD, vascular access procedures, and Medicare spending for alternative modalities of treatment. Am J Kidney Dis 1997;30: S160–77.

[2] Schwab S, Harrington J, Singh A, et al. Vascular access for hemodialysis. Kidney Int 1999; 55:2078–90.

[3] Dixon BS, Novak L, Fangman J. Hemodialysis vascular access survival: upper-arm native arteriovenous fistula. Am J Kidney Dis 2002;39:92–101.

[4] NKF-K/DOQI clinical practical guidelines for vascular access: update 2000. Am J Kidney Dis 2001;29:223–9.

[5] NKF-K/DOQI clinical practical guidelines for vascular access: update 2006. Am J Kidney Dis 2006;48(Suppl 1):S258–63.

[6] Ifudu O, Macey LJ, Homel P, et al. Determinants of type of initial hemodialysis vascular access. Am J Nephrol 1997;17:425–7.

[7] Kalman PG, Pope M, Bhola C, et al. A pratical approach to vascular access for hemodialysis and predictors of success. J Vasc Surg 1999;30:727–33.

[8] Spinowitz BS, Galler M, Golden RA, et al. Subclavian vein stenosis as a complication of subclavian vein catheterization for hemodialysis. Arch Intern Med 1987;147:305–7.

[9] Koskoy C, Kuzu A, Erden I. Predictive value of color Doppler ultrasonography in detecting failure of vascular access grafts. Br J Surg 1995;82:50–2.

[10] Robbin ML, Gallichio MH, Deierhoi MH, et al. US vascular mapping before hemodialysis placement. Radiology 2000;217:83–8.

[11] Silva MB, Hobson RW, Pappas PJ, et al. A strategy for increasing the use of autogenous hemodialysis access procedures: impact of preoperative noninvasive evaluation. J Vasc Surg 1998;27:302–8.

[12] Ascher E, Gade P, Hingorani A, et al. Changes in the practice of angioaccess surgery: impact of the dialysis outcome and quality initiative recommendations. J Vasc Surg 2000;31:84–92.

[13] Mendes RR, Farber MA, Marston WA, et al. Prediction of wrist arteriovenous fistula maturation with preoperative vein mapping with ultrasonography. J Vasc Surg 2002;36:460–3.

[14] Parmley MC, Broughan TA, Jennings WC. Vascular ultrasonography prior to dialysis access surgery. Am J Surg 2002;184:568–72.

[15] Malovrh M. The role of sonography in the planning of arteriovenous fistulas for hemodialysis. Semin Dial 2003;16:299–303.

[16] Tordoir JH, de Bruin HG, Hoeneveld H, et al. Duplex ultrasound scanning in the assessment of arteriovenous fistulas created for hemodialysis access: comparison with digital subtraction angiography. J Vasc Surg 1989;10:122–8.

[17] Glanz S, Bashft B, Gordon DH, et al. Axillary and subclavian vein stenosis: percutaneous angioplasty. Radiology 1988;168:371–3.

[18] Brescia M, Cimino J, Appel K, et al. Chronic hemodialysis using venipuncture and surgically created arteriovenous fistula. N Engl J Med 1966;275:1089–92.

[19] Wolowczyk L, Williams AJ, Donovan KL, et al. The snuffbox arteriovenous fistula for vascular access. Eur J Vasc Endovasc Surg 2000;19:70–6.

[20] Silva MB, Hobson RW, Pappas PJ, et al. Vein transposition in the forearm for autogenous hemodialysis access. J Vasc Surg 1997;26:981–8.

[21] Sparks SR, Vanderlinden JL, Gnanadev DA, et al. Superior patency of perforating antecubital vein arteriovenous fistulae for hemodialysis. Ann Vasc Surg 1997;11:165–7.

[22] Coburn MC, Carney WI. Comparison of basilic vein and polytetrafluoroethylene for brachial arteriovenous fistula. J Vasc Surg 1994;20:896–902.

[23] Taghizadeh A, Dasgupta P, Khan MS, et al. Long-term outcomes of brachiobasilic transposition fistula for haemodialysis. Eur J Vasc Endovasc Surg 2003;26:670–2.

[24] Lay JP, Ashleigh RJ, Tranconi L, et al. Results of angioplasty of Brescia-Cimino haemodialysis fistulae: medium term follow-up. Clin Radiol 1998;53:608–11.

[25] Safa AA, Vaji K, Roberts A, et al. Detection and treatment of dysfunctional hemodialysis access grafts: effects of surveillance program on graft patency and the incidence of thrombosis. Radiology 1996;199:653–7.

[26] Cynamon J, Lakritz P, Wahl S, et al. Hemodialysis graft declotting: description of the "lyse and wait" technique. J Vasc Interv Radiol 1997;8:825–9.

[27] Lumsden AB, MacDonald MJ, Isiklar H, et al. Central venous stenosis in the hemodialysis patient: incidence and efficacy of endovascular treatment. Cardiovasc Surg 1997;5:504–9.

[28] Tokars JI, Light P, Anderson J, et al. A prospective study of vascular access infections at seven outpatient hemodialysis centers. Am J Kidney Dis 2001;37:1232–40.

[29] Schwab DP, Taylor SM, Cull DL, et al. Isolated arteriovenous dialysis access graft segment infection: the results of segmental bypass and partial graft excision. Ann Vasc Surg 2000;14: 63–6.

[30] Ryan JM. Using a covered stent (Wallgraft) to treat pseudoaneurysms of dialysis grafts and fistulas. Am J Radiol 2002;180:1067–71.

[31] Schanzer H, Skadany M, Haimov M. Treatment of angioaccess-induced ischemia by revascularization. J Vasc Surg 1992;16:861–6.

[32] Zanow J, Kruger U, Scholz H. Proximalization of the arterial inflow: a new technique to treat access-related ischemia. J Vasc Surg 2006;43:1216–21.

[33] Riley JT, Miller GA, Wu T, et al. Minimally invasive limited ligation endoluminal revision (MILLER) of arteriovenous fistulas to correct steal syndrome: results and clinical outcomes at one year. Presented at the 2007 Vascular Annual Meeting, Society for Vascular Surgery. Baltimore, MD, June 10, 2007.

ELSEVIER
SAUNDERS

SURGICAL
CLINICS OF
NORTH AMERICA

Surg Clin N Am 87 (2007) 1229–1252

Vena Cava Filters in Surgery and Trauma

LTC Matthew J. Martin, MD, FACS[a,b,*],
Ali Salim, MD, FACS[c,d]

[a]Uniformed Services University of Health Sciences, Bethesda, MD, USA
[b]Department of Surgery, Madigan Army Medical Center,
9040-A Fitzsimmons Avenue, Tacoma, WA 98431, USA
[c]Division of Trauma and Surgical Critical Care, University of Southern California Keck
School of Medicine, 1200 North State Street, Suite 9900, Los Angeles, CA 90017, USA
[d]Los Angeles County Hospital + USC Medical Center, Los Angeles, CA, USA

The concept of interrupting flow in the inferior vena cava (IVC) to prevent pulmonary embolism (PE) has been around since the nineteenth century. Bilateral common femoral vein ligation was suggested as a specific treatment for prevention of recurrent PE in the 1930s and 1940s; however, an unacceptably high incidence of recurrent PE as well as significant lower extremity venous stasis sequelae resulted in abandonment of the procedure. The next approach was ligation of the inferior vena cava. This provided theoretical control of the final common path to the pulmonary circulation for most emboli, and was commonly performed until the late 1960s. The sudden reduction in cardiac output resulted in a high postoperative mortality [1]. In addition, recurrent PE from dilated collateral veins and the venous stasis sequelae were unacceptable outcomes that prompted alternative methods to reduce the risk of PE without causing complete venous occlusion. A variety of surgical methods involving either suture and staple plication or external clips were developed to compartmentalize the vena cava. These techniques provided partial IVC interruption, allowing flow of liquid blood but trapping large emboli. Despite promising early patency rates, high rates of IVC occlusion were noted after brief follow-up [2]. In addition, these techniques required general anesthesia and laparotomy.

The views expressed in this article are those of the authors and do not reflect the official policy of the Department of the Army, the Department of Defense, or the US Government.
* Corresponding author. Department of Surgery, Madigan Army Medical Center, 9040-A Fitzsimmons Avenue, Tacoma, WA 98431.
E-mail address: matthew.martin1@amedd.army.mil (M.J. Martin).

0039-6109/07/$ - see front matter. Published by Elsevier Inc.
doi:10.1016/j.suc.2007.07.008

The next logical step was the development of transvenous approaches with the use of local anesthesia. The first true intravascular device was the Mobin-Uddin umbrella, introduced in 1967 [3]. It was a silicone membrane with small holes allowing for blood flow. It was associated with a high rate of vena caval thrombosis and was subsequently discontinued in 1986. Since then a new generation of devices have been developed that provide the ideal properties for a filter: ease of deployment, clot-trapping effectiveness, and preservation of IVC flow.

Vena cava filters available

Currently, there are two classes of vena cava filters (VCF) in use: permanent and retrievable. Retrievable IVC filters presumably offer the same protection from PE as permanent filters, whereas subsequent retrieval potentially eliminates the long-term complications. For this reason a large number of filters placed today are retrievable. In a multicenter trial coordinated through the American Association for the Surgery of Trauma (AAST), 79% of all filters placed at 21 participating institutions were retrievable [4]. Box 1 lists the current filters approved by the United States Food and Drug Administration. Although each filter design has its device-specific advantages and disadvantages, all filters appear to have roughly comparable effectiveness and overall complication rates.

Indications for vena cava filter placement

The indications and patient selection criteria for VCF placement remain the most controversial and widely debated topics surrounding this

---

Box 1. Currently available vena cava filters

Permanent
Stainless steel Greenfield filter (BostonScientific/Meditech, Boston, Massachusetts)
Titanium Greenfield filter (BostonScientific/Meditech)
Bird's Nest (Cook, Bloomington, Indiana)
Nitinol (Bard, Covington, Georgia)
Vena Tech (B. Braun, Boulogne, France)
TrapEase (Cordis, Europa N.V., L.J. Roden, the Netherlands)
Bard nonrecovery (Bard Peripheral Vascular, Tempe, Arizona)

Retrievable
Günter Tulip (Cook)
Recovery (Bard Peripheral Vascular)
OptEase (Cordis Endovascular, Miami Lakes, Florida)

technology [5–10]. The paucity of prospective controlled trials available for analysis has resulted in the promulgation of a variety of guidelines based on individual interpretation of uncontrolled prospective and retrospective series, literature reviews, consensus panel guidelines, and expert opinion. Without solid data to support a strong evidence-based approach to filter use, the decision to place a VCF is often driven more by individual practice patterns and preferences than actual patient disease and clinical factors.

The one available prospective randomized trial analyzed the utility of VCF in patients who had documented lower extremity deep vein thrombosis (DVT) and no contraindication to anticoagulation [11]. There was a statistically significant decrease in early PE (within 12 days) in the filter group (1.1%) compared with the no filter group (4.8%), but the filter group demonstrated a significant increase in DVT (odds ratio 1.87) that persisted at long-term follow-up [12] and no mortality benefit. From this trial it appears that VCF placement has little value in the average patient who has DVT and who can be safely anticoagulated. There currently exist no other prospective randomized trials to evaluate the multiple other suggested indications for VCF placement.

Current indications for VCF placement can be divided into two broad categories based on the clinical situation: preventive and prophylactic. Preventive indications include medical or surgical patients who have proven venous thromboembolic disease who are now at risk for pulmonary embolism or who have had a documented pulmonary embolism. These have become the most widely accepted and used indications for VCF placement in the United States and worldwide. The goal of VCF placement in this cohort is prevention of an initial clot embolization (known DVT) or additional clot embolizations (known PE). Prophylactic indications involve VCF placement in patients who have no documented DVT or PE, but who are assumed to be at increased risk for the development of venous thromboembolic disease. This scenario is almost universally encountered and reported with surgical and trauma patients, and rarely described or analyzed in medical patients. The creation of these indications has revolved around identifying a set of criteria that reliably predict which patients are at "high risk" of developing a DVT and PE despite standard preventive measures. The utility of VCF placement in this population will thus be highly dependent on the sensitivity and specificity of the criteria used as indications. Other factors that must be taken in to consideration when developing indications for VCF placement are the patient population, presence of any contraindications to standard preventive measures (anticoagulation, compressive devices), the degree and expected duration of disease and immobility, and the ability of the patient to tolerate any adverse pulmonary events ("pulmonary reserve function").

Consensus guidelines

A variety of expert opinion and consensus conference guidelines are available to aid in the decision of whether or not to proceed with VCF placement, although very few of these have focused specifically on surgical and trauma patients [13–20]. Table 1 shows current recommendations from a variety of expert groups and consensus committees. Although the recommendations and supporting evidence vary widely among groups, a common theme is the cited lack of adequate prospective and controlled data to make evidence-based decisions regarding placement of a vena caval filter in all situations. The only Level I recommendation identified is that VCF is not indicated in the patient who has venous thromboembolic disease and who can be anticoagulated [13]. The majority of groups agree that venous thromboembolic disease in the patient who cannot be anticoagulated, has a significant anticoagulation-related complication, or fails anticoagulation are acceptable reasons to consider VCF placement (all Level III recommendations). In the two guidelines focusing solely on trauma patients, no firm conclusions could be drawn, but they advised that VCF should be "considered" only in high-risk trauma patients, especially those who have a contraindication to standard prophylactic dose anticoagulation [17,19,20]. Again, these were noted to be Level III recommendations that are not supported by strong scientific data. Only one guideline addressed cancer patients who have DVT or PE and recommended against routine use of VCF unless another indication was present [13].

Table 2 provides a list of the most commonly cited indications for vena cava filter placement, divided into a small list of widely accepted indications and a longer list of indications that are considered relative or controversial. The remainder of this article focuses on the particular scenarios that are most likely to be encountered by the practicing surgeon.

Trauma

Multiple series have examined the role of prophylactic vena caval filter placement in the "high-risk" trauma patient [4,10,21–31]. These series vary widely in their definitions of "high-risk criteria," as well as patient demographics, indications for placement, type of filter, length of follow up, and methods for determining rates of complications, DVT, and PE. Trauma patients remain one of the highest risk groups for development of venous thromboembolism (VTE), with a reported incidence of DVT as high as 50% and of PE as high as 32% [17,20]. Prolonged immobility, venous stasis and injury, a proinflammatory hypercoagulable state, and the high risk of bleeding all contribute to the increased risk of VTE and the overall poor results with standard thromboprophylaxis seen in severely injured trauma patients [32–36]. This lack of effective VTE prophylaxis options was emphasized in the 2002 Eastern Association for the Surgery of Trauma (EAST) guidelines, with no Level I recommendations for preventing DVT or PE in trauma patients identified [17].

Multiple independent risk factors for VTE in trauma patients have been described, including advanced age, high Injury Severity Score, head injury,

Table 1
Consensus and expert panel reports and recommendations for vena caval filter use

Group	Indications	Recommendations	Level or grade
American College of Physicians & American Academy of Family Physicians	DVT or PE	Insufficient evidence to make recommendations	N/A
British Committee for Standards in Haematology	VTE + contraindication to anticoagulation VTE + anticoagulated PE + anticoagulant failure Free floating thrombus	VCF indicated VCF not indicated Consider VCF only if other options not available VCF not indicated	III (Grade B) IB (Grade A) IV (Grade C) III (Grade B)
American College of Chest Physicians, Consensus Committee on Pulmonary Embolism	DVT or PE in cancer patients	VCF not indicated unless contraindication to anticoagulation	III
American College of Chest Physicians, Consensus Conference on Antithrombotic and Thrombolytic Therapy	DVT + anticoagulation DVT + contraindication to anticoagulation Recurrent VTE + anticoagulation PE + contraindication to anticoagulation	VCF not indicated VCF indicated VCF indicated VCF indicated	IA 2C 2C 2C
International Consensus Conference on Thrombosis	Identical to ACCP Consensus Conference recommendations	See above	See above
Eastern Association for the Surgery of Trauma, Practice Management Guidelines for the Prevention of VTE in Trauma Patients	High-risk trauma patients: contraindication to anticoagulation + injury pattern including: severe head injury spinal cord injury pelvic + long bone multiple long bone	Consider VCF placement	III
Southern California Evidence-Based Practice Center Meta-analysis	Trauma patients (excluding burn, pregnant, and low mechanism elderly) Consider in high-risk group (elderly, spine fractures, spinal cord injury)	No firm conclusions drawn about VCF	III

Abbreviations: ACCP, American College of Chest Physicians; VTE, venous thromboembolism.

Table 2
Accepted and relative indications for vena caval filter placement in surgical patients

Accepted indications	Relative and controversial indications
Known VTE with contraindication to anticoagulation	Known VTE without contraindication to anticoagulation
Known VTE with severe complication of anticoagulation	High-risk trauma:
	severe head injury
Recurrent PE while on therapeutic anticoagulation	spinal cord injury
	vertebral fracture
Progression of DVT while on therapeutic anticoagulation	pelvic and long bone fractures
	prolonged immobility
Recent VTE and operative procedure requiring prolonged withholding of anticoagulation	venous repair
	High risk bariatric patient:
	BMI >50 (superobese)
	elderly
	venous stasis disease
	obesity hypoventilation/sleep apnea
	pulmonary hypertension
	Malignancy
	Free-floating thrombus
	Thrombolysis of DVT
	Known VTE with poor cardiopulmonary reserve
	Chronic thromboembolic pulmonary hypertension
	Hypercoagulable state

Abbreviation: BMI, body mass index.

spinal cord or vertebral injury, pelvic and long bone fractures, venous injury, and multiple transfusions [22,37–40]; however, on careful meta-analysis of available data it appears that only spinal cord and vertebral column injuries are strong independent predictors (Level I recommendation) of VTE, whereas other described risk factors are of marginal or questionable value for reliably identifying a truly high-risk patient who could benefit from VCF placement [17,19,20].

In a 1997 practice pattern survey of 210 United States trauma surgeons (87% from Level I trauma centers) there was overwhelming agreement for vena caval filter placement only in the setting of the traditional indications such as PE while therapeutically anticoagulated (93% agreed) and DVT with a contraindication to anticoagulation (89% agreed) [41]. For all other indications, including standard high-risk trauma criteria, agreement was 50% or less; however, there was a statistically significant trend toward increased filter use for 9 out of 10 relative indications when given the option of choosing a removable VCF. This study also revealed the wide range of VCF use, with 61% of centers inserting 0 to one filters per month, and 13% inserting more than four filters per month. In a subsequent analysis of the National Trauma Data Bank and a survey of 131 participating trauma centers, 86% of VCF appeared to have been placed for prophylactic indications, and 12% were placed in patients who had no identifiable VTE risk factors [37]. Among survey respondents, only 16% stated they would place a VCF for prophylactic indications, with the majority using mechanical compression devices only.

Surgical oncology

Patients who have active malignant disease have long been recognized as a high-risk population for developing venous thromboembolic disease and complications [42–45]. This increased risk can be attributed to various combinations of the prothrombotic state induced by malignant disease, venous stasis caused by mass effect of solid tumors, and the frequent presence of other risk factors (ie, age, immobility) seen in this patient population [46–48]. Aggressive mechanical and chemical prophylaxis is warranted in hospitalized cancer patients, particularly in those who have the added risk of undergoing a surgical procedure. The surgeon must consider not only the factors described for other patient populations, but also must take into account the nature and severity of the malignant process, quality of life, and the estimated duration of survival.

Among cancer patients who have diagnosed VTE, treatment failures and VTE recurrence can be seen in 10% to 20% of cases despite standard anticoagulation therapy, and appear to be significantly higher with oral therapy (warfarin) compared with low molecular weight heparins [49,50]. This has resulted in some authors including malignancy as an indication for VCF placement in patients undergoing major surgical procedures [51–54]. Several series have questioned the validity of malignancy as an indication for VCF placement [49,55–57], however, with one series demonstrating a doubling of the mortality among cancer patients undergoing VCF placement [58]. There remains no consensus opinion or prospective validation data on the use of malignancy as an independent indication for VCF placement.

Bariatrics

With the rapidly spreading "obesity epidemic" and explosion in bariatric surgical procedures worldwide, there has been increasing awareness and debate concerning prevention and management of VTE in the obese surgical patient [40,59–62]. Multiple studies have found obesity to be a strong independent risk factor for the development of DVT, as well as fatal and nonfatal PE. In a prospective study of over 100,000 females, obesity (BMI > 29 kg/m^2) was found to be one of the strongest independent risk factors for PE, with an adjusted relative risk of 2.9 [63]. This risk, combined with the added risk of surgery and difficulties in proper dosing of chemoprophylaxis in obese patients, makes them particularly susceptible to VTE-related morbidity and mortality [64–67].

Efforts to combat the high rate of DVT and PE in this patient population have led some authors to recommend routine preoperative prophylactic IVC filter placement for select patients undergoing bariatric surgery [68]. In one retrospective review of 3861 bariatric procedures there was a low overall incidence of PE identified (0.85%), but mortality in this group was 27%. A prophylactic VCF was used in 145 of these patients, with three postoperative PEs identified (2.1%) in the filter group. Despite this, the study authors' conclusions recommend VCF use in patients who are superobese and who have limited mobility. Ferrell and colleagues [62] retrospectively analyzed 586 patients undergoing gastric bypass and identified 12 who had a VCF placed; 6 of these were prophylactic and 6 were placed for postoperative complications. Despite the identified "technical challenges" of VCF placement in these patients, there were no long-term complications identified, and the study authors recommend VCF placement for patients who have elevated VTE risk factors or patients who have prolonged immobility and ICU stay caused by complications. In another study of 5554 bariatric operations, risk factors for postoperative VTE were identified and recommended as indications for VCF [61]. These included venous stasis disease, body mass index of 60 or greater, truncal obesity, and obesity hypoventilation syndrome. Several recent retrospective studies using similar "high-risk" criteria for patients undergoing bariatric surgery have demonstrated a high technical success rate and a significantly decreased incidence of PE with VCF placement [69,70], with one series demonstrating a 0% rate of PE in patients who received a prophylactic VCF [70].

Contraindication to anticoagulation

One of the most frequently cited reasons for considering or placing a VCF in the surgical patient population is a contraindication to anticoagulation [4,37,41]. In the trauma population this is most commonly secondary to injuries that are high risk for bleeding, such as intracranial hemorrhage, solid organ injuries, or severe pelvic and extremity fractures [71]. In other surgical populations there is often fear of an increased risk of bleeding complications with anticoagulants or the anticipated need to hold anticoagulation for prolonged periods around the time of operation. Although these are certainly valid concerns in many patients, it is the authors' experience that these decisions are often made based on an exaggerated estimate of the bleeding risk associated with pharmacologic anticoagulants, especially when considering prophylactic dose regimens. Prophylactic dose unfractionated heparin and low molecular weight heparins have both been demonstrated to be safe and effective in patients undergoing surgery for cancer, orthopedic surgery, polytrauma, and neurosurgery/neurotrauma, and can usually be started within 24 to 48 hours of injury or surgery [72–77]. Even among patients who have intracranial hemorrhage or solid organ injury being managed nonoperatively, prophylactic dose anticoagulation can usually be safely started after an initial observation period and with no signs of ongoing hemorrhage [72,74,76,78]. In these patients the authors recommend consideration of chemical prophylaxis rather than proceeding directly to prophylactic vena cava filter placement.

Vena cava filter placement techniques

With the increasing use and expanded indications for vena cava filter placement in many centers, the techniques of filter placement and the personnel placing them have undergone significant evolution. Once purely the purvey of interventional radiologists or vascular specialists, vena cava filters are now being placed by a variety of other specialists, including general surgeons and surgical subspecialists, medical internists, and critical care physicians [37,41]. The requirement for specialized personnel and equipment had previously required transfer of the patient to another area of the hospital, which consumes valuable hospital resources and can be hazardous with a critically ill patient. More recently, many series have reported excellent results and significant cost savings with bedside placement of vena cava filters [79–87].

Peripheral venous access and insertion is most commonly obtained via the femoral or internal jugular vein, although antecubital insertion is an option for several filter types [48]. Imaging of the vena cava must then be performed to assess the size and patency of the vena cava, as well as to identify the proper site for filter placement (most commonly below the renal veins) and rule out any anatomic abnormalities such as a duplicated vena cava. This is most commonly done with standard intravenous contrast venography and fluoroscopy. An alternative technique using carbon dioxide as a contrast agent has been described, and may be a promising approach in patients who have contrast allergy or are at risk for contrast induced nepropathy [88–90]. Other recent series have described the use of both transabdominal and intravascular ultrasound (IVUS) to size the vena cava, guide placement, and confirm proper filter positioning [79,80,82,91,92]. One study demonstrated that IVUS was significantly more accurate than contrast venography for the critical steps of sizing the vena cava and determining the optimal site for filter placement, with contrast venography resulting in inaccurate placement and significant overestimation of IVC diameter [93].

Although the ideal and preferred position for VCF placement is in the infrarenal IVC, in cases of anatomic abnormality or proximal thrombus extension, alternative sites must be considered. Placement in the suprarenal vena cava has been analyzed in several series, with outcome measures and rates of migration and caval thrombosis that compare with those with infrarenal positioning [94–96]; however, one should carefully observe these patients for the severe and potentially fatal complication of renal vein thrombosis [97]. Several series have also described placement of VCF in the superior vena cava, typically in the setting of acute upper extremity venous thrombosis and either contraindication to anticoagulation or other high-risk criteria [98–102]. These studies are limited by study quality and relatively small numbers, but generally report low complication rates with high technical success. Complications such as erosion into adjacent structures, superior vena caval thrombosis, migration, and guide wire entrapment are well-described, however, and should be appreciated when considering this option [102–105].

Retrievable filters

Concerns about the permanent nature and long-term complication profile noted with standard vena cava filter designs has led to alterations in filter design that allow for filter removal at a variable time period after placement. Several filter designs are currently available that allow for removal via either the jugular or femoral vein, with technical success rates of 78% to 100% [48,106]. Although initially designed for removal within several weeks of placement, successful delayed removal of many of these filters have been described at time periods of up to 1 year or greater postimplantation [106–108]. These filters may represent a particularly attractive option in the patient who is expected to have only a temporary period of high risk or contraindication to anticoagulation, or for protection during thrombolytic therapy for an established DVT.

Results of vena cava filter placement

Clinical outcomes and results following VCF placement will be highly dependent on multiple factors, such as the patient population, indication for placement, technique of placement, filter type and location, use of concurrent anticoagulation, and the nature and intensity of surveillance and follow-up. Although it is a commonly held misconception that vena cava filters are completely protective for PE, this has not been borne out by clinical experience. There is no question that patients who have vena cava filters remain at risk for PE [5,14,15,109]; the only debate is whether there is a significant benefit in terms of PE reduction with filters, and whether this benefit outweighs the risks of placement. The main outcomes that should be assessed to determine if there exist any benefits of VCF are mortality and the incidence of initial or recurrent pulmonary embolism after filter placement.

Table 3 shows the incidence of recurrent symptomatic PE and several defined complications for a variety of vena cava filters. The majority of studies demonstrate an incidence of symptomatic PE in 2% to 4% of VCF patients, whereas the incidence of asymptomatic PE remains unknown but is undoubtedly higher. The prospective randomized trial by Decousus and colleagues [11] demonstrated a recurrent PE rate of 3.4% and 21.6%

Table 3
Summary of comparison data for Food and Drug Administration-approved inferior vena cava filters

Filter	N	F/U (months)	Recurrent PE	DVT	IVC thromboses	Postphlebitic syndrome
Stainless-steel Greenfield	3184	18 (1–60)	2.6% (0%–9%)	5.9% (0%–18%)	3.6% (0%–18%)	19% (0%–47%)
Titanium-Greenfield	511	5.8 (0–81)	3.1% (0%–3.8%)	22.7% (0%–36%)	6.5% (1%–31%)	14.4% (9%–20%)
Bird's Nest	1426	14.2 (0–60)	2.9% (0%–4.2%)	6% (0%–20%)	3.9% (0%–15%)	14% (4%–41%)
Simon Nitinol	319	16.9 (0–62)	3.8% (0%–5.3%)	8.9% (8%–11%)	7.7% (4%–18%)	12.9% (6%–44%)
Vena-Tech	1050	12 (0–81)	3.4% (0%–8%)	32% (0%–32%)	11.2% (0%–28%)	41% (24%–59%)
Stainless-steel over-the-wire Greenfield	599	26	2.6%	7.3%	1.7%	2% (ulceration)
TrapEase	65	6	0%	45.7%	2.8%	NR
Vena-Tech low-profile	30	2.3	0%	10.3%	0%	NR
Günther Tulip	83	4.5 (0–36)	3.6%	NR	9.6%	NR

Values are given as numbers or percentages as indicated; values in parentheses indicate ranges of reported values.

Abbreviations: F/U, follow-up; NR, not reported.

From Kinney TB. Update on inferior vena cava filters. J Vasc Interv Radiol 2003;14(4):425–40; with permission.

mortality in the filter group compared with 6.3% and 20.1% in the no filter group ($P = $ .16 and 0.65); however, this was for patients who had known DVT who were able to receive anticoagulation, and has limited application to the typical surgical patient in whom a VCF is being considered.

Trauma patients

Analysis of results for VCF placement in trauma patients is mainly limited by the lack of adequate control groups for comparison, with most series using unmatched cohorts or historical data for comparison. A meta-analysis of older series demonstrated a PE incidence of 0.2% with VCF, compared with 1.5% among controls without a VCF and 5.8% for historic controls [19]. Rodriguez and colleagues [110] compared 40 critically injured patients who received a prophylactic VCF with 80 matched historic controls. Only 1 patient (3%) who had a VCF developed PE, compared with 14 (18%) in the control group, four of these being fatal PE. Similar reductions in the incidence of PE with filter use compared with control populations or historical data have been reported in other series [26,111,112]. Rogers and colleagues [28] reported on 132 trauma patients receiving prophylactic VCF with 5-year follow-up data. They found a 2.3% incidence of PE after filter placement and a mortality of 4.4%, with one fatal PE. Carlin and colleagues [113] compared a group of 122 trauma patients who received a therapeutic VCF with 78 patients receiving prophylactic filters. They found a mortality rate of 11% for therapeutic VCF and 3% for prophylactic, and an incidence of recurrent PE of 18% in the therapeutic group versus 0% in the prophylactic group. In addition, they associated a 50% reduction in their overall incidence of PE over a 10-year period with a significant increase in use of VCF. In summary, the majority of series report a decreased incidence of all PE and fatal PE with the use of VCF in appropriately selected patients, but there remains a lack of rigorous control groups for comparison.

Results with retrievable filters in trauma patients

The large majority of experience with retrievable VCF in surgical patients has been in the setting of major trauma. As stated previously, trauma surgeons are more likely to place a VCF if given the option of a retrievable filter [41], and retrievable filters are being increasingly used in many trauma centers [37,114]. Meier and colleagues [115] analyzed the results of prophylactic retrievable VCF placement in 35 trauma patients. Filters were retrieved in 86% of patients, and 36% demonstrated trapped clot or thrombus within the device. The incidence of PE was 3%, which occurred in 1 patient 5 days after VCF removal, and mortality was 3%. Several other series have reported a high technical success rate and low incidence of PE among high-risk trauma patients who received a retrievable VCF [116–118].

In a recently published multicenter study by the AAST, 446 patients received a retrievable VCF, with the majority (76%) placed prophylactically [4]. In this large series, the retrieval rate was only 22%, and only half of patients had postdischarge follow-up reported. The reported rate of "breakthrough" PE in these patients was low at 0.5%, but should be interpreted with caution because of the poor follow-up. Although these filters seem to represent an attractive option for the high-risk trauma patient, they create additional difficult decisions, such as the timing of removal and ensuring adequate follow-up and surveillance. The highest risk for PE is in the early postinjury period, but there remains a significant risk for late PE occurring weeks after injury, which must be considered when timing the removal of a VCF [116,119]. With the expanding use of retrievable filters at many trauma centers, there remains significant debate about their utility, the optimal timing of removal, and the amount and duration of follow-up. These questions will require further prospective data to answer [4,114,116].

Surgical oncology

The prevention and management of VTE in the cancer patient remains problematic, particularly in the perioperative period. In response to concerns about the safety and effectiveness of standard anticoagulant therapy in the cancer patient [49,50,120], many have recommended the consideration of VCF placement in this population [52,55,121,122]. Ghanim and colleagues [123] found no significant difference in overall or in-hospital mortality among 175 patients who had brain tumors and VTE managed with VCF or anticoagulation only, with median survival of 21 weeks and 11 weeks respectively. A study of 166 cancer patients undergoing VCF placement for therapeutic or prophylactic indications demonstrated a median survival time of only 10 months, confirming the overall poor outcomes in this patient population [53]. A series of 116 patients undergoing active treatment of malignant disease found a low procedural complication rate and a low recurrent PE rate of 3% following VCF placement [55]; however, only 14% of patients were alive at 1 year, leading the study authors to conclude that VCF in these patients may be of little clinical benefit. In a retrospective case-control study Schunn and colleagues [56] demonstrated that VCF in cancer patients appeared to be effective at preventing PE, but there was no survival benefit when compared with a matched control population. Similar results have been reported in several other series [58,124,125]. Chau and colleagues [126] used a Markov model of cost effectiveness in comparing VCF or anticoagulation in patients who had malignant brain tumors and DVT. They demonstrated that VCF was not cost-effective in this patient population, but when the model was adjusted to reflect the anticipated 5-year survival for a breast cancer population, VCF appeared to be more effective and less expensive than anticoagulation alone. From the available data it appears that VCF placement will be most effective in cancer patients who have proven VTE and who have good functional status and longer predicted survival times, and should be discouraged in patients who have advanced disease.

Bariatric patients

There are relatively few studies detailing the outcomes from VCF use in the bariatric population, and these are limited to case reports and case series. Piano and colleagues [70] analyzed outcomes from a protocolized approach using a retrievable VCF in 59 patients undergoing bariatric surgery who met high-risk criteria. All filters were placed immediately before surgery, and removal was attempted at 4 weeks postoperatively. There was one postoperative PE (1.7%) in a patient who was not receiving chemical anticoagulation, and no fatal PE or deaths. In another series of patients undergoing open gastric bypass there were 58 prophylactic VCF placed with 100% technical success rate, and no postoperative PE in patients who had VCF, compared with a historic control PE rate of 13% [69]. These results have been similar to those reported in several other smaller series [68,127]; however, interpretation of these results is significantly limited by the lack of prospective data, adequate control populations, standardized approach to chemoprophylaxis, and the small numbers available for analysis. Given the relative infrequency of all PE and fatal PE after bariatric surgery

[128], much larger trials will be required to provide any meaningful data regarding the indications and efficacy of VCF in this patient population.

The argument against vena cava filter efficacy

Although the majority of series cited above have concluded that VCF placement offers a benefit in terms of reduction in PE and PE-related morbidity and mortality, there remains a significant amount of skepticism and ongoing debate. The only prospective randomized trial of VCF demonstrated a reduction in early (within 12 days) PE but no long-term benefit in terms of PE or mortality, and a significantly increased risk of DVT [11]. A large population-based study using discharge data from California hospitals found that there was no reduction in rehospitalization for PE among patients who received a VCF compared with those who had no filter, but that the VCF group had a significantly higher hospital readmission rate for DVT [129]. Spain and colleagues [130] found a low rate of DVT and PE among 2868 trauma patients, 280 of whom were deemed "high-risk" for VTE, despite the use of only one prophylactic VCF over the 2-year study period. There were no diagnosed PE in the low-risk group and no deaths attributable to PE in the high-risk group, leading the study authors to conclude that routine VCF use is a waste of resources with little benefit. The high costs and lack of proven benefit for routine prophylactic VCF use compared with standard prophylactic measures has also been questioned in the population of patients who have acute spinal cord injury [131]. Antevil and colleagues [24] demonstrated a threefold increase in VCF use after introduction of a retrievable filter at their institution, but no significant differences were seen in the incidence of PE or filter-related complications. In addition, only 21% of retrievable filters were successfully removed, which is in agreement with data from a multicenter trial of retrievable VCF [4].

Complications

Surgeons contemplating VCF placement or managing patients who have a VCF should be aware of the potential complications associated with their use. Thrombotic complications associated with VCF include vena caval thrombosis, access site thrombosis, and DVT. Multiple series have confirmed that vena cava filters significantly increase the risk of both initial DVT formation and DVT recurrence [11,12,129], and have prompted recommendations for chemical anticoagulation when possible in patients who have filters [132–134]. In addition to representing a risk for PE, these thrombotic complications can result in renal compromise and extremity postphlebitic symptoms of varying severity [28,97,135–137]. Table 3 lists the incidence of thrombotic complications from a variety of filter types, with DVT and postphlebitic syndromes as high as 46% and 41%

respectively, and vena caval thrombosis demonstrated in up to 11% of patients. Several series in surgical patients have presented significantly lower incidences of these complications, but are generally limited by the duration and intensity of follow-up [4,21,138,139]. Although retrievable filters have been proposed to theoretically avoid some of these long-term thrombotic complications, a large review of retrievable filters published in 1996 found reported complication rates of 6% to 30% for caval thrombosis, 3% to 69% for filter migration, and 5% to 70% for postphlebitic syndrome [106]. Lower complication rates were reported in the AAST multicenter trial of trauma patients receiving retrievable filters [4], but these results are significantly limited by the poor overall follow-up. Filter removal itself is associated with several potential complications that should be considered, including technical failure, bleeding, and access site thrombosis [106,140,141]. In addition, it appears that on average only 25% to 50% of "retrievable" vena cava filters are actually ever removed, which may reflect a conscious decision based on continued VTE risk, or in many cases may represent inadequate planning and follow-up [4,141,142].

Additional rare but potentially serious complications of VCF are filter malposition or migration, filter perforation with hemorrhage or erosion into surrounding structures, and entrapment of guide wires during procedures such as central venous catheter placement [143–152]. Although many of these complications occur at the time of insertion or early in the postprocedure period, the patient who has a VCF does remain at risk for thrombotic and other filter-related complications for the duration of filter placement, and should be evaluated and managed appropriately. In all patients it is critical to incorporate the nature and degree of these potential risks into the decision-making process for VCF placement, particularly when done for prophylactic indications.

Future directions

IVC filters are relatively safe and appear to be effective (at least transiently) in reducing the incidence of PE; however, complications continue to occur and no ideal filter exists that can completely trap all clot and maintain IVC patency. Because venous thromboembolism continues to pose significant problems in all patient populations, other treatment modalities continue to be entertained. Newer anticoagulant agents are continuously developed and studied in an attempt to find the ideal therapy. Although low molecular weight heparin agents are the preferred pharmacological prophylaxis for VTE in trauma patients and other high-risk populations, a number of newer agents are in various stages of development and evaluation. These new anticoagulants can be classified into three groups: (1) inhibitors of activation of coagulation (nematode anticoagulant peptide c2 [NAPc2], derived from the nematode *Ancylostoma canicum*); (2) inhibitors of propagation of coagulation (fondaparinux, idraparinux), and (3) inhibitors of thrombin formation (hirudin, bivalirudin, ximelagatran, mela-gatran) [153,154].

An emerging concept in VTE disease is the role of clot burden. There is evidence that anticoagulant therapy changes clot burden, and that this change influences the long-term frequency of recurrent VTE [155]. Cathe-ter-directed thrombolysis for lower extremity DVT with and without IVC filters has been shown to be safe and effective in treating acute DVT and may actually prevent PE [156]. The actual role of catheter-directed throm-bolysis deserves further evaluation, however promising it may be.

Summary and recommendations

Prevention and management of VTE in surgical patients remains a critical area that has significant implications for patient morbidity and mortality and the health care system as a whole. Although there is a considerable pool of data available for medical preventive and management options, there remains a complete lack of well-controlled data on which to base de-cisions regarding when and how to use vena cava filters [157]. Despite this lack of an evidence-based rationale, the use of vena cava filters, and partic-ularly retrievable vena cava filters placed for prophylactic indications, is rapidly increasing. The increasing use of an unproven technology that is invasive and has a well-defined complication profile should prompt further questioning and analysis.

Based on the available evidence the authors continue to recommend placement of vena cava filters in patients who have established VTE and an absolute contraindication to or significant complication of anticoagula-tion. It should also be considered in patients who have "free-floating" venous thrombus and in patients undergoing thrombolysis, although these are not absolute indications. In the "high-risk" trauma population (severe head injury, pelvic and long bone fractures, spinal cord injury, prolonged immobilization, venous injury) there is little to no evidence to support a practice of routine prophylactic VCF placement, and decisions should be made on an individual basis. The authors believe that most of these patients can be managed with appropriately dosed chemoprophylaxis, and we would consider VCF only in the patient who has a true contraindication to anticoagulation that is expected to persist. Similarly, there are very few data suggesting a benefit of routine prophylactic VCF placement in the bari-atric surgical population or patients who have active malignancy, and these patients may be at higher risk for VCF associated complications; however, in patients who have multiple risk factors and other considerations, such as poor cardiopulmonary reserve or relative contraindications to anticoagula-tion, an individual risk-to-benefit analysis should be performed when decid-ing on VCF placement. If a decision is made to place a retrievable VCF, then particular attention should be paid to ensuring the filter is left in place for the duration of the period of increased risk, and appropriate follow-up should be arranged and ensured for subsequent filter removal. Large, well-controlled trials using the currently available devices as well as alternative methods of VTE treatment and prophylaxis are critically needed to determine if there is any true benefit of vena cava filter placement over standard management, and which patient populations would maximally benefit.

References

[1] Alberts WM, Tonner JA, Goldman AL. Echocardiography in planned interruption of the inferior vena cava. South Med J 1989;82(6):772–4.

[2] Goldhaber SZ, Buring JE, Lipnick RJ, et al. Interruption of the inferior vena cava by clip or filter. Am J Med 1984;76(3):512–6.

[3] Menzoian JO, LoGerfo FW, Weitzman AF, et al. Clinical experience with the Mobin-Uddin vena cava umbrella filter. Arch Surg 1980;115(10):1179–81.

[4] Karmy-Jones R, Jurkovich GJ, Velmahos GC, et al. Practice patterns and outcomes of retrievable vena cava filters in trauma patients: an AAST multicenter study. J Trauma 2007;62(1):17–24 [discussion: 24–5].

[5] Chiou AC, Biggs KL, Matsumura JS. Vena cava filters: why, when, what, how? Perspect Vasc Surg Endovasc Ther 2005;17(4):329–39.

[6] Cooper JM, Silberzweig J, Mitty HA. Vena cava filters: available devices and current practices. Mt Sinai J Med 1996;63(3–4):273–81.

[7] Cotroneo AR, Di Stasi C, Cina A, et al. Venous interruption as prophylaxis of pulmonary embolism: vena cava filters. Rays 1996;21(3):461–80.

[8] Decousus H, Julliard-Delsart D, Mismetti P. [Current indications of cava filters]. Rev Med Interne 1997;18(Suppl 6):646s–50s.

[9] Deshpande KS, Hatem C, Karwa M, et al. The use of inferior vena cava filter as a treatment modality for massive pulmonary embolism. A case series and review of pathophysiology. Respir Med 2002;96(12):984–9.

[10] Erstad BL. Venous thromboembolism in multiple trauma patients. Pharmacotherapy 1998; 18(5):1011–23.

[11] Decousus H, Leizorovicz A, Parent F, et al. A clinical trial of vena caval filters in the prevention of pulmonary embolism in patients with proximal deep-vein thrombosis. Prevention du Risque d'Embolie Pulmonaire par Interruption Cave Study Group. N Engl J Med 1998;338(7):409–15.

[12] Eight-year follow-up of patients with permanent vena cava filters in the prevention of pulmonary embolism: the PREPIC (Prevention du Risque d'Embolie Pulmonaire par Interruption Cave) randomized study. Circulation 2005;112(3):416–22.

[13] Opinions regarding the diagnosis and management of venous thromboembolic disease. ACCP Consensus Committee on Pulmonary Embolism. American College of Chest Physicians. Chest 1998;113(2):499–504.

[14] Baglin TP, Brush J, Streiff M. Guidelines on use of vena cava filters. Br J Haematol 2006; 134(6):590–5.

[15] Bick RL, Haas SK. International consensus recommendations. Summary statement and additional suggested guidelines. European Consensus Conference, November 1991. American College of Chest Physicians consensus statement of 1995. International Consensus Statement, 1997. Med Clin North Am 1998;82(3):613–33.

[16] Buller HR, Agnelli G, Hull RD, et al. Antithrombotic therapy for venous thromboembolic disease: the Seventh ACCP Conference on Antithrombotic and Thrombolytic Therapy. Chest 2004;126(Suppl 3):401S–28S.

[17] Rogers FB, Cipolle MD, Velmahos G, et al. Practice management guidelines for the prevention of venous thromboembolism in trauma patients: the EAST practice management guidelines work group. J Trauma 2002;53(1):142–64.

[18] Snow V, Qaseem A, Barry P, et al. Management of venous thromboembolism: a clinical practice guideline from the American College of Physicians and the American Academy of Family Physicians. Ann Fam Med 2007;5(1):74–80.

[19] Velmahos GC, Kern J, Chan LS, et al. Prevention of venous thromboembolism after injury: an evidence-based report—Part II: Analysis of risk factors and evaluation of the role of vena caval filters. J Trauma 2000;49(1):140–4.

[20] Velmahos GC, Kern J, Chan LS, et al. Prevention of venous thromboembolism after injury: an evidence-based report—Part I: Analysis of risk factors and evaluation of the role of vena caval filters. J Trauma 2000;49(1):132–8 [discussion: 139].

[21] Johns JS, Nguyen C, Sing RF. Vena cava filters in spinal cord injuries: evolving technology. J Spinal Cord Med 2006;29(3):183–90.

[22] Imberti D, Ageno W. A survey of thromboprophylaxis management in patients with major trauma. Pathophysiol Haemost Thromb 2005;34(6):249–54.

[23] Gonzalez RP, Cohen M, Bosarge P, et al. Prophylactic inferior vena cava filter insertion for trauma: intensive care unit versus operating room. Am Surg 2006;72(3):213–6.

[24] Antevil JL, Sise MJ, Sack DI, et al. Retrievable vena cava filters for preventing pulmonary embolism in trauma patients: a cautionary tale. J Trauma 2006;60(1):35–40.

[25] Offner PJ, Hawkes A, Madayag R, et al. The role of temporary inferior vena cava filters in critically ill surgical patients. Arch Surg 2003;138(6):591–4 [discussion: 594–5].

[26] Khansarinia S, Dennis JW, Veldenz HC, et al. Prophylactic Greenfield filter placement in selected high-risk trauma patients. J Vasc Surg 1995;22(3):231–5 [discussion: 235–6].

[27] Greenfield LJ, Proctor MC, Michaels AJ, et al. Prophylactic vena caval filters in trauma: the rest of the story. J Vasc Surg 2000;32(3):490–5 [discussion: 496–7].

[28] Rogers FB, Strindberg G, Shackford SR, et al. Five-year follow-up of prophylactic vena cava filters in high-risk trauma patients. Arch Surg 1998;133(4):406–11 [discussion: 412].

[29] Rogers FB, Shackford SR, Ricci MA, et al. Prophylactic vena cava filter insertion in selected high-risk orthopaedic trauma patients. J Orthop Trauma 1997;11(4):267–72.

[30] Brasel KJ, Borgstrom DC, Weigelt JA. Cost-effective prevention of pulmonary embolus in high-risk trauma patients. J Trauma 1997;42(3):456–60 [discussion 460–2].

[31] Gosin JS, Graham AM, Ciocca RG, et al. Efficacy of prophylactic vena cava filters in high-risk trauma patients. Ann Vasc Surg 1997;11(1):100–5.

[32] Kinasewitz GT, Yan SB, Basson B, et al. Universal changes in biomarkers of coagulation and inflammation occur in patients with severe sepsis, regardless of causative micro-organism [ISRCTN74215569]. Crit Care 2004;8(2):R82–90.

[33] Sanchez CM, Suarez MA, Nebra A, et al. [Early activation of coagulation and fibrinolysis in traumatic brain injury and spontaneous intracerebral hemorrhage: a comparative study]. Neurologia 2004;19(2):44–52.

[34] Stein SC, Chen XH, Sinson GP, et al. Intravascular coagulation: a major secondary insult in nonfatal traumatic brain injury. Neurosurgery 2002;97(6):1373–7.

[35] Velmahos GC. The current status of thromboprophylaxis after trauma: a story of confusion and uncertainty. Am Surg 2006;72(9):757–63.

[36] Velmahos GC, Nigro J, Tatevossian R, et al. Inability of an aggressive policy of thrombo-prophylaxis to prevent deep venous thrombosis (DVT) in critically injured patients: are current methods of DVT prophylaxis insufficient? J Am Coll Surg 1998;187(5):529–33.

[37] Knudson MM, Ikossi DG. Venous thromboembolism after trauma. Curr Opin Crit Care 2004;10(6):539–48.

[38] Levy ML, Granville RC, Hart D, et al. Deep venous thrombosis in children and adolescents. J Neurosurg 2004;101(Suppl 1):32–7.

[39] Grandas OH, Klar M, Goldman MH, et al. Deep venous thrombosis in the pediatric trauma population: an unusual event: report of three cases. Am Surg 2000;66(3):273–6.

[40] Cushman M. Epidemiology and risk factors for venous thrombosis. Semin Hematol 2007; 44(2):62–9.

[41] Quirke TE, Ritota PC, Swan KG. Inferior vena caval filter use in US trauma centers: a practitioner survey. J Trauma 1997;43(2):333–7.

[42] Ho WK, Hankey GJ, Lee CH, et al. Venous thromboembolism: diagnosis and management of deep venous thrombosis. Med J Aust 2005;182(9):476–81.

[43] Lin J, Proctor MC, Varma M, et al. Factors associated with recurrent venous thromboembolism in patients with malignant disease. J Vasc Surg 2003;37(5):976–83.

[44] Semrad TJ, O'Donnell R, Wun T, et al. Epidemiology of venous thromboembolism in 9489 patients with malignant glioma. J Neurosurg 2007;106(4):601–8.

[45] Piccioli A, Prandoni P, Goldhaber SZ. Epidemiologic characteristics, management, and outcome of deep venous thrombosis in a tertiary-care hospital: the Brigham and Women's Hospital DVT registry. Am Heart J 1996;132(5):1010–4.

[46] Falanga A, Donati MB. Pathogenesis of thrombosis in patients with malignancy. Int J Hematol 2001;73(2):137–44.

[47] Falanga A, Rickles FR. Pathophysiology of the thrombophilic state in the cancer patient. Semin Thromb Hemost 1999;25(2):173–82.

[48] Kinney TB. Update on inferior vena cava filters. J Vasc Interv Radiol 2003;14(4):425–40.

[49] Lee AY, Levine MN. Management of venous thromboembolism in cancer patients. Oncology (Williston Park) 2000;14(3):409–17, 421 [discussion: 422, 425–6].

[50] Lee AY, Levine MN, Baker RI, et al. Low-molecular-weight heparin versus a coumarin for the prevention of recurrent venous thromboembolism in patients with cancer. N Engl J Med 2003;349(2):146–53.

[51] Streiff MB. Vena caval filters: a comprehensive review. Blood 2000;95(12):3669–77.

[52] Streiff MB. Vena caval filters: a review for intensive care specialists. J Intensive Care Med 2003;18(2):59–79.

[53] Greenfield LJ, Proctor MC, Saluja A. Clinical results of Greenfield filter use in patients with cancer. Cardiovasc Surg 1997;5(2):145–9.

[54] Marcy PY, Magne N, Gallard JC, et al. Cost-benefit assessment of inferior vena cava filter placement in advanced cancer patients. Support Care Cancer 2002;10(1):76–80.

[55] Jarrett BP, Dougherty MJ, Calligaro KD. Inferior vena cava filters in malignant disease. J Vasc Surg 2002;36(4):704–7.

[56] Schunn C, Schunn GB, Hobbs G, et al. Inferior vena cava filter placement in late-stage cancer. Vasc Endovascular Surg 2006;40(4):287–94.

[57] Ihnat DM, Mills JL, Hughes JD, et al. Treatment of patients with venous thromboembolism and malignant disease: should vena cava filter placement be routine? J Vasc Surg 1998;28(5):800–7.

[58] Rosen MP, Porter DH, Kim D. Reassessment of vena caval filter use in patients with cancer. J Vasc Interv Radiol 1994;5(3):501–6.

[59] Davidson BL, Buller HR, Decousus H, et al. Effect of obesity on outcomes after fondaparinux, enoxaparin, or heparin treatment for acute venous thromboembolism in the Matisse trials. J Thromb Haemost 2007;5(6):1191–4.

[60] DeMaria EJ, Portenier D, Wolfe L. Obesity surgery mortality risk score: proposal for a clinically useful score to predict mortality risk in patients undergoing gastric bypass. Surg Obes Relat Dis 2007;3(2):134–40.

[61] Hamad GG, Bergqvist D. Venous thromboembolism in bariatric surgery patients: an update of risk and prevention. Surg Obes Relat Dis 2007;3(1):97–102.

[62] Ferrell A, Byrne TK, Robison JG. Placement of inferior vena cava filters in bariatric surgical patients—possible indications and technical considerations. Obes Surg 2004; 14(6):738–43.

[63] Goldhaber SZ, Grodstein F, Stampfer MJ, et al. A prospective study of risk factors for pulmonary embolism in women. JAMA 1997;277(8):642–5.

[64] Michota F, Merli G. Anticoagulation in special patient populations: are special dosing considerations required? Cleve Clin J Med 2005;72(Suppl 1):S37–42.

[65] Schwiesow SJ, Wessell AM, Steyer TE. Use of a modified dosing weight for heparin therapy in a morbidly obese patient. Ann Pharmacother 2005;39(4):753–6.

[66] Spruill WJ, Wade WE, Huckaby WG, et al. Achievement of anticoagulation by using a weight-based heparin dosing protocol for obese and nonobese patients. Am J Health Syst Pharm 2001;58(22):2143–6.

[67] Prystowsky JB, Morasch MD, Eskandari MK, et al. Prospective analysis of the incidence of deep venous thrombosis in bariatric surgery patients. Surgery 2005;138(4):759–63 [discussion: 763–5].

[68] Frezza EE, Wachtel MS. A simple venous thromboembolism prophylaxis protocol for patients undergoing bariatric surgery. Obesity (Silver Spring) 2006;14(11):1961–5.

[69] Gargiulo NJ 3rd, Veith FJ, Lipsitz EC, et al. Experience with inferior vena cava filter placement in patients undergoing open gastric bypass procedures. J Vasc Surg 2006;44(6): 1301–5.

[70] Piano G, Ketteler ER, Prachand V, et al. Safety, feasibility, and outcome of retrievable vena cava filters in high-risk surgical patients. J Vasc Surg 2007;45(4):784–8 [discussion: 788].

[71] Nathens AB, McMurray MK, Cuschieri J, et al. The practice of venous thromboembolism prophylaxis in the major trauma patient. J Trauma 2007;62(3):557–62 [discussion: 562–3].

[72] Cothren CC, Smith WR, Moore EE, et al. Utility of once-daily dose of low-molecular-weight heparin to prevent venous thromboembolism in multisystem trauma patients. World J Surg 2007;31(1):98–104.

[73] Leonardi MJ, McGory ML, Ko CY. A systematic review of deep venous thrombosis prophylaxis in cancer patients: implications for improving quality. Ann Surg Oncol 2007; 14(2):929–36.

[74] Payen JF, Faillot T, Audibert G, et al. [Thromboprophylaxis in neurosurgery and head trauma]. Ann Fr Anesth Reanim 2005;24(8):921–7.

[75] Kleindienst A, Harvey HB, Mater E, et al. Early antithrombotic prophylaxis with low molecular weight heparin in neurosurgery. Acta Neurochir (Wien) 2003;145(12):1085–90 [discussion: 1090–1].

[76] Kurtoglu M, Buyukkurt CD, Kurtoglu M, et al. [Venous thromboembolism prophylaxis with low molecular weight heparins in polytraumatized patients in intensive care unit (extended series)]. Ulus Travma Acil Cerrahi Derg 2003;9(1):37–44.

[77] Thaler HW, Roller RE, Greiner N, et al. Thromboprophylaxis with 60 mg enoxaparin is safe in hip trauma surgery. J Trauma 2001;51(3):518–21.

[78] Alejandro KV, Acosta JA, Rodriguez PA. Bleeding manifestations after early use of low-molecular-weight heparins in blunt splenic injuries. Am Surg 2003;69(11):1006–9.

[79] Passman MA, Dattilo JB, Guzman RJ, et al. Bedside placement of inferior vena cava filters by using transabdominal duplex ultrasonography and intravascular ultrasound imaging. J Vasc Surg 2005;42(5):1027–32.

[80] Corriere MA, Passman MA, Guzman RJ, et al. Comparison of bedside transabdominal duplex ultrasound versus contrast venography for inferior vena cava filter placement: what is the best imaging modality? Ann Vasc Surg 2005;19(2):229–34.

[81] Rosenthal D, Wellons ED, Levitt AB, et al. Role of prophylactic temporary inferior vena cava filters placed at the ICU bedside under intravascular ultrasound guidance in patients with multiple trauma. J Vasc Surg 2004;40(5):958–64.

[82] Garrett JV, Passman MA, Guzman RJ, et al. Expanding options for bedside placement of inferior vena cava filters with intravascular ultrasound when transabdominal duplex ultrasound imaging is inadequate. Ann Vasc Surg 2004;18(3):329–34.

[83] Sing RF, Heniford BT. Bedside insertion of the inferior vena cava filter in the intensive care unit. Am Surg 2003;69(8):660–2.

[84] Gamblin TC, Ashley DW, Burch S, et al. A prospective evaluation of a bedside technique for placement of inferior vena cava filters: accuracy and limitations of intravascular ultrasound. Am Surg 2003;69(5):382–6.

[85] Wellons ED, Matsuura JH, Shuler FW, et al. Bedside intravascular ultrasound-guided vena cava filter placement. J Vasc Surg 2003;38(3):455–7 [discussion: 457–8].

[86] Pignataro ED. Bedside insertion of inferior vena cava filters. Int J Trauma Nurs 1998;4(2): 44–7.

[87] Sing RF, Smith CH, Miles WS, et al. Preliminary results of bedside inferior vena cava filter placement: safe and cost-effective. Chest 1998;114(1):315–6.

[88] Holtzman RB, Lottenberg L, Bass T, et al. Comparison of carbon dioxide and iodinated contrast for cavography prior to inferior vena cava filter placement. Am J Surg 2003; 185(4):364–8.

[89] Sing RF, Cicci CK, Lequire MH, et al. Bedside carbon dioxide cavagrams for inferior vena cava filters: preliminary results. J Vasc Surg 2000;32(1):144–7.

[90] Sing RF, Stackhouse DJ, Cicci CK, et al. Bedside carbon dioxide (CO2) preinsertion cavagram for inferior vena cava filter placement: case report. J Trauma 1999;47(6): 1140–1.

[91] Chiou AC. Intravascular ultrasound-guided bedside placement of inferior vena cava filters. Semin Vasc Surg 2006;19(3):150–4.

[92] Matsuura JH, White RA, Kopchok G, et al. Vena caval filter placement by intravascular ultrasound. Cardiovasc Surg 2001;9(6):571–4.

[93] Ashley DW, Gamblin TC, Burch ST, et al. Accurate deployment of vena cava filters: comparison of intravascular ultrasound and contrast venography. J Trauma 2001;50(6): 975–81.

[94] Greenfield LJ, Proctor MC. Suprarenal filter placement. J Vasc Surg 1998,28(3):432–8 [discussion: 438].

[95] Burov VP, Kapranov SA. Temporary placement of the cava filter to the suprarenal segment of the inferior vena cava. Angiol Sosud Khir 2005;11(2):45–7.

[96] Matchett WJ, Jones MP, McFarland DR, et al. Suprarenal vena caval filter placement: follow-up of four filter types in 22 patients. J Vasc Interv Radiol 1998;9(4):588–93.

[97] Marcy PY, Magne N, Frenay M, et al. Renal failure secondary to thrombotic complications of suprarenal inferior vena cava filter in cancer patients. Cardiovasc Intervent Radiol 2001; 24(4):257–9.

[98] Nadkarni S, Macdonald S, Cleveland TJ, et al. Placement of a retrievable Gunther Tulip filter in the superior vena cava for upper extremity deep venous thrombosis. Cardiovasc Intervent Radiol 2002;25(6):524–6.

[99] Watanabe S, Shimokawa S, Shibuya H, et al. Superior vena caval placement of a temporary filter: a case report. Vasc Surg 2001;35(1):59–62.

[100] Ascher E, Hingorani A, Tsemekhin B, et al. Lessons learned from a 6-year clinical experience with superior vena cava Greenfield filters. J Vasc Surg 2000;32(5):881–7.

[101] Ascher E, Hingorani A, Mazzariol F, et al. Clinical experience with superior vena caval Greenfield filters. J Endovasc Surg 1999;6(4):365–9.

[102] Ascer E, Gennaro M, Lorensen E, et al. Superior vena caval Greenfield filters: indications, techniques, and results. J Vasc Surg 1996;23(3):498–503.

[103] Cousins GR, DeAnda A Jr. Images in cardiothoracic surgery. Superior vena cava filter erosion into the ascending aorta. Ann Thorac Surg 2006;81(5):1907.

[104] Hussain SM, McLafferty RB, Schmittling ZC, et al. Superior vena cava perforation and cardiac tamponade after filter placement in the superior vena cava—a case report. Vasc Endovascular Surg 2005;39(4):367–70.

[105] Sheikh MA, Topoulos AP, Deitcher SR. Isolated internal jugular vein thrombosis: risk factors and natural history. Vasc Med 2002;7(3):177–9.

[106] Imberti D, Ageno W, Carpenedo M. Retrievable vena cava filters: a review. Curr Opin Hematol 2006;13(5):351–6.

[107] Bovyn G, Ricco JB, Reynaud P, et al. Long-duration temporary vena cava filter: a prospective 104-case multicenter study. J Vasc Surg 2006;43(6):1222–9.

[108] Binkert CA, Sasadeusz K, Stavropoulos SW. Retrievability of the recovery vena cava filter after dwell times longer than 180 days. J Vasc Interv Radiol 2006;17(2 Pt 1): 299–302.

[109] Cherian J, Gertner E. Recurrent pulmonary embolism despite inferior vena cava filter placement in patients with the antiphospholipid syndrome. J Clin Rheumatol 2005;11(1): 56–8.

[110] Rodriguez JL, Lopez JM, Proctor MC, et al. Early placement of prophylactic vena caval filters in injured patients at high risk for pulmonary embolism. J Trauma 1996;40(5): 797–802 [discussion: 802–4].

[111] Rogers FB, Shackford SR, Ricci MA, et al. Routine prophylactic vena cava filter insertion in severely injured trauma patients decreases the incidence of pulmonary embolism. J Am Coll Surg 1995;180(6):641–7.

[112] Langan EM 3rd, Miller RS, Casey WJ 3rd, et al. Prophylactic inferior vena cava filters in trauma patients at high risk: follow-up examination and risk/benefit assessment. J Vasc Surg Sep 1999;30(3):484–8.

[113] Carlin AM, Tyburski JG, Wilson RF, et al. Prophylactic and therapeutic inferior vena cava filters to prevent pulmonary emboli in trauma patients. Arch Surg 2002;137(5):521–5 [discussion: 525–7].

[114] Morris CS, Rogers FB, Najarian KE, et al. Current trends in vena caval filtration with the introduction of a retrievable filter at a level I trauma center. J Trauma 2004;57(1):32–6.

[115] Meier C, Keller IS, Pfiffner R, et al. Early experience with the retrievable OptEase vena cava filter in high-risk trauma patients. Eur J Vasc Endovasc Surg 2006;32(5):589–95.

[116] Greene FL, Sing RF, Mostafa G, et al. Retrievable vena cava filter use in trauma population. J Trauma 2005;58(5):1091.

[117] Rosenthal D, Wellons ED, Lai KM, et al. Retrievable inferior vena cava filters: early clinical experience. J Cardiovasc Surg (Torino) 2005;46(2):163–9.

[118] Grande WJ, Trerotola SO, Reilly PM, et al. Experience with the recovery filter as a retrievable inferior vena cava filter. J Vasc Interv Radiol 2005;16(9):1189–93.

[119] Sing RF, Camp SM, Heniford BT, et al. Timing of pulmonary emboli after trauma: implications for retrievable vena cava filters. J Trauma 2006;60(4):732–4 [discussion: 734–5].

[120] Debourdeau P, Meyer G, Sayeg H, et al. [Classical anticoagulant treatment of venous thromboembolic disease in cancer patients. Apropos of a retrospective study of 71 patients]. Rev Med Interne 1996;17(3):207–12.

[121] Andrea N, Ansell J. Management of thrombosis in the cancer patient. J Support Oncol 2003;1(4):235–8, 240–32 [discussion: 239–0, 243–5].

[122] Yonezawa K, Yokoo N, Yamaguchi T. Effectiveness of an inferior vena caval filter as a preventive measure against pulmonary thromboembolism after abdominal surgery. Surg Today 1999;29(8):821–4.

[123] Ghanim AJ, Daskalakis C, Eschelman DJ, et al. A five-year, retrospective, comparison review of survival in neurosurgical patients diagnosed with venous thromboembolism and treated with either inferior vena cava filters or anticoagulants. J Thromb Thrombolysis 2007, in press.

[124] Schwarz RE, Marrero AM, Conlon KC, et al. Inferior vena cava filters in cancer patients: indications and outcome. J Clin Oncol 1996;14(2):652–7.

[125] Wallace MJ, Jean JL, Gupta S, et al. Use of inferior vena caval filters and survival in patients with malignancy. Cancer 2004;101(8):1902–7.

[126] Chau Q, Cantor SB, Caramel E, et al. Cost-effectiveness of the bird's nest filter for preventing pulmonary embolism among patients with malignant brain tumors and deep venous thrombosis of the lower extremities. Support Care Cancer 2003;11(12):795–9.

[127] Keeling WB, Haines K, Stone PA, et al. Current indications for preoperative inferior vena cava filter insertion in patients undergoing surgery for morbid obesity. Obes Surg 2005; 15(7):1009–12.

[128] Carmody BJ, Sugerman HJ, Kellum JM, et al. Pulmonary embolism complicating bariatric surgery: detailed analysis of a single institution's 24-year experience. J Am Coll Surg 2006; 203(6):831–7.

[129] White RH, Zhou H, Kim J, et al. A population-based study of the effectiveness of inferior vena cava filter use among patients with venous thromboembolism. Arch Intern Med 2000; 160(13):2033–41.

[130] Spain DA, Richardson JD, Polk HC Jr, et al. Venous thromboembolism in the high-risk trauma patient: do risks justify aggressive screening and prophylaxis? J Trauma 1997; 42(3):463–7 [discussion: 467–9].

[131] Maxwell RA, Chavarria-Aguilar M, Cockerham WT, et al. Routine prophylactic vena cava filtration is not indicated after acute spinal cord injury. J Trauma 2002;52(5):902–6.

[132] Anderson RC, Bussey HI. Retrievable and permanent inferior vena cava filters: selected considerations. Pharmacotherapy 2006;26(11):1595–600.

[133] Yale SH, Mazza JJ, Glurich I, et al. Recurrent venous thromboembolism in patients with and without anticoagulation after inferior vena caval filter placement. Int Angiol 2006; 25(1):60–6.

[134] Gomes MP, Kaplan KL, Deitcher SR. Patients with inferior vena caval filters should receive chronic thromboprophylaxis. Med Clin North Am 2003;87(6):1189–203.

[135] Paton BL, Jacobs DG, Heniford BT, et al. Nine-year experience with insertion of vena cava filters in the intensive care unit. Am J Surg 2006;192(6):795–800.

[136] Sing RF, Cicci CK, Smith CH, et al. Bedside insertion of inferior vena cava filters in the intensive care unit. J Trauma 1999;47(6):1104–7.

[137] Greenfield LJ, Proctor MC. Recurrent thromboembolism in patients with vena cava filters. J Vasc Surg 2001;33(3):510–4.

[138] Giannoudis PV, Pountos I, Pape HC, et al. Safety and efficacy of vena cava filters in trauma patients. Injury 2007;38(1):7–18.

[139] Hoff WS, Hoey BA, Wainwright GA, et al. Early experience with retrievable inferior vena cava filters in high-risk trauma patients. J Am Coll Surg 2004;199(6):869–74.

[140] Mismetti P, Rivron-Guillot K, Quenet S, et al. A prospective long-term study of 220 patients with a retrievable vena cava filter for secondary prevention of venous thromboembolism. Chest 2007;131(1):223–9.

[141] Ray CE Jr, Mitchell E, Zipser S, et al. Outcomes with retrievable inferior vena cava filters: a multicenter study. J Vasc Interv Radiol 2006;17(10):1595–604.

[142] Kirilcuk NN, Herget EJ, Dicker RA, et al. Are temporary inferior vena cava filters really temporary? Am J Surg 2005;190(6):858–63.

[143] Brzezinski M, Schmidt U, Fitzsimons MG. Acute and massive hemorrhage due to caval perforation by an inferior vena cava filter—absolute indication for surgery? Case report and review of literature. Burns 2006;32(5):640–3.

[144] Herbstreit F, Kuhl H, Peters J. A cemented caval vein filter: case report. Spine 2006;31(24): E917–9.

[145] Ganguli S, Tham JC, Komlos F, et al. Fracture and migration of a suprarenal inferior vena cava filter in a pregnant patient. J Vasc Interv Radiol 2006;17(10):1707–11.

[146] Schweitzer M, Steele KE, Lidor A, et al. Acute vena cava thrombosis after placement of retrievable inferior vena cava filter before laparoscopic gastric bypass. Surg Obes Relat Dis 2006;2(6):661–3.

[147] Sakai Y, Masuda H, Arai G, et al. Accidental dislocation of an intracaval temporary filter into the heart in a case of renal cell carcinoma extending into the vena cava. Int J Urol 2006; 13(8):1118–20.

[148] Epstein NE. Retrievable inferior vena cava filter embolizes to right ventricle/pulmonary outflow tract. Spine J 2006;6(1):94–5.

[149] Hayes JD, Stone PA, Flaherty SK, et al. TrapEase vena cava filter: a case of filter migration and pulmonary embolism after placement. Ann Vasc Surg 2006;20(1):138–44.

[150] Albino P, Goncalves D, Sobrinho G, et al. [Phlegmasia caerulea dolens: therapeutic considerations]. Rev Port Cir Cardiotorac Vasc 2005;12(1):41–5.

[151] Chattar-Cora D, Tutela RR Jr, Tulsyan N, et al. Inferior vena cava filter ensnarement by central line guide wires—a report of 4 cases and brief review. Angiology 2004;55(4):463–8.

[152] Kaufman JL, Berman JA. Accidental intraaortic placement of a Greenfield filter. Ann Vasc Surg 1999;13(5):541–4.
[153] Agnelli G, Becattini C. New anticoagulants. Semin Thromb Hemost 2006;32(8):793–802.
[154] Agnelli G. New pharmacologic strategies for arterial and venous thromboembolism. Haematologica 2001;86(11 Suppl 2):58.
[155] Hull RD, Marder VJ, Mah AF, et al. Quantitative assessment of thrombus burden predicts the outcome of treatment for venous thrombosis: a systematic review. Am J Med 2005; 118(5):456–64.
[156] Bandyopadhyay T, Martin I, Lahiri B. Combined thrombolysis and inferior vena caval interruption as a therapeutic approach to massive and submassive pulmonary embolism. Conn Med 2006;70(6):367–70.
[157] Girard P, Stern JB, Parent F. Medical literature and vena cava filters: so far so weak. Chest 2002;122(3):963–7.

SURGICAL
CLINICS OF
NORTH AMERICA

Surg Clin N Am 87 (2007) 1253–1265

Endovenous Laser Treatment of Varicose Veins

Kathleen D. Gibson, MD[a,b,*], Brian L. Ferris, MD[a,b],
Daniel Pepper, MD[a,b]

[a]Lake Washington Vascular Surgeons, Kirkland, WA, USA
[b]Lake Washington Vascular Surgeons, 1135 116th Avenue NE,
Suite 305, Bellevue, WA 98104, USA

Venous insufficiency is one of the most common conditions seen in a vascular surgery practice, causing leg fatigue, pain, and swelling in millions of patients. Epidemiologic prevalence estimates of varicose veins vary widely depending on the population studied, but are highest in Western populations with 20% to 25% of women and 7% to 15% of men having visible varicosities [1,2]. Incompetence of the great saphenous vein (GSV) is the most common cause of varicose veins; however, the small saphenous vein (SSV) has valvular insufficiency in up to 20% of affected limbs [3].

Until the past decade, truncal saphenous incompetence was most commonly treated with high ligation and stripping. Although an effective treatment, surgical ligation and stripping requires general or spinal anesthesia. Postoperatively patients often have significant discomfort and bruising and routinely require narcotic analgesia. A desire to offer patients who have varicose veins a less painful treatment alternative to stripping, with a faster return to work and normal activities, led to the development of endovenous thermal ablation techniques. Critical advances in venous imaging and endovascular techniques made the application of this technology clinically successful. Endovenous laser treatment (EVLT) and radiofrequency ablation (RF) are rapidly becoming a standard of care in the treatment of varicose veins, because they can offer treatment in an outpatient setting and patients can return to normal activity levels almost immediately.

---

* Corresponding author. Lake Washington Vascular Surgeons, 1135 116th Avenue NE, Suite 305, Bellevue, WA 98104.
E-mail address: drgibson@lkwv.com (K.D. Gibson).

0039-6109/07/$ - see front matter © 2007 Elsevier Inc. All rights reserved.
doi:10.1016/j.suc.2007.07.017   *surgical.theclinics.com*

Development and application of endovenous laser treatment

In 1999 RF was the first endovenous technique that gained Federal Drug Administration (FDA) approval for treatment of the GSV [4] (VNUS Medical Technologies, Sunnydale, CA). The first report describing EVLT was by Carlos Boné in 1999 [5], and the first English-language citation was published in 2001 by Navarro and colleagues [6]. FDA approval for EVLT using an 810-nm device was granted in January of 2002 (Diomed, Andover, MA) [7]. The mechanism of action of laser ablation is to cause a nonthrombotic occlusion of the vein by delivery of laser energy (heat) endoluminally. The endothelium is destroyed and the vessel contracts and ultimately fibroses. Follow-up duplex ultrasound imaging of a successfully ablated vein shows a bright structure with no lumen. Several manufacturers sell consoles that produce lasers and disposable laser catheters and sheaths. Currently consoles delivering lasers in wavelengths of 810, 940, 980, 1319, and 1320 nm are commercially available (Table 1).

Endovenous laser therapy of the GSV has been proven to be safe, with long-term results comparable or superior to traditional high ligation and stripping [8–10]. Closure of the GSV by duplex ultrasound was 93% in a study of 499 limbs 2 years post-EVLT [8], and in a series of 990 limbs followed for 3 years only 3.3% of limbs showed recanalization of the GSV. Multiple studies have demonstrated that both endothermal techniques, RF and EVLT, are safe and effective. Each procedure has its own proponents, with supporters of EVLT citing higher recanalization rates with RF, and proponents of RF citing greater patient discomfort than with EVLT. As would be expected, literature reports cited by industry tend to quote studies most favorable to their product and most disparaging to their competition. Both procedures offer significantly decreased pain and bruising compared with stripping, with an earlier return to normal activities [10,11]. The authors consider the decision to use RF versus EVLT a personal preference of the treating physician. Having tried both methods, the authors prefer EVLT because of its wider applicability (4 French sheath with EVLT versus 6 French with RF), ease of use, speed of pullback (although recent changes in RF technology have decreased its pullback time), and

Table 1
Commercially available laser consoles

Company	Wavelength	Trade name	Website
Diomed, Andover, MA	810 nm	EVLT	www.evlt.com
Vascular Solutions, Minneapolis, MN	810 nm	Vari-Lase	www.vascularsolutions.com
Dornier MedTech, Kennesaw, GA	940 nm	Dornier D940	www.varicosecenter.com
Angiodynamics, Queensbury, NY	980 nm	Venacure	www.angiodynamics.com
Biolitec AG, Jena, Germany	980 nm	ELVeS	www.biolitec.com
Sciton, Palo Alto, CA	1319 nm	Pro-V	www.sciton.com
Cooltouch, Roseville, CA	1320 nm	Cooltouch	www.cooltouch.com

decreased cost of disposable catheters. Table 2 [12–19] compares EVLT, RF, and surgical stripping from a sampling of available studies.

All wavelengths of endovenous laser seem to be safe and effective. Kabnick randomized 51 patients to treatment with either an 810- or 980-nm wavelength laser. Both groups had similar outcomes and a paucity of complications. The 980-nm group had less bruising at 1 week and the 810-nm group had less itching at 3 weeks [20]. Proebstle and colleagues performed a nonrandomized comparison of 113 patients treated with a 940-nm diode laser at 15 W of power, 136 patients with 30 W of power, and 33 patients with a 1320-nm Nd:YAG laser set at 8 W of power. There was a statistically significant difference in pain and need for analgesics between the 1320-nm group and the 940-nm group with power set at 30 W [21]. The power level of 30 W, however, is significantly higher than that used by most other investigators and higher than what the authors use in our own practice (980 nm laser set at 12–15 W, dependent on diameter of treated vein). The authors have been using our 980-nm laser for nearly 4 years and have been pleased with the efficacy of this device and have not had undue problems with bruising or postprocedure pain. Advertising of 'painless' EVLT or RF treatment is misleading and likely to disappoint patients, however. We advise all of our patients to expect 12 to 14 days of discomfort in the path of the endoluminally treated vein, and to expect a 'string-like' pulling sensation for 1 to 2 months after. NSAIDS suffice for pain control for almost all patients.

Most published studies focus on EVLT of the GSV. The authors routinely perform laser ablation of the SSV and of accessory saphenous branches. Any vein branches that are sufficiently large (at least 2.0–2.5 mm), straight, and can be "pushed" to a depth of 1 cm below the skin surface with tumescence are amenable to laser ablation. Concerns about damage to the sural nerve with SSV ablation are unfounded when appropriate and sufficient tumescence fluid is delivered within the fascial envelope, and efficacy is similar to that achieved with GSV treatment. In the authors' series

Table 2
Comparison of endovenous laser treatment versus radiofrequency ablation versus surgical stripping of the great saphenous vein

	EVLT	RF	Ligation and stripping
Location of treatment	Office	Office	Hospital or outpatient
Catheter cost/size	$100[a]/4–5 Fr	$700[a]/6–8 Fr	N/A
Clinical success (%)			
Immediate	98–100 [8,9,13]	83–98 [11,13,18]	65–77 [11,12,17]
1–6 months	94 [13]	89–91 [11,13,18]	
1–4 years	93–97 [8,9,20]	67–96 [12,18]	
DVT (%)	0–8 [8,9,29]	0–16 [11–14]	5 [15]
Bruising/hematoma (%) (1 week)	24 [8]	33 [11]	65 [11]
Paresthesias (%)	0–8 [8,9,20,32]	0–23 [11,19]	14–40 [11,16]

[a] Approximate cost rounded to nearest $10 quoted to Lake Washington Vascular, PLLC, May 2007.

of 210 limbs, 1.6% had numbness at the lateral malleolus postprocedure and successful SSV closure was demonstrated in 100% of limbs at 1 week and 96% of limbs at a mean follow-up of 4 months. Thrombus extension into the popliteal vein was seen in 5.7% of limbs, with limbs lacking a Giacomini extension branch at highest risk [22]. Other investigatord have confirmed the efficacy of EVLT of the SSV and the paucity of serious complications [9,23].

A newer application of endovenous therapy for venous disease is the treatment of incompetent perforating veins (IPV). Increasing numbers of IPVs have been shown to increase CEAP (clinical severity, etiology, anatomy, physiology) clinical severity class in a linear fashion [24]. Alternatives for perforator treatment include open surgical ligation, subfascial endoscopic perforator ligation (SEPS) and ultrasound-guided foam sclerotherapy. The SEPS procedure was shown in a nationwide registry to decrease symptoms of chronic venous insufficiency and to promote ulcer healing [25]; however, the SEPS procedure requires a general anesthetic and multiple incisions. Given the rapid evolution in the treatment of venous insufficiency, the next step in perforator ligation is the development of a safe and durable procedure that can be performed in an office setting. "Stab and hook" phlebectomy can be performed in the office under local anesthesia with ultrasound guidance, but is most difficult in areas such as lipodermatosclerotic skin (CEAP clinical severity class 4 through 6). Recently, ablation of IPVs with RF has been described [26]. Because the laser fiber has a smaller diameter than the RF device, it seems logical that it should also be effective in ablating IPVs. A case report describing EVLT of IPVs has been published [27], and the authors have successfully tried this technique in our practice also. Further clinical study is necessary to determine if widespread application of EVLT for treatment of IPVs is feasible, safe, and effective.

Technique

Successful treatment of varicose veins with EVLT requires careful preoperative planning. A thorough history and physical examination is the first step. Patients should be queried regarding any previous vein procedures (sclerotherapy, previous ablation, or stripping), history of deep venous thrombosis (DVT), superficial thrombophlebitis, or personal or family history of thrombophilia. The authors treat patients who have a history of thrombophilia or previous DVT with prophylactic enoxaparin peri-procedurally. Patients taking Coumadin for medical indications are left on their anticoagulation. Because the GSV is a common conduit for coronary artery bypass, an assessment of risk factors for current or future coronary artery disease should be made. If the patient has active coronary disease or has significant risk factors, the risks and benefits of ablating the GSV should be carefully weighed and discussed with the patient and their primary care doctor or cardiologist. Care must also be taken with patients who have peripheral arterial disease; therefore, pedal pulses should always be palpated during the initial physical examination. The physical examination should assess the presence, distribution, and size of varicosities. The presence or absence of edema, skin changes, or ulceration should be assessed. In the authors' practice all patients have digital photographs of their legs taken before and after treatment. The authors consider photographic documentation to be a vital part of the medical record of a patient who has venous disease.

The second step in preoperative planning is a duplex ultrasound examination. A detailed "roadmap" of incompetent saphenous trunks and other sources of varicose veins is important. Failure to address non-saphenous sources of varicosities, such as perforators, accessory branches, and pelvic veins, can lead to immediate or early treatment failure and patient dissatisfaction. An assessment of the deep system is particularly important in patients who have a history of DVT, edema, skin changes, or ulceration (CEAP clinical severity classes 3 through 6) or in young patients who have severe varicosities and suspicion for Klippel-Trenaunay syndrome. Precise near-field resolution is the most important feature for diagnostic imaging and treatment of varicose veins. The authors' practice uses a GE Logic 9 machine with a 12-MHz "hockey stick" probe and a 10-MHz linear probe for preoperative mapping.

Following vein mapping, a treatment plan can be made. The authors' practice routinely uses EVLT to treat incompetent GSVs, SSVs, and accessory branches. An incompetent anterolateral branch from the saphenofemoral junction is a common cause of lateral thigh and calf varicosities. These varicosities often terminate into an incompetent lateral calf perforator. The anterolateral branch often has a fairly long, straight subfascial origin that can be treated with EVLT. Depending on the distribution and size of side branches, adjunctive treatments such as microphlebectomy, perforator ligation, and foam sclerotherapy can be considered and performed at the same time as the EVLT. The treatment plan and risks and expectations are then discussed with the patient and an informed consent is obtained.

EVLT can be performed in a hospital or in an outpatient clinic setting. Although EVLT can be performed without conscious sedation, the authors find that most of our patients prefer or request light sedation. Any conscious sedation performed in a clinic setting requires expertise on the part of the treating physician with airway management and emergent reversal of sedation. Reversal agents, oxygen, and emergency airway supplies should be readily available. Patients under conscious sedation should have continuous pulse oximetry monitoring and frequent checks of blood pressure and heart rate. Conscious sedation in the clinic setting is safest if a trained individual (such as an RN) administers the sedation and monitors the patient while the physician performs the EVLT.

In the authors' practice, EVLT is performed with sterile technique. After the patient is positioned (supine for the GSV, prone for the SSV), the limb is prepped and draped in sterile fashion. The desired venous access site is identified with ultrasound. Although in many practices the physician holds the ultrasound probe with one hand and accesses the vein with another, the authors' team includes a registered vascular technologist (RVT), and they hold the probe during the procedure. We find this two-person approach increases the speed and efficiency of the procedure and we also find it to be less ergonomically fatiguing than holding the probe ourselves. We gain access with a micropuncture kit (19-g reflective tip access needle, 0.018-in short wire, and 4 French micro-sheath) while visualizing the target vein on the ultrasound screen image provided by the 12-MHz hockey stick probe. The excellent near-field resolution of the probe makes access of even small veins possible. The authors have found accessing the vein initially in cross section and then switching to a longitudinal view for wire placement works well (Fig. 1).

Our initial enthusiasm for EVLT focused on the less invasive nature of the procedure and the ability to offer comprehensive vein treatment in our office. We soon realized, however, the unanticipated but enormous benefit of real-time high quality ultrasound guidance by sterile-sheathed linear probes during the procedure. This benefit cascades into the microphlebectomy and sclerotherapy adjuncts also, when compared with the pre-EVLT preoperative marking of perforators by a vascular technologist who would not be present during the operation.

Expedient access of the vein is the most important part of the procedure. If the vein is punctured with a needle but wire access fails, the vein invariably goes into venospasm at that location and a more proximal access point needs to be found. After access with the micropuncture sheath is confirmed, a 0.035-mm wire is passed. The wire should be visualized to cross the saphenofemoral junction (SFJ) into the common femoral vein for the GSV (unless there has been previous SFJ ligation) or through the saphenopopliteal junction (SPJ) for the SSV if there is a connection between the SSV and the popliteal vein. A 4- (preferably) or 5-French sheath that has been flushed with heparinized saline is then passed over the wire, the wire is removed, and a laser fiber placed through the sheath. The tip of the laser fiber should be positioned back at least 2 cm from the SFJ or SPJ. If a superficial epigastric

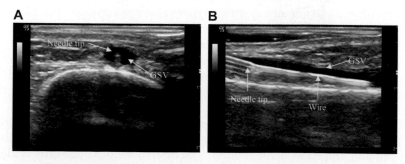

Fig. 1. Cross-sectional (*A*) and longitudinal (*B*) views of venous access.

or external pudendal vein or competent Giacomini vein are present at the SFJ or SPJ, the authors recommend positioning the laser tip distal (ie, caudal) to these branches to keep them open (Fig. 2). This may keep the junction open and make clot extension into the deep vein less likely. In the authors' practice, the RVT and the surgeon must agree that the tip is adequately distal (caudal) to the SFJ or SPJ before proceeding. Attention to leg position is important, because a laser fiber entering the GSV below the knee and positioned 2 cm caudal to the SFJ while the knee is in extension may easily protrude into the common femoral vein during knee flexion done to facilitate tumescent injections. Failure to appreciate and recognize this movement of the laser tip could lead to laser ablation of the CFV with permanent serious detrimental consequences.

A tumescent solution consisting of 500 ml of normal saline, 50 ml of 1% lidocaine with epinephrine, and 50 ml of 8.4% sodium bicarbonate is prepared. Using a micropuncture needle, the solution is injected just above and parallel to the sheath to create a layer of tumescence surrounding the sheath and laser fiber. The ultrasound probe is held in longitudinal view during tumescence. A cross-sectional view verifies adequate tumescence around a collapsed vein. If the vein is under a fascial layer, the cross-sectional view of the laser fiber and sheath within the vein after tumescence should look like an "eye" (Fig. 3). The purpose of the tumescence is fourfold. First, it helps to push blood out of the vein and collapse the vein wall onto the laser, preventing a layer of blood from "protecting" the vein wall from the intentional thermal injury. Second, it pushes surrounding tissue away from the vein, including saphenous or sural nerve fibers. Third, the lidocaine anesthetizes the surrounding soft tissues; and finally, it provides a "heat sink" around the vein to dilute and dissipate the heat from the laser energy. The layer of tumescence should "push" the vein down so that it is at least 1 cm below the surface of the skin. The tumescent solution may be delivered with hand injections using a traditional syringe, an autofill syringe, or by use

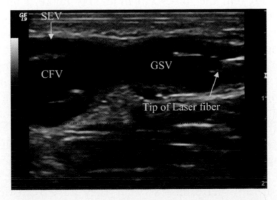

Fig. 2. Position of laser fiber distal to the superficial epigastric vein.

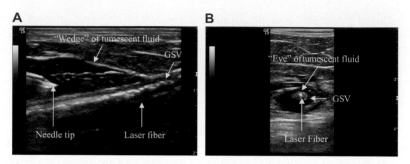

Fig. 3. Longitudinal (*A*) and cross-sectional (*B*) views during tumescence.

of a peristaltic pump (such as a Klein pump, HK Surgical, San Clemente, CA). In our practice, the authors have found that use of the peristaltic pump decreases procedure time, reduces hand fatigue, more adequately empties and compresses the target vein, and provides a larger column of fluid around the vein than can be achieved with manual injections. The pump speed can be varied depending on the size of the vein.

The patient is placed in the Trendelenburg position before tumescent anesthesia. It is important to have the vein as empty as possible, using tumescence and positioning to drain the vein of blood. After appropriate protective eyewear is placed on the patient and all personnel, the laser is activated and slowly pulled back. Pullback rate and watts of power used vary depending on which laser device is used, and inexperienced users should follow the manufacturer's instructions. With experience, one may wish to vary energy delivered and pullback speed depending on the diameter of the vein being treated and the depth of the vein from the skin.

Patients undergoing EVLT may undergo concomitant procedures, such as microphlebectomy, perforator ligation, or foam sclerotherapy. Timing these interventions during the case (before or after the laser ablation) should take into account that the tumescent fluid may make it impossible to see branch varicosities or perforator veins adjacent to the GSV or SSV. One may wish to access these veins with an angiocatheter or butterfly needle before tumescence if foam sclerotherapy is planned. In general, the further a branch varicosity lies away from the saphenous trunk that is treated, the less likely it is to be nonvisible after treatment. For example, anterior and lateral thigh and calf veins bulge less after EVLT of the GSV, but are likely still visible and cosmetically bothersome. Concomitant treatment of such veins with microphlebectomy or sclerotherapy yields a better cosmetic result and improved patient satisfaction. Based on the distribution of varicosities, during the preoperative visit the patient should be counseled about the likelihood that visible varicosities will still exist after EVLT if there is no concomitant therapy performed so that they have realistic expectations about the procedure outcome.

At the completion of the procedure, the SFJ and SPJ are inspected with duplex ultrasound to make sure there is no thrombus extending into the common femoral or popliteal veins. In the authors' practice, if we believe we see thrombus in the SFJ or SPJ on completion (when tumescence or laser induced steam bubbles often obscure a clear view), we may administer a subcutaneous dose of low molecular weight heparin (LMWH) on the procedure table, with a follow-up duplex evaluation the next day. In most of those patients, no thrombus is identified on that second visit. When the procedure is completed, the laser access site is covered with a steri-strip and a transparent dressing. Microphlebectomy and perforator ligation incisions are likewise dressed. Any veins treated with foam sclerotherapy are covered with compression pads. The authors place absorbent pads over the pathway of the vein treated with EVLT to absorb any tumescent fluid that might leak out of the skin. A class II or III compression stocking is then placed over the limb. The stocking is worn constantly for 2 to 4 days without removal, and then removed for bathing, but then otherwise worn for the next 2 weeks. The patient immediately ambulates and is instructed to try to walk regularly for the next several days.

Postoperatively the patient has another check of the SFJ or SPJ within the first week to assess for clot extension into deep veins, which we refer to as endovenous heat-induced thrombosis (EHIT; as termed by Kabnick and colleagues [28]). Patients generally return to normal activity levels within days after the procedure. Unless extensive microphlebectomies have been done, most patients do not require narcotic analgesics and do well with NSAIDs for pain control. The most common postprocedure complaints are an aching discomfort in the path of the laser lasting 12 to 14 days and a tight pulling sensation along the course of the treated vein for up to 2 months. In the authors' practice, patients are seen in follow-up at 2 weeks and 6 to 8 weeks postprocedure. Photo documentation of the appearance of the limb after treatment is taken at the final follow-up visit.

Complications

Serious complications following EVLT are uncommon. Pulmonary emboli are extremely rare with only one literature report found in the authors' review [9]. Extension of clot into deep veins has been noted by many investigators, with an incidence of 0% to 8% for the GSV [8,9,29] and 0% to 5.7% for the SSV [9,22,23]. The variability in the observation of deep vein thrombus is likely accounted for by different techniques, learning curve, the sensitivity of the equipment used to detect the thrombus, and the time interval between EVLT and imaging to look for thrombus. In our clinical experience, the authors have discovered several EHITs 3 days post-EVLT that are no longer present 1 week post-EVLT with only daily aspirin treatment. The authors agree with Kabnick and colleagues that EHITs do not behave like de novo DVT. Kabnick's abstract suggested that clots flush with the SFJ or SPJ do not need anticoagulation and clots extending into the SFJ or SPJ filling less than 50% of the diameter of the deep vein be treated with LMWH until the thrombus recedes out of the deep vein. Clots filling greater than 50% of the diameter of the deep vein or occlusive clots are treated with standard DVT treatments [28]. The authors use a similar algorithm as that proposed by Kabnick and colleagues with some modification. In our practice, the authors also observe "tails" of thrombus extending into the SFJ or SPJ by 0.5 cm or less if they are not occupying a significant cross-sectional diameter of the deep vein (although the significance of the filling is left to the discretion of the treating physician). The authors have found it helpful for our vascular technologists to sketch out a longitudinal and cross-sectional drawing of the EHIT for help in assessing whether this is merely a "tail" of the GSV or SSV thrombus, versus a significant clot impeding venous return and threatening occlusion. These patients are observed with serial ultrasound and are placed on LMWH if the clot extends under observation. The authors find that most thin tails of thrombus recede quickly, with many patients requiring observation or anticoagulation for only days or weeks. Although neither Kabnick's nor the authors' algorithm has been clinically tested, in our practice with an experience of treating approximately 1800 limbs over three and a half years we have had no pulmonary emboli or significant clot extensions.

When the technique of EVLT was being developed, manufacturers recommended that ablation be performed in the above-knee portion of the GSV only. This recommendation was driven by concerns about saphenous and sural nerve injury. Saphenous neuralgia is a common complication after GSV stripping, especially below the knee [16,30,31]. Injury to the sural nerve [32–34] and even the tibial nerve [35] has been reported with SSV stripping. The preponderance of published reports show that paresthesias following ELVT GSV [8,9,20,36] and the SSV are uncommon [9,22,23]. The authors routinely treat the SSV and the GSV to the distal calf, and start some GSV ablations just above the medial malleolus and some SSV ablations at or below the lateral malleolus, always maintaining an adequate tumescence column. In the authors' practice the most common manifestation of nerve injury is numbness, and actual neurogenic pain is rare. In most patients, the numbness is self-limited, improving over a period of months, and few patients find it to be bothersome.

Many studies describe the incidence of bruising and discomfort following EVLT, but in the authors' experience these are self-limited issues and severe bruising and pain are not common. Certainly we have found, as demonstrated by others [8,11], that endovenous therapies have significantly less postprocedure discomfort and bruising as compared with traditional surgical therapies. The authors have seen no clinically significant infections caused specifically by EVLT (excepting erythema at the access site treated with oral antibiotics) but have had three infections requiring incisions and drainage in areas of perforator ligation and sclerotherapy performed as concomitant procedures. There is one literature report of a phlegmonous infection of a limb treated with surgical drainage and antibiotics [37]. Hyperpigmentation along the course of the treated vein can be seen, especially if the vein is above the fascial level and in thin individuals. In the authors' experience, the SSV is invariably surrounded by a fascial sheath and we have not seen hyperpigmentation following SSV EVLT. Although not clinically proven, adequate tumescence to empty the vein of blood and depress it away from the skin and patient compliance with adequate compression may decrease the chance of hyperpigmentation. In all but the most severe cases, which are rare, the authors have seen hyperpigmented areas gradually fade to the point that they are no longer noticeable over a period ranging from a few months to a year.

Summary

Advances in imaging and catheter technology made the development of EVLT possible. EVLT offers patients a fast outpatient procedure with minimal downtime and discomfort. The procedure is durable and safe. It is versatile and allows the practitioner to treat incompetence of the saphenous trunks and accessory branches. In combination with concomitant treatments such as microphlebectomy and foam sclerotherapy aided by real-time high resolution ultrasound, excellent cosmetic and functional results can be achieved in most patients. Incorporating EVLT into the authors' practice has increased the satisfaction of our patients and has enabled us to treat a wider variety of patients with a more efficient procedure compared with traditional techniques.

References

[1] Sisto T, Reunanen A, Laurikka J, et al. Prevalence and risk factors of varicose veins in lower extremities: mini-Finland health survey. Eur J Surg 1995;161(6):405–14.

[2] Callam MJ. Epidemiology of varicose veins. Br J Surg 1994;81(2):167–73.

[3] Englehorn CA, Englehorn AL, Cassou MF, et al. Patterns of saphenous reflux in women with varicose veins. J Vasc Surg 2005;41(4):645–51.

[4] Goldman MP. Closure of the greater saphenous vein with endoluminal radiofrequency thermal heating of the vein wall in combination with ambulatory phlebectomy: preliminary 6-month follow-up. Dermatol Surg 2000;26(5):452–6.

[5] Boné C. Tratamiento endoluminal de las varices con laser de diodo; estudio reliminary. Rev Patol Vasc 1999;5:35–46.

[6] Navarro L, Min R, Boné C. Endovenous laser: a new minimally invasive treatment for varicose veins—preliminary observations using an 810 nm diode laser. Dermatol Surg 2001;27:117–22.

[7] New Device Approval. Available at: http://www.fda.gov/cdrh/pdf/p990021a.pdf. Accessed April 2007.

[8] Min RJ, Khilnani N, Zimmet SE. Endovenous laser treatment of saphenous vein reflux: long-term results. J Vasc Interv Radiol 2003;14:991–6.

[9] Ravi R, Rodriguez-Lopez JA, Traylor EA, et al. Endovenous ablation of incompetent saphenous veins: a large single-center experience. J Endovasc Ther 2006;13:244–8.

[10] de Medeiros CA, Luccas GC. Comparison of endovenous treatment with an 810 nm laser versus conventional stripping of the great saphenous vein in patients with primary varicose veins. Dermatol Surg 2005;31(12):1685–94.

[11] Lurie F, Creton D, Eklof B, et al. Prospective randomized study of endovenous radiofrequency obliteration (closure procedure) versus ligation and stripping in a selected patient population (EVOLVeS Study). J Vasc Surg 2003;38(2):207–14.

[12] Perala J, Rautio T, Biancari F. Radiofrequency endovenous obliteration versus stripping of the long saphenous vein in management of primary varicose veins: 3 year outcome of a randomized study. Ann Vasc Surg 2005;19(5):669–72.

[13] Puggioni A, Kalra M, Carmo M, et al. Endovenous laser therapy and radiofrequency ablation of the great saphenous vein: analysis of early efficacy and complications. J Vasc Surg 2005;42(3):488–93.

[14] Higorani AP, Ascher E, Markevich N. Deep venous thrombosis after radiofrequency ablation of greater saphenous vein: a word of caution. J Vasc Surg 2004;40(3):500–4.

[15] van Rij AM, Chai J, Hill GB, et al. Incidence of deep vein thrombosis after varicose vein surgery. Br J Surg 2004;91(12):1582–5.

[16] Subramonia S, Lees T. Sensory abnormalities and bruising after long saphenous vein stripping: impact on short-term quality of life. J Vasc Surg 2005;42(3):510–4.

[17] Jones L, Braithwaite BD, Selwyn D, et al. Neovascularisation is the principal cause of varicose vein recurrence: results of a randomized trial of stripping the long saphenous vein. Eur J Vasc Endovasc Surg 1996;12(4):442–5.

[18] Merchant RF, Pichot O, Myers KA. Four-year follow-up on endovascular radiofrequency obliteration of great saphenous reflux. Dermatol Surg 2005;31(2):129–34.

[19] Vasquez MA, Wang J, Mahathanaruk M, et al. The utility of the Venous Clinical Severity Score in 682 limbs treated by radiofrequency saphenous vein ablation. J Vasc Surg 2007; 45(5):1008–15.

[20] Kabnick LS. Outcome of different endovenous laser wavelengths for great saphenous vein ablation. J Vasc Surg 2006;43(1):88–93.

[21] Proebstle TM, Moehler T, Gul D, et al. Endovenous treatment of the great saphenous vein using a 1,320 nm Nd:YAG laser causes fewer side effects than using a 940 nm diode laser. Dermatol Surg 2005;31(12):1678–84.

[22] Gibson KD, Ferris BF, Polissar N, et al. Endovenous laser treatment of the small saphenous vein: efficacy and complications. J Vasc Surg 2007;45(4):795–803.

[23] Proebstle TM, Gul D, Kargl A, et al. Endovenous laser treatment of the lesser saphenous vein with a 940-nm diode laser: early results. Dermatol Surg 2003;29(4):357–61.

[24] Stuart WP, Adam DJ, Allan PL, et al. The relationship between the number, competence, and diameter of medial calf perforating veins and the clinical status in healthy subjects and patients with lower-limb venous disease. J Vasc Surg 2000;32(1):138–43.

[25] Gloviczki P, Bergan JJ, Rhodes JM, et al. Mid-term results of endoscopic perforator vein interruption for chronic venous insufficiency: lessons learned from the North American subfascial endoscopic perforator surgery registry. North American Study Group. J Vasc Surg 1999;29(3):489–502.

[26] Peden E, Lumsden A. Radiofrequency ablation of incompetent perforating veins. Perspect Vasc Surg Endovasc Ther 2007;19(1):73–7.

[27] Uchino IJ. Endovenous laser closure of the perforating vein of the leg. Phlebology 2007; 22(2):80–2.

[28] Kabnick LS, Ombrellino M, Agis H, et al. Endovenous heat induced thrombus (EHIT) at the superficial-deep venous junction: a new post-treatment clinical entity, classification and potential treatment strategies. Abstract presented at American Venous Forum 18th Annual Meeting. Miami (FL), February 23, 2006.

[29] Mozes G, Kalra M, Carmo M, et al. Extension of saphenous thrombus into the femoral vein: a potential complication of new endovenous ablation techniques. J Vasc Surg 2005;41:130–5.

[30] Holme JB, Skajaa K, Holme K. Incidence of lesions of the saphenous nerve after partial or complete stripping of the long saphenous vein. Acta Chir Scand 1990;156(2):145–8.

[31] Morrison C, Dalsing MC. Signs and symptoms of saphenous nerve injury after greater saphenous vein stripping: prevalence, severity and relevance for modern practice. J Vasc Surg 2003;38(5):886–90.

[32] Mondelli M, Reale F, Cavallaro T. Neuroma of the sural nerve as a complication of stripping of the small saphenous vein. Surg Neurol 1997;48(4):330–2.

[33] Seror P. Sural nerve lesions: a report of 20 cases. Am J Phys Med Rehabil 2002;81(11): 876–80.

[34] Simonetti S, Bianchi S, Martinoli C. Neurophysiological and ultrasound findings in sural nerve lesions following stripping of the small saphenous vein. Muscle Nerve 1999;22(12): 1724–6.

[35] Prandl EC, Schintler M, Scharnagl E, et al. Severing of the tibial nerve with stripping of the lesser saphenous vein—a rare complication of surgery for varicosity [abstract]. Chirurg 2006; 77(9):856–7.

[36] Siani A, Flaishman I, Rossi A, et al. Indications and result of endovenous laser treatment (EVLT) for greater saphenous incompetence. Our experience. Minerva Cardioangiol 2006;54(3):369–76.

[37] Dunst KM, Huemer GM, Wayand W, et al. Diffuse phlegmonous phlebitis after endovenous laser treatment of the greater saphenous vein. J Vasc Surg 2006;43(5):1056–8.

ELSEVIER
SAUNDERS

SURGICAL
CLINICS OF
NORTH AMERICA

Surg Clin N Am 87 (2007) 1267–1284

Endovenous Radiofrequency Ablation of Superficial and Perforator Veins

Steven M. Roth, MD, MS[a,b,*]

[a]*Vein Care Pavilion of the South, 447 North Belair Road, Suite 103, Evans, GA 30809, USA*
[b]*University Surgical Associates, 818 St. Sebastian Way, Augusta, GA 30901, USA*

In general, the overall lack of enthusiasm for the treatment of chronic venous insufficiency in the past stemmed from less objective testing methods and more invasive surgical procedures that were fraught with increased patient morbidity and dissatisfaction. Primary venous insufficiency and varicose veins are important vascular conditions that affect 25 million people in Western civilization [1]. The management of superficial and perforator venous reflux disease has progressed to encompass more objective diagnostic methods, including venous duplex scanning and treatment procedures that are more simplified by minimally invasive, endovenous techniques. One such endovascular procedure called radiofrequency ablation (RFA) has been accepted in recent years as a favorable alternative to conventional surgery.

The successful treatment of lower extremity chronic venous insufficiency includes the elimination of all sources of venous reflux. The most common sources of reflux are superficial veins, which may or may not include the deep or perforator venous systems [2–4]. The primary objective in the treatment of superficial and perforator venous reflux disease is elimination of the refluxing veins from the venous circulation. The traditional surgical approach for saphenous vein reflux has been saphenous vein ligation at the saphenofemoral junction with ligation of all tributary vessels, with or without removal of the refluxing saphenous vein. Sclerotherapy of the incompetent saphenous vein has been found to be short lived and is not a recommended technique [5]. Reducing venous hypertension in this manner was not usually enough to eliminate truncal varicosities, and frequently required stab phlebectomy at the same time or later by sclerotherapy. Eliminating perforator vein reflux required open (Linton procedure) or endoscopic interruption of

* Vein Care Pavilion of the South, 447 North Belair Road, Suite 103, Evans, GA 30809.
E-mail address: vascularman40@yahoo.com

0039-6109/07/$ - see front matter © 2007 Elsevier Inc. All rights reserved.
doi:10.1016/j.suc.2007.07.009
surgical.theclinics.com

abnormal venous flow (subfascial endoscopic perforator vein surgery or SEPS), and sclerotherapy with or without ultrasound guidance. With world-wide clinical experience increasing, endovenous RFA has become the most common alternative approach to superficial and perforator venous reflux disease [5].

Radiofrequency ablation mechanism of action

Endovenous RFA, also referred to as the VNUS Closure procedure (VNUS Medical Technologies Inc., San Jose, California) is a catheter-based endovascular intervention. The direction of RF energy into tissue to cause its destruction is safer and more controllable than other mechanisms used for this purpose. With RF energy delivered in continuous or sinusoidal-wave mode, there is no stimulation of neuromuscular cells when a high frequency (between 200 and 3000 kHz) is used. The mechanism by which RF current heats tissue is resistive (or ohmic) heating of a narrow rim of tissue that is in direct contact with the electrode. Deeper tissue planes are then slowly heated by conduction from the small region of volume heating. Heat is dissipated from the region by further heat conduction into normo-thermic tissue. By regulating the degree of heating, subtle gradations of either controlled collagen contraction or total thermocoagulation of the vein wall can be achieved. The heat produced during RFA is caused by the resistance of the tissue in the veins wall allowing passage of the current. Therefore, during this resistive heating, the heat is generated in the vein wall and not in the catheter tip. A thermocouple on one of the electrodes applied to the vein wall measures the temperature, which can be kept constant by negative feedback. Clinically, the device produces precise tissue destruction with endothelial denudation, denaturing of the media and intramural collagen, with subsequent fibrotic seal of the vein lumen with minimal formation of thrombus and coagulum. Bipolar electrodes are used to heat the vein wall. The net effect is venous spasm and collagen shrinkage that produce maximal physical contraction [6]. The selective insulation of the electrodes results in a preferential delivery of the radiofrequency energy to the vein wall and minimal heating of the blood within the vessel, which eliminates vessel perforation.

The thermal effect on the vein wall is directly related to the treatment temperature and the treatment time, the latter being a function of catheter pullback speed. With a treatment temperature of 85° to 90°C at a pullback speed of 3 to 4 cm /min, the thermal effect induced sufficient collagen contraction to occlude the lumen, while limiting heat penetration to perivenous tissue. In an in vitro model measuring changes in adventitial temperature along the vein, the highest temperature measured was 64°C, and after a 2 mm tumescent fluid layer, this decreased to 51°C. This emphasizes one of the benefits of tumescent fluid infiltration during the clinical procedure [7].

The other endovenous catheter-based thermoablation technique employs a laser system. Several companies now make laser systems that use variable wavelengths (810 nm–1320 nm). With laser, heat is generated by the action of the laser on the chromophore (substance that absorbs the laser light). It is thought that the mechanism of damage to the vein wall is the generation of a steam bubble around the laser tip from the blood still within the vein. This steam then transmits its heat to the vein wall via the high temperature gradient. The major chromophore at shorter wavelengths is hemoglobin, and longer wavelengths may have more of an action on water and collagen. The laser is fired and the vein wall is heated, probably via the steam bubble that is produced (boiling blood). There is no feedback, so control is by the amount of energy put into the fiber, the number and length of the pulses per centimeter if pulsed treatment is used, or the rate of pullback of the fiber if continuous laser energy is used. Thus there have been concerns that the variability of the amount of blood within the vein itself, the variability of the thickness of the vein wall, and the lack of any feedback information during treatment mean that it is difficult to know if one is under- or overtreating. Because this variability is more likely with laser and not RFA, laser treatment is, in the author's opinion, less likely to give consistently reproducible results and more likely to cause vessel perforation and patient discomfort and ecchymosis [8,9].

The Closure system and radiofrequency ablation technique

Radiofrequency ablation is performed using the Closure catheter noted above. There are currently three types of catheters: (1) ClosurePLUS in both 6 Fr and 8 Fr for saphenous veins and accessory branches (Fig. 1); (2) radiofrequency system ClosureRFS and ClosurePLEX catheters for perforator veins (Fig. 2); and (3) the newly released ClosureFAST catheter for saphenous veins and accessory branches (Fig. 3). The ClosurePLUS catheter is designed for delivery of controlled RF to shrink vein wall collagen, and includes collapsible catheter electrodes around which the vein may shrink, and a central lumen to allow a guide wire or fluid delivery structured within a 5 Fr (1.7 mm) catheter. This design permits treatment of veins as small as 2 mm and as large as 24 mm. The thermocouple on the electrode measures temperature and provides feedback to the RF generator. The control unit displays power, impedance, temperature, and elapsed time so that precise temperature control is obtained. The RF generator delivers the minimum power necessary to maintain the desired electrode temperature (Fig. 4).

Detailed procedure techniques have been described elsewhere [10,11]. The patient may be given oral or intravenous sedation and placed in a supine position on an adjustable table. The course of the greater saphenous vein (GSV) from the saphenofemoral junction to the knee, the lesser saphenous vein (LSV) from its junction with the gastrocnemic, popliteal, or other deep

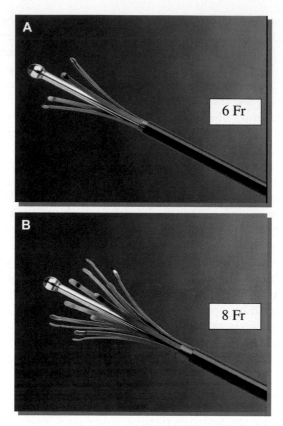

Fig. 1. VNUS ClosurePLUS 6 Fr catheter (*A*) and 8 Fr catheter (*B*). (*Courtesy of* VNUS Medical Technologies, San Jose, California; with permission.)

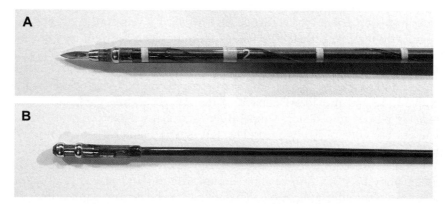

Fig. 2. VNUS ClosureRFS catheter (*A*) and VNUS ClosurePLEX catheter (*B*). (*Courtesy of* VNUS Medical Technologies, San Jose, California; with permission.)

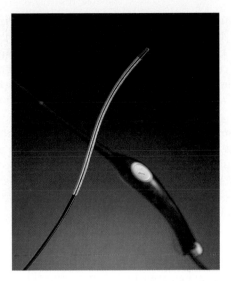

Fig. 3. VNUS ClosureFAST catheter. (*Courtesy of* VNUS Medical Technologies, San Jose, California; with permission.).

vein to the mid calf, and accessory branch (ie, anterior lateral branch) from its origin to the knee is mapped 6 to 8 cm apart using duplex ultrasound (Logic e, GE Medical Systems Ultrasound and Primary Care Diagnostics LLC, Milwaukee, Wisconsin) and marked with indelible ink. A patch of nitropaste may be applied to the planned access site before sterile surgical preparation to help dilate the vein and prevent venospasm (which can make percutaneous access difficult). Other venous dilation techniques may be applied as well (heating pad, tourniquet, reverse Trendelenburg position, and the like). After sterile preparation, the access sites and those sites marked previously are infiltrated with 1% buffered xylocaine without epinephrine. The vein is accessed using ultrasound guidance in transverse or longitudinal view with a 21 gauge needle that can accommodate a .018" wire. The smaller needle and wire are much more forgiving in causing

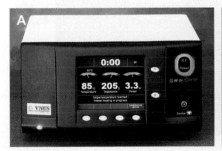
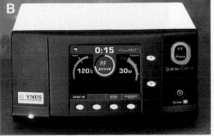

Fig. 4. Radiofrequency generator (RFG) PLUS screen with ClosurePLUS (*A*) and ClosureFAST (*B*). (*Courtesy of* VNUS Medical Technologies, San Jose, California; with permission.)

venospasm than an 18 gauge needle and .035" guide wire. Using the Sel-denger technique, the introducer sheath (6 Fr or 8 Fr) is advanced into the vein. A 6 or 8 Fr catheter is advanced up to the appropriate end point. For the GSV, the catheter is delivered 1 cm below the ostium of the super-ficial epigastric vein. This position is confirmed by ultrasound (Fig. 5). The patient is placed into significant Trendelenberg position, and approximately 200 to 400 mL of tumescent fluid (normal saline, 1% xylocaine with epi-nephrine, bicarbonate) is injected directly, under ultrasound guidance, into the saphenous compartment from the insertion site up to 3 cm below the saphenofemoral junction. The tumescent solution provides local anes-thetic, protects the surrounding tissues from heat-related damage, and com-presses the vein around the catheter electrodes, ensuring complete vein wall treatment. The final position of the tip of the catheter is confirmed by ultra-sound and the final injection of tumescent fluid is injected into the tissue sur-rounding the proximal 3 cm of the GSV where visualization will now be more obscured. To optimize exsanguination of the vein a circumferentially placed Esmark wrap can be applied. External compression to ensure contact between the vein wall and the electrodes and to maintain the temperature of the tip of the catheter at 85° to 90°C can be achieved manually with the ul-trasound probe. The withdrawal rate varies with desired treatment temper-ature. At conclusion of the procedure, the patency of the common femoral artery and common femoral vein, (popliteal, tibial, and gastrocnemic veins with the LSV), successful contraction of the GSV with a residual diameter of

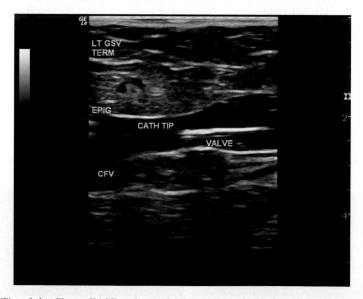

Fig. 5. Tip of the ClosureFAST catheter (CATH TIP) at the saphenofemoral junction 1 cm distal to the origin of the lateral superficial epigastric vein (EPIG). CFV, common femoral vein; GSV, greater saphenous vein.

less than 2 mm, and flow through the saphenofemoral junction (SFJ) into the lateral epigastric vein are confirmed by duplex examination (Fig. 6). Patients are then placed in elastic wrap bandages, and asked to wear graduated compression stockings with at least 30 mm/Hg of compression and to walk at least 30 minutes per day. They are told to resume normal activity immediately and encouraged to resume aerobic exercise, but to avoid weight lifting for the next 2 or 3 days. A duplex ultrasound scan should be performed within 72 hours postoperatively to rule out any evidence of deep vein thrombosis (DVT). The procedure is commonly performed on an outpatient basis in an office setting, minor procedure room, ambulatory surgical center, or a traditional operating room.

The technique required for perforator vein RFA requires more detailed mapping than for superficial veins. Because the perforator veins are typically not linear in orientation like the superficial veins, and are more curvilinear and angulated throughout their course, adequate visualization with duplex ultrasound to allow for easy access can be challenging. Once an adequate approach angle has been identified and the access site marked, similar preparations are made as noted above. A rigid radiofrequency stylet (Closure RFS) catheter or more flexible catheter (ClosurePLEX) may be used. The perforator vein is accessed directly with the ClosureRFS catheter using duplex ultrasound. A 21 gauge access needle and .018" guide wire are used to access the perforator vein using the Seldinger technique when the ClosurePLEX is used. Either catheter is advanced to the level of the muscular fascia.

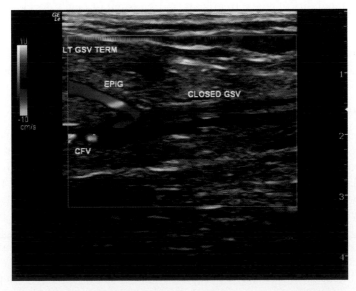

Fig. 6. Flow from common femoral vein (CFV) through terminal greater saphenous vein (LT GSV TERM) and the lateral superficial epigastric vein (EPIG), greater saphenous vein (GSV) diameter <2 mm, and no flow demonstrated through the GSV (CLOSED GSV).

When the stylet is removed, the catheter tip of the ClosureRFS catheter will be in the proper position (5–10 mm from the fascia), whereas the Closure-PLEX should be pulled back 5 to 10 mm. The tip of the catheter is held in this position, tumescent fluid infiltration introduced above and below the catheter tip, and the patient placed in Trendelenberg position. The treatment temperature can be 85° to 90° C for 5 minutes, pulling back 1 to 10 mm during the last 1 minute. During the first 4 minutes the catheter tip is rotated to the 12, 6, 3, and 9 o'clock positions, each for 1 minute of treatment. An alternative technique uses a 12 gauge angiocatheter to initially access the perforator vein with duplex ultrasound and act as a portal for the ClosureRFS or ClosurePLEX catheters. Once the treatment is completed, the deep veins and arteries are assessed for patency, the catheters removed, and pressure is applied. Patients have a stretch wrap applied to the leg with a graduated compression stocking of at least 30 mm/Hg, and are asked not to remove it for 3 to 4 days. Patients are expected to resume normal activity just as with the superficial veins, and a follow-up scan is done within 72 hours.

Although SEPS has recently been the most common way to treat incompetent perforator veins, there are several potential advantages of using ultrasound-guided endovenous RFA. The first is that the intervention is truly a minimally invasive procedure that can be performed in the office. Unlike SEPS, the approach is not limited by the perforating vein location. With RFA technique, the physician can access the incompetent perforator veins (IPVs)at various positions including the more proximal locations (Boyd's, Dodd's, Hunter's, lateral perforators, perimalleolar). The procedure also allows the flexibility of repeat treatment for persistent or newly developed IPVs. The use of RFA is generally reserved for patients who have advanced chronic venous insufficiency with clinical, etiologic, anatomic, and pathophysiologic (CEAP) classes 4 to 6, although it can be performed as part of the primary treatment for varicose veins, and is useful for treating recurrent varicose veins.

Radiofrequency ablation safety

The VNUS Closure system received US Food and Drug Administration (FDA) approval in March 1999. To date, there have been over 100,000 RFA procedures performed worldwide, and its safety has been carefully reported [12–14]. Most impressively, a clinical registry was established in 1998 to monitor procedure safety and treatment outcomes. More than 30 centers worldwide contributed data, and RFA has the largest collection of published data in endovenous surgery, including registry data regarding endovenous therapy with 5 year follow-up, and both single center data and multicenter randomized trials comparing RFA with vein stripping.

Modifications in the RFA procedure were made as data were reported. Tumescent infiltration was initiated to reduce the risk of skin burns, which are rarely observed now. DVT is a potential risk for any surgical procedure. In the setting of RFA, DVT can originate from the treated superficial or perforator vein and extend into the deep venous system. Attention is drawn to careful tip positioning to ensure that treatment begins a short distance from the SFJ, and to preserve the physiological blood flow from the superficial epigastric tributary. Immediate and sufficient ambulation is encouraged in addition to the follow-up ultrasound scan within 72 hours. The DVT rates were reported to be 0% to 1% in most series that have been published. In one series [15], DVT was detected in 12 of 73 limbs (16.4%), which is felt to be an aberrancy from the experiences of others [16,17].

Paresthesia was reported to occur in 9% to 19% of limbs within 1 week after the procedure [12–14,18–27], and gradually resolved over time [25]. Limiting treatment to the above-knee segment decreases the risk of paresthesia because 90% of the time the saphenous nerve travels within the saphenous compartment from the groin to the knee, and then travels superficial to this compartment, and thus is more susceptible to injury with heat in the below-knee location despite tumescent fluid infiltration. Similarly, with RFA treatment of the LSV, the peroneal nerve and superficial branches of the sural nerve emerge around mid-calf level and should be avoided [7].

Treatment efficacy and outcomes

Pichot and colleagues [28] have described the morphological and hemodynamic outcomes following RFA using detailed duplex ultrasound. There is a sonographic progression observed in the pathologic sequelae of the treated vein. Veins closed completely were initially hypoechogenic compared with the surrounding tissue, and progressed into a hyperechogenic state and finally became isoechogenic, indicating a healing process. Approximately 60% of veins were hypoechogenic and 40% were hyperechogenic at 1 week. At 6 months, they became either hyperechogenic or isoechogenic. Weiss [19] demonstrated the sonographic disappearance of the saphenous vein in 90% of limbs after 2 years.

Anatomical failure is defined as partial or nonocclusion of a treated vein resulting from incomplete treatment or subsequent recanalization. It has been demonstrated that even with anatomical failure, clinical improvement was often demonstrated in patients [25]. The strong possibility of later recurrence in these patients was also evident.

Morphologic differences in the SFJ following RFA have been studied. Four types of SFJ morphologies were identified [25,28,29]. The three most common include: J-1, defined as complete SFJ obliteration with no SFJ flow; J-2 as patent SFJ tributaries draining toward the femoral vein with or without a short saphenous stump; and J-3 as terminal GSV competence with normal antegrade flow coming from both tributaries and the saphenous vein above a limited GSV obliteration. Two years after RFA, the most common findings were either complete SFJ obliteration or a 5 cm or less patent terminal stump conducting antegrade tributary flow through the SFJ, accounting for approximately 90% of the limbs treated [25,29].

The clinical significance of a short patent SFJ stump was analyzed by Merchant and colleagues [25]. A total of 319 limbs (286 patients) in the clinical registry were followed up at 1 week, 6 months, 1 year, and 2 years, with 121 limbs having 2-year data. Symptom improvement and varicose vein absence demonstrated no statistically significant differences between patients who have complete SFJ obliteration and those who have a short patent SFJ stump at any follow-up time points. Although the distal trunk is occluded, SFJ competence is often restored, even with a short patent stump. A patent stump can serve a conduit and preserve the normal physiologic flow from one or more patent tributaries, such as those draining blood from abdominal and pudendal areas. Preservation of this physiological flow has been considered to be an advantage of endovenous procedures over traditional veins stripping because it causes less hemodynamic disturbance. More hemodynamic disturbance is thought to be one of the factors responsible for stimulating neovascularization following vein stripping.

RFA treatment results for large veins were studied by Merchant and colleagues [30]. In the 5-year registry data, there were 39 veins with diameter greater than 12 mm (maximum diameter 24 mm). Vein occlusion rate was 97% within 1 week and 92.6% at 6 months and 1 year. The author has had similar experience (Fig. 7).

The efficacy of RFA treatment has been reported by several groups [19–27]. The largest study with the longest follow-up is the clinical registry series. A 90% reflux-free rate was reported at 2 years [15]. The latest available results with 5-year follow-up data demonstrated RFA treatment efficacy of 84% compared with 89% at 1 year, showing the durability of the treatment. It is important to note that in the registry the patients who have longer follow-ups are those treated at the very early stages of RFA. Because the RFA procedure technique has improved compared with earlier treatments, treatment efficacy has improved.

Patient symptom relief has been reported by several studies. Approximately 85%, 79%, and 39% of limbs had pain, fatigue, or edema, respectively, before the procedure; these decreased to 29%, 7%, and 8% within 1 week after the procedure. A further decrease of the percentage of symptomatic limbs was observed at 6 months, and the symptom improvement remained stable over 5 years. Pullback speed less than 3 cm/min and body mass index (BMI) greater than 25 m/kg^2 were identified as risk factors for anatomical failure. These results have established the long-term treatment outcomes of RFA in eliminating saphenous reflux and alleviating patient symptoms.

Endovenous radiofrequency ablation versus vein stripping

The premise behind both RFA and traditional vein stripping is to remove the incompetent vein from the venous circulation to reduce the venous hypertension, with subsequent resolution of symptoms without significant morbidity. The advantages of RFA over vein stripping are demonstrated

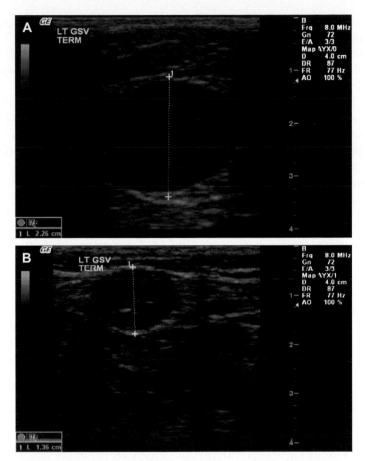

Fig. 7. (*A*) Before VNUS Closure was performed on large greater saphenous vein (GSV), it measured 22.6 mm. (*B*) Three months after VNUS closure, the terminal GSV (LT GSV TERM) had no flow and measured 13.6 mm.

in three randomized comparative trials. Rautio and colleagues [20] reported significantly less postoperative pain, quantitated with a visual analog scale, in the RFA group than in the stripping group at rest, on standing, and on walking, with the most distinct differences between the 5th to the 14th post-operative days. The analgesics needed in the RFA patients were statistically less for the stripping group. Sick leaves were also significantly shorter in the RFA group, and physical function was restored faster in the RFA patients, measured with the RAND-36 generic health-related quality of life (QOL) questionnaire. All the operations were successful and the complications were similar between the two groups in this study. These patients were fol-lowed-up at 3 years [31]. Venous clinical severity scores (VCSS) were similar for both groups. None of the RFA-occluded GSVs were recanalized. Vari-cose vein recurrence rate was documented in 5 of 15 limbs (33%) in the RFA group and 3 of 13 limbs (23%) in the stripping group, and the difference was not statistically significant. Similarly, Stötter and colleagues [21], in their randomized trial in Germany, reported a significantly lower pain score in the RFA group versus the stripping group within 6 weeks following the procedure.

RFO and vein stripping were further compared on bilaterally recurrent patients [32]. Sixteen patients who had bilateral recurrent GSV reflux were randomly treated with RFA on one leg and with vein stripping on the other leg. The RFA was faster (25 minutes versus 40 minutes), associated with significantly less postoperative pain and bruising, and had higher patient preference. It was concluded that RFA should be the treatment of choice for recurrent saphenous vein reflux.

The VNUS company sponsored a multicenter prospective randomized trial called EndoVenous Obliteration versus Ligation and Vein Stripping (EVOLVES). The early follow-up (within 4 months) focused on the comparison of the procedure related complications, patient recuperation, and quality of life outcomes between the two treatment procedures, and the procedure impact on the hemodynamic and clinical outcomes was demonstrated through 1 and 2 year follow-up evaluations [22,23]. Patients who had symptomatic varicose veins and GSV incompetence were randomized into either the RFA or the vein stripping group. RFA was performed on 44 limbs and stripping on 36 limbs. There were no differences between the groups in patient demographics, VCSS, or CEAP clinical class distribution before the treatment [25,33]. The most significant differences seen between the two groups were on patient recovery. The mean time to return to normal activity was 1.15 days for the RFA patients compared with 3.89 days ($P = .02$) for vein stripping. There were 80.5 % of RFA patients who returned to routine activities within 1 day, versus 46.9% of patients with stripping ($P < .01$). Mean values for the time to return to work were 4.7 days in the RFA group and 12.4 days in the stripping group ($P = .05$). Of note, there were significantly fewer complications and adverse advents observed in the RFA group through 3 weeks postoperatively, mostly because of higher rates of tenderness, ecchymosis, and hematoma following vein stripping. The postoperative VCSS were significantly different at 72 hours and 1 week, but the difference disappeared at later follow-up. The QOL surveys (CIVIQ2 questionnaire) showed clearly superior patient QOL in the RFA patients; the most significant differences were seen in global, pain, and physical scores. The pain score improvement form pretreatment baseline was significantly better in RFO than in the stripping patients at all the follow-up time points out to 2 years. The differences observed in global scores were statistically significant at 72 hours and 1 week, and surprisingly also at 1 and 2 years. Clinical and hemodynamic outcomes were similar for both groups at 2 years. There were no differences in patient symptoms and signs, and no differences on varicose vein recurrence rates. Duplex ultrasound examination revealed 91.7% and 89.7% of limbs free of reflux in the RFA and vein stripping groups, respectively. At 2 years, neovascularization was reported in 1 RFA limb (2.8%) and 4 vein stripping limbs (13.8%) ($P > .05$) [25,33].

The lower incidence of neovascularization with RFA was also reported by Pichot and colleagues [29]. Sixty three limbs were studied with ultrasound scan protocol and found to have no evidence of neovascularization at 2 years after the treatment. Two advantages of RFA that are thought to account for the low incidence of neovascularization are: (1) no incision and surgical dissection of the groin, and (2) minimal hemodynamic disturbance because of preservation of physiologic abdominal wall drainage. Recurrence can refer to either clinical recurrence (ie, varicose vein recurrence) or hemodynamic recurrence (ie, SFJ reflux). Varicose vein recurrence rates after vein stripping have been reported between 20% and 50% at 2 to 5 years [34–41] and up to 70% by 10 years [42]. The varicose vein recurrence rate is more subjective; the recurrence of SFJ reflux is a more objective measure and provides important hemodynamic information that permits detection and prediction of clinical recurrence. It was reported that 87% of limbs were free from reflux at 2 years and 71% were reflux free at 5 years after vein stripping [40]. Vein ligation without stripping achieved only 58% freedom from reflux at 2 years, and only 29% freedom from reflux at 5 years. Fischer and colleagues [43] studied 125 limbs after ligation of the true saphenofemoral junction and its related tributaries, and found that 60% of limbs had SFJ reflux at mean follow-up of 3.4 years.

New technology with endovenous ablation

The VNUS ClosureFAST catheter is the next generation of closure catheter that was developed to improve the procedure speed and the ease of use compared with the current Closure catheter. The catheter consists of a flexible catheter shaft and a 7 cm long distal heating element. The heating element has a fixed diameter and is covered with a glide cover to prevent sticking after heating. Good contact between the catheter and the vein wall is established by tumescent infiltration, Trendelenberg position, and external compression, and is monitored by an external thermocouple on the catheter and the computer software in the RF generator. The temperature of the heating element is monitored and controlled by a temperature sensor that regulates the amount of energy delivered during the treatment. Unlike the current Closure and endovenous laser devices that involve continuous pull-back, the ClosureFAST catheter uses segmental heating approach. Once the catheter is positioned and the vein appropriately compressed, the heating element is activated with RF energy for the duration of the 20-second heating cycle. The 7 cm element heats to 120°C, allowing for a 0.5 cm overlap between each treated segment to ensure complete treatment along the length. The new catheter does not require a saline drip, which is different from the previous VNUS catheters, and it appears to completely eliminate the high impedance issues caused by coagulum buildup with the previous catheter. After completion of the 20-second heating cycle, the catheter is positioned to the next segment, guided by the shaft markers, and treatment starts again. Accurate pullback is facilitated by positioning the sheath to align with one of the 6.5 cm markers on the catheter shaft. Two heating cycles are applied to the first segment near the SFJ to ensure sufficient treatment of this important segment (Fig. 8) [44].

The clinical experience with the ClosureFAST catheter comes from Europe. More than 200 limbs were treated, with the longest follow-up being 6 months. All treated veins remained closed at the latest follow-up, confirmed by ultrasound examinations. There were no DVTs, skin burns, or other serious adverse events. The average treatment time was 2.2 minutes, with an average treatment length of 37 cm. The average time from catheter insertion to catheter removal was approximately 16 minutes [44].

The new procedure is well-tolerated by patients, and there was no noticeable difference in patient reaction to this procedure compared with the current Closure procedure. Postprocedural recovery continued to be benign;

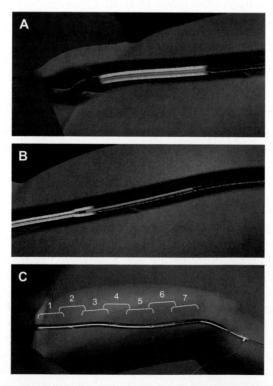

Fig. 8. (*A*) ClosureFAST catheter stationary during treatment at sapheno-femoral junction. (*B*) Slight overlap between treatments. (*C*) Vein treated stepwise along the length. (*Courtesy of* VNUS Medical Technologies, San Jose, California; with permission.)

79% of limbs experienced no pain and 87% experienced no tenderness. The experience of Lumsden and Peden [44] reported results that concurred with those of the European study. This is an important distinction between RFA and endovenous laser (EVL). After EVL, 67% to 100% of patients reported to have some degree of pain, with more than 50% of patients requiring analgesics for pain management, and a 10% to 33% rate of thrombophlebitis. The pain, bruising, and thrombophlebitis are thought to be the result of vein wall perforation and the thrombotic mechanism associated with EVL [45–47].

With the new device, a 40 cm-long vein segment can be treated stepwise in less than 3 minutes, which is equal to or faster than EVL protocols. The rate of immediate vein occlusion at the saphenofemoral junction is 100%, a value not reached previously by most users of laser and RFA. The limited number of side effects is clearly the same as with previous RFA procedures, but not nearly as high as with laser treatment.

Comparison of endoluminal techniques

Endovenous radiofrequency ablation is a new endoluminal treatment for those patients who have superficial and perforator venous reflux disease. These endoluminal techniques are challenging the traditional methods of open surgery that have been used for decades in treating primary varicose vein disease and venous stasis ulcer disease. The other endoluminal technique, EVL, can only be used for superficial venous reflux disease and cannot be used safely for perforator venous reflux disease. EVL has not been studied as thoroughly as RFA in comparing the endoluminal technique with open surgery [48,49]. The longest follow-up with clinical results after EVL has been 2 years, whereas detailed results are available at 5-year follow-up for RFA. There is no randomized controlled trial comparing RFA with EVL or sclerotherapy with endoluminal thermal obliteration; however, a randomized controlled trial comparing RFA to EVL demonstrated better primary obliteration and less postoperative pain and bruising with RFA [50]. In terms of thromboembolic events after endoluminal treatment, RFA and EVL presented an approximate equal rate of 0.5%. Vein closure after RFA was 87.2% in a multicenter study, and varicose vein recurrence was 27.4% at 5 year follow-up; vein obliteration after EVL was reported by various groups to be 76% to 96.8% at 1- to 2-year follow-up [50].

One of the advantages usually credited to EVL treatment is that the duration of the procedure is shorter than that for RFA because of the faster pullback speed. The new VNUS ClosureFAST catheter has eliminated this advantage. A cost comparison of the two techniques indicates that although the EVL fiber is cheaper than the RF catheter, the cost of the generator is less for the RF procedure [51].

Summary

Endovenous radiofrequency obliteration has become the favored alternative choice in the treatment of superficial and perforator venous reflux disease. RFA not only outperforms traditional vein stripping and perforator interruption with regard to morbidity and outcome, it reduces the incidence of neovascularization that is frequently blamed for the higher recurrence rates with vein stripping. RFA has been shown to have fewer postprocedural complications than laser treatment. Some of the previous shortcomings of the VNUS ClosurePLUS catheter, including high impedance failure, coagulum buildup, and slower pullback speed, have been eliminated with the new ClosureFAST catheter. This new catheter system is an important advancement that combines the faster withdrawal speed of laser treatment with the fewer side effects and high ablation rate commonly seen with RFA.

Acknowledgments

The author would like to recognize the help of Mr. Ralph Roper, RVT for his assistance with the preparation of the ultrasound images, as well as all the staff of the Vein Care Pavilion of the South and the Vein Care Pavilion of America.

References

[1] Callam MJ. Epidemiology of varicose veins. Br J Surg 1994;81:167–73.
[2] Ruckley CV, Evans CJ, Allan PL, et al. Chronic venous insufficiency: clinical and duplex correlations. The Edinburgh Vein Study of Venous Disorders in the General Population. J Vasc Surg 2002;36:520–5.
[3] Labropoulos N, Delis K, Nicolaides AN, et al. The role of the distribution and anatomic extent of reflux in the development of signs and symptoms in chronic venous insufficiency. J Vasc Surg 1996;23(3):504–10.
[4] Weiss RA. RF-mediated endovenous occlusion. In: Weiss RA, Feied CF, Weiss MA, editors. Vein diagnosis and treatment: a comprehensive approach. New York: McGraw-Hill Medical Publishing Division; 2001. p. 211–21.
[5] Bergan JJ. Endovenous sphenous vein obliteration. In: Whittmore AD, Bandyk DF, editors. Advances in vascular surgery, vol. 9. Chicago: Mosby-Year Book; 2001. p. 123–32.
[6] Nicolaides AN, Griffin MB, Lennox AF, et-al. Endovenous vein closure. In: Greenhalgh RM Becquemin JP Raithel D, et-al, editors. Vascular and endovascular surgical techniques. 4th edition. Philadelphia: WB Saunders; 2001. p. 507–10.
[7] Zikorus AW, Mirizzi MS. Evaluation of setpoint temperature and pullback speed on vein adventitial temperature during endovenous radiofrequency energy delivery in an in-vitro model. Vasc Endovascular Surg 2004;38:167–74.
[8] Min RJ, Zimmet SE, Isaacs MN, et al. Endovenous laser treatment of the incompetent greater saphenous vein. J Vasc Interv Radiol 2001;12:1167–71.
[9] Proebstle TM. Comments on "Comparison of endovenous radiofrequency versus 810 nm diode laser occlusion of large veins in animal model." Dermatol Surg 2002;28: 596–600.

[10] Weiss RA. RF-mediated endovenous occlusion. In: Weiss RA, Feied CF, Weiss MA, editors. Vein diagnosis and treatment: a comprehensive approach. 1st edition. St. Louis (MO): Quality Medical Publishing; 1999. p. 217–24.

[11] Weiss RA. Radiofrequency endovenous occlusion (Closure Technique). In: Frenek HS, editor. Fundamentals of phlebology: venous disease for clinicians. 2nd edition. London: Royal Society of Medicine Press Ltd.; 2002. p. 101–4.

[12] Manfrini S, Gasbarro V, Danielsson G, et al. Endovenous management of saphenous vein reflux. J Vasc Surg 2000;32:330–42.

[13] Chandler JG, Pichot O, Sessa C, et al. Treatment of primary venous insufficiency by endovenous saphenous vein obliteration. Vasc Surg 2000;34:201–14.

[14] Dauplaise TL, Weiss RA. Duplex-guided endovascular occlusion of refluxing saphenous veins. Journal of Vascular Technology 2001;25:79–82.

[15] Sybrandy JEM, Wittens CHA. Initial experiences in endovenous treatment of saphenous vein reflux. J Vasc Surg 2002;36:1207–12.

[16] Hingorani AP, Ascher E, Markevich N, et al. Deep venous thrombosis after radiofrequency ablation of greater saphenous vein: a word of caution. J Vasc Surg 2004;40(3):500–4.

[17] Subramonia S, Lees T. Regarding "Deep vein thrombosis after radiofrequency ablation of greater saphenous vein: a word of caution." J Vasc Surg 2005;41(5):915–6.

[18] Chandler JG, Pichot O, Sessa C, et al. Defining the role of extended saphenofemoral junction ligation: a prospective comparative study. J Vasc Surg 2000;32:941–53.

[19] Weiss RA, Weiss MA. Controlled radiofrequency endovenous occlusion using a unique radiofrequency catheter under duplex guidance to eliminate saphenous varicose vein reflux: a 2-year follow-up. Dermatol Surg 2002;28:38–42.

[20] Rautio T, Ohinmaa A, Perälä J, et al. Endovenous obliteration versus conventional stripping operation in the treatment of primary varicose veins: a randomized controlled trial with comparison of costs. J Vasc Surg 2002;35:958–65.

[21] Stötter L, Schaaf I, Bockelbrink A, et al. [Radiofrequency obliteration, invagination, or cryostripping: which is the best tolerated by the patients?]. Phlebologie 2005;34:19–24 [in German].

[22] Lurie F, Creton D, Eklof B, et al. Prospective Randomized Study of Endovenous Radiofrequency Obliteration (Closure) versus Ligation and Stripping in a selected patient population (EVOLVES study). J Vasc Surg 2003;38:207–14.

[23] Lurie F, Creton D, Eklof B, et al. Prospective Randomised Study of Endovenous Radiofrequency Obliteration (Closure) Versus Ligation and Vein Stripping (EVOLVeS): two-year follow-up. Eur J Vasc Endovasc Surg 2005;29(1):67–73.

[24] Goldman MP, Amiry S. Closure of the greater saphenous vein with endoluminal radiofrequency thermal heating of the vein wall in combination with ambulatory phlebectomy: 50 patients with more than 6-month follow-up. Dermatol Surg 2002;28:29–31.

[25] Merchant RF, DePalma RG, Kabnick LS. Endovascular obliteration of saphenous reflux: a multicenter study. J Vasc Surg 2002;35(6):1190–6.

[26] Rautio TT, Perälä JM, Wiik HT, et al. Endovenous obliteration with radiofrequency-resistive heating for greater saphenous vein insufficiency: a feasibility study. J Vasc Interv Radiol 2002;13:569–75.

[27] Gale SS, Dosick SM, Seiwert AJ, et al. Regarding "Deep venous thrombosis after radiofrequency ablation of greater saphenous vein." J Vasc Surg 2005;41(2):374.

[28] Pichot O, Sessa C, Chandler JG, et al. Role of duplex imaging in endovenous obliteration for primary venous insufficiency. J Endovasc Ther 2000;7:451–9.

[29] Pichot O, Kabnick LS, Creton D, et al. Duplex ultrasound scan findings two years after great saphenous vein radiofrequency endovenous obliteration. J Vasc Surg 2004;39:189–95.

[30] Merchant RF, Pichot O, Mayers KA. Four-year follow-up on endovascular radiofrequency obliteration of great saphenous reflux. Dermatol Surg 2005;31:129–34.

[31] Perala J, Rautio T, Biancari F, et al. Radiofrequency endovenous obliteration versus stripping of the long saphenous vein in the management of primary varicose veins: 3-year outcome of a randomized study. Ann Vasc Surg 2005;19:1–4.

[32] Hinchliffe RJ, Ubhi J, Beech A, et al. A prospective randomised controlled trial of VNUS closure versus surgery for the treatment of recurrent long saphenous varicose veins. Eur J Vasc Endovasc Surg 2006;31(2):212–8.

[33] Kistner RL, Eklof B, Masuda EM. Diagnosis of chronic venous disease of the lower extremities: the "CEAP" classification. Mayo Clin Proc 1996;71:338–45.

[34] Dwerryhouse S, Davies B, Harradine K, et al. Stripping the long saphenous vein reduces the rate of reoperation for recurrent varicose veins: five-year results of a randomized trial. J Vasc Surg 1999;29:589–92.

[35] Rutgers PH, Kitslaar PJ. Randomized trial of stripping versus high ligation combined with sclerotherapy in the treatment of the incompetent greater saphenous vein. Am J Surg 1994; 168:311–5.

[36] Neglen P, Einarsson E, Eklof B. The functional long-term value of different types of treatment for saphenous vein incompetence. J Cardiovasc Surg (Torino) 1993;34:295–301.

[37] Munn SR, Morton JB, Macbeth WA, et al. To strip or not to strip the long saphenous vein? A varicose veins trial. Br J Surg 1981;68:426–8.

[38] Hammarsten J, Pedersen P, Cederlund CG, et al. Long saphenous vein saving surgery for varicose veins. A long-term follow-up. Eur J Vasc Surg 1990;4:361–4.

[39] Jones L, Braithwaite BD, Selwyn D, et al. Neovascularisation is the principal cause of varicose vein recurrence: results of a randomised trial of stripping the long saphenous vein. Eur J Vasc Endovasc Surg 1996;12:442–5.

[40] van Rij AM, Jiang P, Solomon C, et al. Recurrence after varicose vein surgery: a prospective long-term clinical study with duplex ultrasound scanning and air plethysmography. J Vasc Surg 2003;38:935–43.

[41] Kostas T, Ioannou CV, Touloupakis E, et al. Recurrent varicose veins after surgery: a new appraisal of a common and complex problem in vascular surgery. Eur J Vasc Endovasc Surg 2004;27:275–82.

[42] Campbell WB, Vijay Kumar A, Collin TW, et al. The outcome of varicose vein surgery at 10 years: clinical findings, symptoms and patient satisfaction. Randomised and economic analysis of conservative and therapeutic interventions for varicose veins study. Ann R Coll Surg Engl 2003;85:52–7.

[43] Fischer R, Linde N, Duff C, et al. Late recurrent saphenofemoral junction reflux after ligation and stripping of the greater saphenous vein. J Vasc Surg 2001;34(2):236–40.

[44] Lumsden AB, Peden EK. Clinical use of the new VNUS ClosureFAST radiofrequency catheter. Endovascular Today 2007;(Suppl):7–10.

[45] Proebstle TM, Lehr HA, Kargl A, et al. Endovenous treatment of the greater saphenous vein with a 940-nm diode laser: thrombotic occlusion after endoluminal thermal damage by laser-generated steam bubbles. J Vasc Surg 2002;35:729–36.

[46] Proebstle TM, Krummenauer F, Gul D, et al. Nonocclusion and early reopening of the great saphenous vein after endovenous laser treatment is fluence dependent. Dermatol Surg 2004; 30:174–8.

[47] Kabnick LS. Outcome of different endovenous laser wavelengths for great saphenous vein ablation. J Vasc Surg 2006;43:88–93.

[48] de Medeiros CA, Luccas GC. Comparison of endovenous treatment with an 810-nm laser versus conventional stripping of the great saphenous vein in patients with primary varicose veins. Dermatol Surg 2005;31:1685–94.

[49] Vuylsteke M, Van den Bussche D, Audenaert EE, et al. Endovenous laser obliteration for the treatment of primary varicose veins. Phlebology 2006;21:80–7.

[50] Morrison N. Saphenous ablation: what are the choices, laser or RF energy. Semin Vasc Surg 2005;18:15–8.

[51] Perrin M. Endoluminal treatment of lower-limb varicose veins by radiofrequency and endovenous laser. Endovascular Today 2007;(Suppl):22–4.

SURGICAL
CLINICS OF
NORTH AMERICA

Surg Clin N Am 87 (2007) 1285–1295

Foam Sclerotherapy for the Treatment of Superficial Venous Insufficiency

Kathleen D. Gibson, MD*, Brian L. Ferris, MD,
Daniel Pepper, MD

*Lake Washington Vascular Surgeons, 1135 116th Avenue NE,
Suite 305, Bellevue, WA 98104, USA*

Sclerotherapy has been in use for nearly a century to treat both telangiectasias and varicose veins. The widespread use of foam sclerotherapy has evolved over the past decade. Foam sclerotherapy (FST) offers a number of advantages over traditional "liquid" sclerotherapy, and allows a skilled practitioner to treat veins of larger diameter, including saphenous trunks. The ease of use, low complication rate, and high rate of efficacy make foam sclerotherapy an important tool in the treatment of varicose veins and venous ulcerations. It is readily performed in an outpatient clinic setting, requires no procedural sedation, and patients return to normal activity levels very quickly with minimal discomfort. In many cases, foam sclerotherapy may replace traditional "stab and hook" phlebectomy. It is an emerging minimally invasive alternative to endovenous laser (EVLT) or radiofrequency ablation (RFA) of saphenous veins, and recent data demonstrate that in experienced hands, FST is a viable alternative treatment to traditional ligation and stripping of the saphenous trunks [1].

Development of foam sclerotherapy

Foam sclerosants are produced by forcibly mixing a liquid with a gas through a small aperture, producing small sclerosant encapsulated gas bubbles. Air and carbon dioxide (CO_2) are typical gases, and the most common choices of sclerosant include polidocanol (POL) and sodium tetradecyl

---

Dr. Gibson is a principal investigator, and Dr. Pepper and Dr. Ferris are coinvestigators of the Varisolve trial sponsored by BTG corporation, West Conshohocken, Pennsylvania.

* Corresponding author.
E-mail address: drgibson@lkwv.com (K.D. Gibson).

0039-6109/07/$ - see front matter
doi:10.1016/j.suc.2007.07.001   *surgical.theclinics.com*

sulfate (STS). Foam sclerotherapy differs from liquid sclerotherapy in that, once injected into a vein, foam pushes blood out of the way and completely fills the vein, rather than being diluted by blood and "washing" through the vessel. In this manner it is in contact with the vessel wall for a longer period of time, which increases the efficacy in comparison to liquid sclerotherapy. Volume and concentration of the sclerosing agent can therefore be decreased as the active contact time is increased with FST. On duplex ultrasound one can observe the treated vessel rapidly go into vasospasm.

The first published description of mixing air with a sclerosant was in 1944, by Orbach [2]. This technique, however, was not widely adopted. In the 1990s several papers were published regarding the use of foam sclerosants. Juan Cabrera of Spain was next to describe the creation of sclerosant foam to treat varicose veins in the early 1990s, with a paper published in 1997 [3]. Monfreux [4] in the same year published a technique for creating a foam sclerosant using a glass syringe and a sterile plug. Other methods using different techniques and gases were proposed. Tessari in 2000 [5] proposed the method to create foam sclerosants that is most widely used today. This simple and inexpensive technique uses two syringes and a three-way stopcock. Such "homemade" foam is of course not standardized, and although not yet available nor US Food and Drug Administration (FDA)-approved, commercially produced foam sclerosants are in development. Standardized commercial products should provide more consistent foam characteristics (bubble size, sclerosant strength) and sterility.

Only sclerosant solutions classified as "detergents" can be used to make foam. Worldwide, POL and STS (Sotradecol, Bioniche Pharma, Bogart, Georgia) are the most common agents used for the production of foamed sclerosant. In the United States, only STS has FDA approval; however, Phase II clinical trials are underway evaluating the safety of foamed POL (Varisolve, BTG corporation, West Conshohocken, Pennsylvania) [6].

Foam sclerotherapy has a number of applications. It can be used to treat reticular veins, varicose vein side branches in conjunction with EVLT or RFA, recurrent or residual varicosities after saphenous vein treatment, or as a "stand alone" treatment to ablate saphenous veins. In general FST is less applicable for the treatment of telangectasias, and in the authors' practice we still often treat telangectasias with liquid sclerosants. Several authors have reported excellent results in the treatment of venous ulcerations with FST. The authors have found, as have others, that FST works well to obliterate the nests of small varicosities that are seen in areas of lipodermatosclerosis and venous ulcers [7]. Successful treatment of venous angiomata and Klippel-Trenaunay syndrome has also been reported [8].

Techniques

As with all other varicose vein treatments, much of the ultimate success of foam sclerotherapy is proper pretreatment workup. In the authors' practice, duplex ultrasound is an indispensable tool for working up and treating patients who have varicose veins. All patients seeking treatment of varicose veins should undergo a duplex ultrasound to determine and map out the source of the varicosities. Treatment of varicosities without understanding their source, (eg, incompetent saphenous trunks, perforators, or pelvic sources) can result in undertreatment of the problem, which may lead to failure or recurrence. We believe identification of incompetent perforator veins is especially important when treating venous stasis and ulceration. Of the features currently available on duplex ultrasound machines from various manufacturers, the authors have found that the most important feature for the planning and treatment of varicose veins is precise near-field resolution. In our practice we use a GE Logic 9 machine (General Electric Healthcare, Waukesha, Wisconsin) with a 12 MHz "hockey stick" probe. The excellent near-field resolution makes cannulation of even relatively small varicosities straightforward.

Following pretreatment workup and informed consent, digital photographs are taken of the patient's limbs for "before and after" comparisons. We then mark the varicosities with an indelible marker. Reticular veins and small surface varicosities can be accessed without ultrasound guidance; however, we usually use ultrasound-guided injection for larger varicose veins. Although other authors have described accessing the veins with the patient standing, we prefer ultrasound-guided access with the patient lying down.

Branch veins can be accessed with an angiocatheter or a hypodermic or butterfly needle. Foam is created before accessing the vein using Tessari's technique. The authors use a 3 cc syringe, a 10 cc syringe, and a three-way stopcock. We agitate 2 cc of liquid sclerosant with 8 cc of air (4:1 ratio air to liquid). The liquid is then rapidly exchanged between the two syringes until thick white foam is produced (about 20 exchanges). No bubbles should be visible in the foam (Fig. 1). The foam should be used immediately because it will start to separate within minutes. Stability of the foam depends on concentration (higher concentrations are more stable [7]) and which solution is used. The concentration of the liquid sclerosant used depends on the size of the vessel to be treated (Table 1). The foam is injected and followed with ultrasound to fill the desired vein. Volumes injected into side branches should be small (1 to 2 cc) and distance of injection from the saphenofemoral or saphenopopliteal junction or major perforator veins should be noted to prevent inadvertent entry of large volumes of foam into deep veins. Gentle massage can help to work the foam further along the vein. Further injections may be needed to fill all of the veins. On duplex ultrasound imaging, the veins should be observed to go into intense vasospasm (Fig. 2).

Incompetent saphenous veins can be directly accessed with an angiocatheter, or the foam can be directed into the vein through a major tributary. When treating the greater saphenous vein (GSV), the saphenofemoral junction is compressed with digital or transducer pressure to prevent migration of foam into the common femoral vein [1,8]. Boutouroglou and

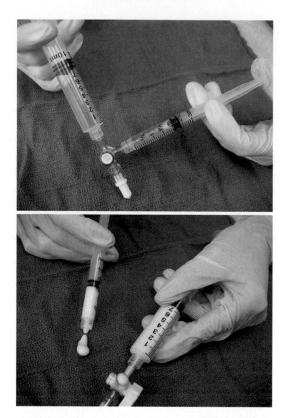

Fig. 1. Tessari method to create foamed sclerosant.

colleagues [9] have suggested ligation of the saphenofemoral junction at the same time as foam injection of the GSV. This technique could potentially prevent foam embolization. This study, however, suggests that the rationale behind SFJ ligation at the same time as FST is to decrease recanalization rates rather than to decrease the risk of embolization. The pressure on the saphenofemoral junction is continued until spasm and lack of flow in the GSV is verified with ultrasound.

Following injection, compression pads are placed over the path of the vein and secured with tape. The patient is then placed in a compression

Table 1
Recommended concentration of solution for creation of foam

Vein size	STS	POL
Telangectasia	0.1%	0.25%–0.75%
Reticular veins	0.2%	0.5%–1.0%
Small varicose veins	0.3%–1.0%	1.0%
Large varicose and saphenous veins	1.0%–3.0%	1.0%–3.0%

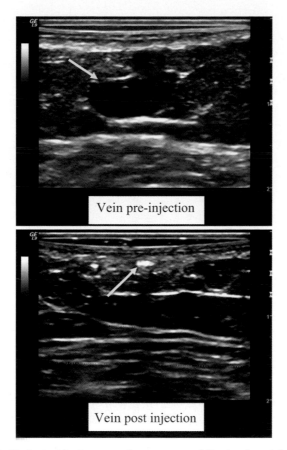

Fig. 2. Varicose vein demonstrating vasospasm following foam injection.

stocking (Class II or III), which is worn constantly for at least 48 hours. After 2 days, the authors allow the patient to take off the stocking and remove the compression pads. Other than bathing, we recommend that the patient continue wearing compression stockings for 2 to 3 weeks. Injections are performed without the need for sedation, and the majority of patients are very comfortable during the follow-up interval. Patients will occasionally complain of tenderness over the treated veins, and nonsteroidal anti-inflammatory medications are usually all that is required for relief.

Results

A number of studies regarding the efficacy of foam sclerotherapy have been published. The techniques used, type of veins treated, clinical severity of limbs treated and clinical outcomes studied vary widely. Table 2 summarizes a sampling of published data. Efficacy reports vary depending on the

Table 2
Summary of published data

Author	Year	Soln	N	Study summary	Results
Hamel-Desnos et al [10]	2003	POL	88	Prospective randomized trial comparing FST versus liquid sclerotherapy of GSV. Endpoint elimination of reflux in treated veins.	3 wks and 6 mos: 84% and 80% of FST group showed elimination of reflux, compared with 40% and 26% treated with liquid sclerotherapy
Barrett et al [11]	2004	STSandPOL	100	Retrospective review of GSV or SSV treatment. Endpoint elimination of reflux and quality of life (QOL) questionnaire	Mean follow-up of 22.5 months, 97% complete saphenous occlusion or fibrosis with "minimal flow"; 94% patients reported improved QOL
Kakkos et al [15]	2005	STS	38	Treated recurrent varicose veins in 45 limbs. Endpoint elimination of reflux in treated veins.	Endpoint reached in 87% limbs: 58% required 1 session only; 11% needed ≥3 sessions.
Bergan et al[a] [8]	2006	POL	56	77 limbs, CEAP 4–6 treated. Comparison groups compression only, and crossovers that failed compression. Endpoints relief of pain and inflammation, and ulcer healing.	10/22 ulcers in compression group healed at 6 weeks. All FST and crossovers healed at 6 weeks. VCSS improvement greatest in FST group (P < 0.041)
Bergan et al[a] [8]	2006	POL	261	328 limbs, CEAP 2 and 3. Endpoint "abolishment of reflux and obliteration of varicose clusters"	Endpoint reached in 79.8% of limbs.
Wright et al [1]	2006	POL	710	Randomized trial comparing FST with "alternative" treatment (sclerotherapy or surgery) in phlebologist and vascular surgeon groups. Endpoint occlusion of trunk veins and elimination of reflux	Success of FST at 3 and 12 mos was 93.8% and 89.6% respectively in phlebology group, and 68.2% and 63.1% in the vascular surgeon group.
Boutouroglou et al [9]	2006	STS	60	Randomized trial comparing GSV ligation and stripping with SFJ ligation plus FST. Endpoint elimination of reflux.	Short-term success with FST 87%. Decreased operative time and return to work with FST.
Darke and Baker [23]	2006	POL	181	220 limbs treated, GSV, SSV, or side branches. Endpoint closure of saphenous vein or closure of 85% of varicosities.	Endpoints reached after one treatment in 163 limbs, two in 32 limbs, and three in one limb (91% success).

Abbreviations: CEAP, Clinical, Etiologic, Anatomic, and Pathophysiologic score; SSV, small saphenous veins; VCSS, Venous Clinical Severity Score.
[a] Two different patient groups, results in same paper.

number of injection sessions required and on the defined endpoint. Comparisons of FST compared with liquid sclerosants have demonstrated significantly better efficacy of FST in ablating GSV reflux [10]. Efficacy of closure or elimination of reflux of saphenous veins ranges from 63% to 97% in a time range of 3 months to 22 months. In many studies, however, a substantial percentage of patients required more than one session of treatment to adequately treat the saphenous veins. In a series of 100 patients published by Barrett and colleagues [11], the number of sessions required to achieve elimination of reflux ranged from one to five sessions, with a mean of 2.1 sessions.

The concentration of sclerosant used varies depending on author. A recently published randomized trial of 80 patients compared the outcome and side effects of treatment of the GSV with 1% versus 3% POL. The 3% group had a 1-year GSV occlusion rate of 80.1% compared with 69.5% in the 1% group, but this difference was not statistically significant. The 3% group had higher rates of thrombophlebitis and hyperpigmentation, but again, statistical significance was not seen [12]. Although these results are interesting, the small sample size precludes any definitive conclusions about the ideal concentration of foam sclerosant to use. Future investigations should clarify the trade-off between rates of complications and efficacy.

Boutouroglou and colleagues [9], comparing traditional ligation and stripping to saphenofemoral ligation plus FST, showed that both length of time to return to "normal physical activity" and operative time is substantially shorter with FST. Time to return to work or normal physical activities ranged from 0 to 6 days for the FST group and 5 to 20 days in the ligation and stripping group. This study did not include a comparison of recovery and operative time in patients treated with endovenous thermal techniques.

Recurrent varicose veins are common (up to 25% at 5 years) after ligation and stripping [13,14]. "Re-do" operations can have increased morbidity, and often the nature of the recurrence precludes endovenous thermal ablation techniques, because both require relatively straight segment of veins to facilitate treatment. Foam sclerotherapy is ideally suited to treat recurrent varicosities. A recent study shows reflux was eliminated in 87% of limbs treated for recurrent varicose veins. Fifty-eight percent of limbs required one session of sclerotherapy, and 11% required three or more sessions [15].

Venous ulceration represents the "end-stage" of venous insufficiency, and historically has been a challenging problem to treat. Compression therapy, antibiotics for infection, and meticulous and diligent wound care remain essential components for healing. Perforator vein incompetence can be demonstrated in 50% to over 80% of patients presenting for surgical therapy of primary varicose veins [16,17]. Increasing numbers of incompetent perforator veins (IPV) have been shown to increase clinical, etiologic, anatomic, and pathophysiologic (CEAP) class (clinical severity of venous insufficiency) in a linear fashion [18]. Historically, open perforator ligation (Linton procedure, introduced in the 1930s) involved long, cosmetically unacceptable incisions. Subfascial endoscopic perforator ligation (SEPS procedure), introduced in the 1990s, offered smaller incisions, less morbidity, and shorter hospital stays than the Linton procedure [19]. The SEPS procedure was shown in a nationwide registry to decrease symptoms of chronic venous insufficiency and promote ulcer healing [20]. Nonetheless, the SEPS procedure requires a general anesthetic and multiple incisions, and the most distal perforators are often the most difficult to visualize, yet the most critical to interrupt. Direct perforator ligation through areas of lipodermatosclerosis can be difficult and poses healing problems. Several authors have shown that ultrasound-guided FST can be successfully used to treat incompetent perforator and truncal varicosities in patients who have venous ulceration. A series by Cabrera and colleagues [21] showed complete ulcer healing in 83% of patients treated with FST at 6 months, with a mean number of 3.6 treatments. Pascarella and colleagues [7] demonstrated that patients who have venous ulceration treated with FST and compression therapy had statistically faster healing of their ulceration than patients treated with compression therapy alone.

Long-term data (beyond several years) do not exist on recanalization of GSV segments treated with FST. A randomized trial conducted over 30 years ago by Hobbs comparing surgical treatment of the GSV to liquid sclerotherapy showed excellent results with sclerotherapy initially (95% "cured" at 1 year), but extremely high failure rates by 6 years (5% "cured") [22]. Although these data are outside of what we might expect with more recent studies, both in the exceptionally high success rates at 1 year and failure rates at 6 years, they do suggest that until more long-term data are available regarding FST, recanalization remains a concern. Boutouroglou and colleagues [9] have suggested that recanalization rates might be decreased with SFJ ligation; however, this theory has yet to be proven.

Although a number of studies compare FST of the GSV to traditional surgical techniques [1,9], no published reports exist comparing FST to endovenous thermal ablation techniques such as RFA and EVLT. Many studies have been published comparing EVLT and RF to traditional ligation and stripping. In general, RFA and EVLT have compared favorably with surgery in terms of efficacy, and offer faster and less painful recovery. Foam sclerotherapy offers advantages over EVLT and RFA in that it is simpler to perform and does not require expensive catheters and laser or RF generators. Additionally, FST can be used to treat veins that are too tortuous for an RF or laser fiber to negotiate. If FST of truncal saphenous reflux is to replace endovenous thermal ablation techniques, however, long-term durability will need to be as good as that seen with RFA and EVLT.

Complications

In experienced hands, foam sclerotherapy is a safe procedure, and serious complications are rare. Superficial thrombophlebitis is the most common complication [8,15], but is usually minor and self-limited in the authors' experience. Patients who have trapped coagulum in a closed vein segment often have decreased tenderness over the veins after expression of the coagulum. This can be readily accomplished during a follow-up visit using a small wheal of local anesthetic, and then puncture and drainage of the coagulum with an 18-gauge needle or the tip of an 11 blade. In the study by Bergan and colleagues [8], trapped coagulum was drained in 37.8% of limbs treated with FTS. Skin pigmentation following FST is also common, and patients should be counseled regarding the possibility before treatment. In most cases, the pigmentation will gradually fade over a period of months. The Bergan and colleagues study showed that 32.9% of patients had skin discoloration at 60 days, and 7.2% had it at 1 year. Inadequate compression is theorized to increase the risk of skin pigmentation [8]. Other less common complications include skin necrosis causing ulceration or blistering [15,23], and telangectasia matting [11].

A number of authors have reported transient side effects during and immediately following foam sclerotherapy. Dry cough, transient scotoma, migraine, chest discomfort, and other self-limited visual and neurologic disturbances have been noted [8,11,24,25]. In 6395 FTS sessions recorded in a multicenter registry, 19 episodes (0.3%) of visual disturbance were noted. All resolved with observation without any long-term sequelae [25]. Several of the authors' patients have reported initiation of migraines during FST, all resembling their usual migraine symptoms.

More serious complications such as deep venous thrombosis (DVT) have been reported [8,11,24,25]. Rates of DVT have ranged from 0% to 1.8% [8,15]. The most common sites noted for DVT are gastrocnemius and calf veins. In most of these cases, these clots do not require anticoagulation and may be followed with serial duplex scans. In the above-mentioned multicenter registry, one femoral DVT was noted in 6395 sessions [25].

One of the gravest complications reported was a single case report of stroke following foam sclerotherapy. This occurred in a patient later found to have a patent foramen ovale (PFO). The stroke occurred after foam treatment of the GSV and of note, the volume of foam used was substantial (20 cc). Although this is an isolated report, it does demonstrate the embolic potential of foam sclerosant, and the need to use caution in terms of volumes injected [26]. The current Varisolve trial is specifically investigating the safety of foam sclerotherapy treatment of the GSV in patients who have known PFO [6].

Summary

Multiple investigations have demonstrated the safety and efficacy of FST in the treatment of venous disorders. It offers advantages over alternative treatments in decreased cost, ease of treatment, and decreased post-treatment discomfort and recovery time. Disadvantages of FST include the need in many patients for more than one session of treatment, and possibly decreased efficacy compared with traditional surgery, especially in physicians inexperienced with sclerotherapy. Because efficacy rates vary a great deal depending on the case series, comparisons with traditional techniques are somewhat difficult. It is possible that the variability in results depends on the experience of the practitioners and the "nonuniformity" of homemade foam. It will be interesting to see if future studies with commercial grade foam demonstrate more consistent results. One of the most widely used agents worldwide, POL, has not yet gained approval for use in the United States by the FDA. Safety studies (in progress) and future efficacy studies of this agent should provide valuable data. Despite these evolving studies, it is clear that FST is an important tool in the treatment of varicose veins and venous ulcerations. After decades of little change in the treatment of venous insufficiency, with open surgical treatment representing the norm, the age of minimally invasive vein therapy is truly upon us.

References

[1] Wright D, Gobin JP, Bradbury AW, et al. Varisolve® polidocanol microfoam compared with surgery or sclerotherapy in the management of varicose veins in the presence of trunk vein incompetence: European randomized controlled trial. Phlebology 2006;21(4):180–90.

[2] Orbach EJ. Sclerotherapy of varicose veins: utilization of an intravenous air block. Am J Surg 1944;66:362–6.

[3] Cabrera Garrido JR, Cabrera Garcia-Olmedo JR, Garcia-Olmedo Dominguez MA. Elargissement des limites de la schlerotherapie: nouveaux produirs sclerosants. Phlebologie 1997;50:181–8 [in French].

[4] Monfreux A. Traitement sclerosant des troncs saphenies et leurs collaterals de gros caliber par le methode MUS. Phlebologie 1997;50:355–60 [in French].

[5] Tessari L. Nouvelle technique d'obtention de la sclero-mousse. Phlebologie 2000;53:129 [in French].

[6] Safety study of Varisolve® procedure for treatment of varicose veins in patients with right-to-left cardiac shunt, April 2007, Available at: http://clinicaltrials.gov/show/NCT00442364. Accessed April 2007.

[7] Pascarella L, Bergan JJ, Mekenas LV. Severe chronic venous insufficiency treated by foamed sclerosant. Ann Vasc Surg 2006;20:83–91.

[8] Bergan J, Pascarella L, Mekenas L. Venous disorders:treatment with sclerosant foam. J Card Surg 2006;47:115–24.

[9] Boutouroglou DG, Azzam M, Kakkos SK, et al. Ultrasound-guided foam sclerotherapy combined with sapheno-femoral ligation compared to surgical treatment of varicose veins: early results of a randomized controlled trial. Eur J Vasc Endovasc Surg 2006;31:93–100.

[10] Hamel-Desnos C, Desnos P, Wollman JC, et al. Evaluation of the efficacy of polidocanol in the form of foam compared with liquid form in sclerotherapy of the greater saphenous vein: initial results. Dermatol Surg 2003;29(12):1170–5.

[11] Barrett JM, Allen B, Ockelford A, et al. Microfoam ultrasound-guided sclerotheray of varicose veins in 100 legs. Dermatol Surg 2004;30:6–12.

[12] Cuelen RPM, Bullens-Goessens Y, Sebastien JA, et al. Outcomes and side effects of duplex-guided sclerotherapy and treatment of great saphenous veins with 1% versus 3% polidocanol foam: results of a randomized controlled trial with 1-year follow-up. Dermatol Surg 2007;33:276–81.

[13] Hartmann K, Klode J, Pfister R, et al. Recurrent varicose veins: sonography-based re-examination of 210 patients 14 years after ligation and saphenous vein stripping. Vasa 2006;35(1):21–6.

[14] Allegra C, Antignani PL, Carlizza A. Recurrent varicose veins following surgical treatment: our experience with five years follow-up. Eur J Vasc Endovasc Surg 2007;33(6):751–6.

[15] Kakkos SK, Bountouroglou DG, Azzam M. Effectiveness and safety of ultrasound-guided foam sclerotherapy for recurrent varicose veis: immediate results. J Endovasc Ther 2006;13: 357–64.

[16] Blomgren L, Johansson G, Dahlberg-Akerman A, et al. Changes in superficial and perforating vein reflux after varicose vein surgery. J Vasc Surg 2005;42(2):315–20.

[17] Danielsson G, Eklof B, Grandinetti A, et al. Deep axial reflux, an important contributor to skin changes or ulcer in chronic venous disease. J Vasc Surg 2003;38(6):1336–41.

[18] Stuart WP, Adam DJ, Allan PL, et al. The relationship between the number, competence and diameter of medial calf perforating veins and the clinical status in healthy subjects and patients with lower-limb venous disease. J Vasc Surg 2000;32(1):138–43.

[19] Stuart WP, Adam DJ, Bradbury AW, et al. Subfascial endoscopic perforator surgery is associated with significantly less morbidity and shorter hospital stay than open operation (Linton's procedure). Br J Surg 1997;84(10):1364–5.

[20] Gloviczki P, Bergan JJ, Rhodes JM, et al. Mid-term results of endoscopic perforator vein interruption for chronic venous insufficiency: lessons learned from the North American subfascial endoscopic perforator surgery registry. North American Study Group. J Vasc Surg 1999;29(3):489–502.

[21] Cabrera J, Redondo P, Becerra A, et al. Ultrasound-guided injection of polidocanol microfoam in management of venous leg ulcers. Arch Dermatol 2004;140(6):667–73.

[22] Hobbs JT. Surgery and sclerotherapy in the treatment of varicose veins. A random trial. Arch Surg 1974;109(6):793–6.

[23] Darke SG, Baker SJA. Ultrasound-guided foam sclerotherapy for the treatment of varicose veins. Br J Surg 2006;93(8):969–74.

[24] Guex JJ, Allaert FA, Gellet JL, et al. Immediate and midterm complications of sclerotherapy: report of a prospective multicenter registry of 12,173 sclerotherapy sessions. Dermatol Surg 2005;31(2):123–8.

[25] Tessari L, Cavezzi A, Frullini A. Preliminary experience with a new sclerosing foam in the treatment of varicose veins. Dermatol Surg 2001;27:58–60.

[26] Forlee MV, Grouden M, Moore DJ, et al. Stroke after varicose vein foam injection sclerotherapy. J Vasc Surg 2006;43:162–4.

ELSEVIER
SAUNDERS

Surg Clin N Am 87 (2007) 1297–1307

SURGICAL
CLINICS OF
NORTH AMERICA

Index

Note: Page numbers of article titles are in **boldface** type.

0039-6109/07/$ - see front matter © 2007 Elsevier Inc. All rights reserved.
doi:10.1016/S0039-6109(07)00137-5   *surgical.theclinics.com*